Nutraceuticals in Human Health

Nutraceuticals in Human Health

Special Issue Editors

Alessandra Durazzo
Massimo Lucarini
Antonello Santini

MDPI • Basel • Beijing • Wuhan • Barcelona • Belgrade • Manchester • Tokyo • Cluj • Tianjin

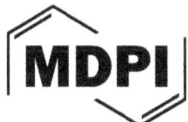

Special Issue Editors
Alessandra Durazzo
CREA-Research Centre for Food and Nutrition
Italy

Massimo Lucarini
CREA-Research Centre for Food and Nutrition
Italy

Antonello Santini
Department of Pharmacy
University of Napoli Federico II
Italy

Editorial Office
MDPI
St. Alban-Anlage 66
4052 Basel, Switzerland

This is a reprint of articles from the Special Issue published online in the open access journal *Foods* (ISSN 2304-8158) (available at: https://www.mdpi.com/journal/foods/special_issues/nutraceuticals_human_health).

For citation purposes, cite each article independently as indicated on the article page online and as indicated below:

LastName, A.A.; LastName, B.B.; LastName, C.C. Article Title. *Journal Name* **Year**, *Article Number*, Page Range.

ISBN 978-3-03936-457-2 (Hbk)
ISBN 978-3-03936-458-9 (PDF)

© 2020 by the authors. Articles in this book are Open Access and distributed under the Creative Commons Attribution (CC BY) license, which allows users to download, copy and build upon published articles, as long as the author and publisher are properly credited, which ensures maximum dissemination and a wider impact of our publications.

The book as a whole is distributed by MDPI under the terms and conditions of the Creative Commons license CC BY-NC-ND.

Contents

About the Special Issue Editors vii

Alessandra Durazzo, Massimo Lucarini and Antonello Santini
Nutraceuticals in Human Health
Reprinted from: *Foods* **2020**, *9*, 370, doi:10.3390/foods9030370 1

Analía A. Lu Martínez, Juan G. Báez González, Minerva Bautista Villarreal, Karla G. García Alanis, Sergio A. Galindo Rodríguez and Eristeo García Márquez
Studied of Defatted Flour and Protein Concentrate of *Prunus serotine* and Applications
Reprinted from: *Foods* **2020**, *9*, 29, doi:10.3390/foods9010029 5

Samee Ullah, Anees Ahmed Khalil, Faryal Shaukat and Yuanda Song
Sources, Extraction and Biomedical Properties of Polysaccharides
Reprinted from: *Foods* **2019**, , 304, doi:10.3390/foods8080304 27

Monika Swat, Iga Rybicka and Anna Gliszczyńska-Świgło
Characterization of Fulvic Acid Beverages by Mineral Profile and Antioxidant Capacity
Reprinted from: *Foods* **2019**, *8*, 605, doi:10.3390/foods8120605 51

Massimo Lucarini, Alessandra Durazzo, Johannes Kiefer, Antonello Santini, Ginevra Lombardi-Boccia, Eliana B. Souto, Annalisa Romani, Anja Lampe, Stefano Ferrari Nicoli, Paolo Gabrielli, Noemi Bevilacqua, Margherita Campo, Massimo Morassut and Francesca Cecchini
Grape Seeds: Chromatographic Profile of Fatty Acids and Phenolic Compounds and Qualitative Analysis by FTIR-ATR Spectroscopy
Reprinted from: *Foods* **2020**, *9*, 10, doi:10.3390/foods9010010 63

Su Cheol Baek, Ki Hong Nam, Sang Ah Yi, Mun Seok Jo, Kwang Ho Lee, Yong Hoon Lee, Jaecheol Lee and Ki Hyun Kim
Anti-adipogenic Effect of β-Carboline Alkaloids from Garlic (*Allium sativum*)
Reprinted from: *Foods* **2019**, *8*, 673, doi:10.3390/foods8120673 77

Wan-Ning Liu, Jia Shi, Yu Fu and Xin-Huai Zhao
The Stability and Activity Changes of Apigenin and Luteolin in Human Cervical Cancer Hela Cells in Response to Heat Treatment and Fe^{2+}/Cu^{2+} Addition
Reprinted from: *Foods* **2019**, *8*, 346, doi:10.3390/foods8080346 89

Samy Sayed, Mohamed Ahmed, Ahmed El-Shehawi, Mohamed Alkafafy, Saqer Al-Otaibi, Hanan El-Sawy, Samy Farouk and Samir El-Shazly
Ginger Water Reduces Body Weight Gain and Improves Energy Expenditure in Rats
Reprinted from: *Foods* **2020**, *9*, 38, doi:10.3390/foods9010038 105

Besma Omri, Marwen Amraoui, Arbi Tarek, Massimo Lucarini, Alessandra Durazzo, Nicola Cicero, Antonello Santini and Mounir Kamoun
Arthrospira Platensis (Spirulina) Supplementation on Laying Hens' Performance: Eggs Physical, Chemical, and Sensorial Qualities
Reprinted from: *Foods* , *8*, 386, doi:10.3390/foods8090386 119

Besma Omri, Nadir Alloui, Alessandra Durazzo, Massimo Lucarini, Alessandra Aiello, Raffaele Romano, Antonello Santini and Hedi Abdouli
Egg Yolk Antioxidants Profiles: Effect of Diet Supplementation with Linseeds and Tomato-Red Pepper Mixture before and after Storage
Reprinted from: *Foods* **2019**, *8*, 320, doi:10.3390/foods8080320 131

Besma Omri, Ben Larbi Manel, Zemzmi Jihed, Alessandra Durazzo, Massimo Lucarini, Raffaele Romano, Antonello Santini and Hédi Abdouli
Effect of a Combination of Fenugreek Seeds, Linseeds, Garlic and Copper Sulfate on Laying Hens Performances, Egg Physical and Chemical Qualities
Reprinted from: *Foods* **2019**, *8*, 311, doi:10.3390/foods8080311 147

Denise Beconcini, Francesca Felice, Angela Fabiano, Bruno Sarmento, Ylenia Zambito and Rossella Di Stefano
Antioxidant and Anti-Inflammatory Properties of Cherry Extract: Nanosystems-Based Strategies to Improve Endothelial Function and Intestinal Absorption
Reprinted from: *Foods* **2020**, *9*, 207, doi:10.3390/foods9020207 157

Carolina Fredes, Alejandra Parada, Jaime Salinas and Paz Robert
Phytochemicals and Traditional Use of Two Southernmost Chilean Berry Fruits:
Murta (*Ugni molinae* Turcz) and Calafate (*Berberis buxifolia* Lam.)
Reprinted from: *Foods* **2020**, *9*, 54, doi:10.3390/foods9010054 179

Ming-Yue Ji, Agula Bo, Min Yang, Jin-Fan Xu, Lin-Lin Jiang, Bao-Chang Zhou and Min-Hui Li
The Pharmacological Effects and Health Benefits of *Platycodon grandiflorus*—A Medicine Food Homology Species
Reprinted from: *Foods* **2020**, *9*, 142, doi:10.3390/foods9020142 195

About the Special Issue Editors

Alessandra Durazzo was awarded a Master's degree in Chemistry and Pharmaceutical Technology cum laude in 2003, and a PhD in Horticulture in 2010. Since 2005, she has been a researcher at the CREA-Research Centre for Food and Nutrition. The core of her research is the study of chemical, nutritional and bioactive components of food, with particular regard to the wide spectrum of substances classes and their nutraceutical features. For several years, she was involved in national and international research projects on the evaluation of several factors (agronomic practices, processing, etc.) that affect food quality, the levels of bioactive molecules and the total antioxidant properties, as well as their possible impact on the biological role played by bioactive components in human physiology. Her research activities are addressed also towards developing, managing and updating the Food Composition Database, as well as Bioactive Compounds and Food Supplements databases; particular attention is given towards the harmonization of analytical procedures and classification and codification of food supplements.

Massimo Lucarini received a Master's degree in Industrial Chemistry cum laude of the University of Rome "La Sapienza", Italy (1992) and a PhD in Chemistry also of the University of Rome "La Sapienza". His research activity is mainly aimed at the evaluation of nutrient content, molecules with biological and anti-nutrient activity in foods and diets, studies of stability of technological treatments of food products using specific process markers. Particular interest is addressed to the evaluation of the nutritional quality of foods, the bioavailability of nutrients and bioactive components and their interaction with the food matrix (using in vitro models and cellular models), and to applications in the nutraceutical field; recent attention focuses on the exploitation of waste from the agri-food industry, with a view to sustainable agri-food production. In relation to the study of bioactive molecules, the experience gained in this field is wide ranging from carotenoids to phenolic substances, and from caseinophosphopeptides (CPP) to the components of dietary fiber. An integral part of the research carried out is linked to institutional activity, including food composition tables, guidelines for healthy nutrition, and evaluation of fraud risk in the agri-food system. In relation to the production system, the effects of technological treatments on molecules of nutritional interest are also evaluated. He is also interested in using natural substances with strong antioxidant properties to improve the shelf-life of food products. The research activity is also aimed at the development of new analytical methods, the exchange of scientific information and the acquisition of new skills both at the national and international level, through training courses, participation in congresses and seminars. The dissemination activity is carried out through the production of scientific articles, interviews released in national journals and broadcasting systems, the creation of web pages, participation in congresses, educational and informative activities.

Antonello Santini, Ph.D., is Professor of Food Chemistry and Food Chemistry and Analysis of Food and Nutraceuticals at the Departments of Pharmacy and at the Department of Agriculture of the University of Napoli Federico II, Napoli, Italy. He is also visiting professor at the Albanian University of Tirana, Albania. He holds a PhD in Chemical Sciences. His research areas of interest are substantiated by many international collaborations, mainly in the field of food; food chemistry, nutraceuticals, functional food; supplements; recovery of natural compounds bioactive using eco sustainable and environment friendly techniques from agro-food byproducts; nanocompounds; nanonutraceuticals; food risk assessment, safety and contaminants; mycotoxins and secondary metabolites; food analysis; chemistry and food education. He is responsible for funded research projects and responsible for general cultural agreements established between the University of Napoli Federico II and many Universities worldwide. His research activity is substantiated by more than 200 papers in peer reviewed reputed international Journals. He is member of the European Food Safety Authority EFSA, ERWG, Parma, Italy; member of the Italian Authority for Food Safety (CNSA), Italian Ministry of Health, Rome Italy; member of Managing Board, Italian Chemistry Society (SCI) Division of Teaching (DD-SCI), Rome, Italy, as well as an expert member for Chemistry, EurSchool, European Commission, Bruxelles, Belgium.

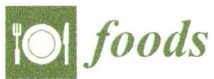

Editorial

Nutraceuticals in Human Health

Alessandra Durazzo [1,*], Massimo Lucarini [1,*] and Antonello Santini [2,*]

1. CREA-Research Centre for Food and Nutrition, Via Ardeatina 546, 00178 Rome, Italy
2. Department of Pharmacy, University of Napoli Federico II, Via D. Montesano 49, 80131 Napoli, Italy
* Correspondence: alessandra.durazzo@crea.gov.it (A.D.); massimo.lucarini@crea.gov.it (M.L.); asantini@unina.it (A.S.); Tel.: +39-(0)6-51494430 (A.D.); +39-(0)6-51494446 (M.L.); +39-(0)81-253-9317 (A.S.)

Received: 13 March 2020; Accepted: 17 March 2020; Published: 23 March 2020

Abstract: The combined and concerted action of nutrient and biologically active compounds is flagged as an indicator of a "possible beneficial role" for health. The use and applications of bioactive components cover a wide range of fields, in particular the nutraceuticals. In this context, the Special Issue entitled "Nutraceuticals in Human Health" is focused on the all aspects around the nutraceuticals, ranging from analytical aspects to clinical trials, from efficacy studies to beneficial effects on health status.

Keywords: nutraceuticals; bioactive compounds; medicinal food; safety; health; regulation; clinical tests; efficacy; analysis; formulation

---

Introduction

The combined and concerted action of nutrient components and biologically active compounds is flagged as indicator of a "possible beneficial role" for health. The use and applications of bioactive components cover a large range of fields, in particular nutraceuticals ones [1–3].

Nutraceuticals are obtained from foods of vegetal or animal origin, and the current interest and ongoing worldwide research aims to shed light and fully clarify their mechanism of action, their safety and efficacy by substantiating their role by means of clinical data [4,5]. An effort to clarify their mechanism of action will in fact open a door to a next generation of therapeutic agents that do not propose themselves as an alternative to drugs, but, instead, can be helpful to: (i) prevent a cluster of conditions that could occur together (metabolic syndrome), e.g. heart disease, stroke, and type 2 diabetes; (ii) to complement a pharmacological therapyespecially for those individuals who do not qualify for a conventional pharmacological therapy [6,7].

This Special Issue is dedicated to the role and perspectives of nutraceuticals in human health, examined from different angles, ranging from analytical aspects to clinical trials, from efficacy studies to beneficial effects on health conditions.

Concerning the study of functional ingredients and applications, Lu Martínez et al. [8] have studied and proposed the use of *Prunus* serotine defatted flour without hydrogen cyanide risk in cookies and protein concentrate in emulsion stability. Ullah et al. [9] well reviewed and summarized the biomedical properties of polysaccharides as therapeutical agents. It is worth mentioning the work of Swat et al. [10] on characterization of fulvic acid beverages available on the global market. Alternative functional ingredients obtained from waste/side products from industrial grape manufacturing, i.e., grape seeds, were investigated by Lucarini et al. [11].

Studies on evaluation of beneficial effects of nutraceuticals in vitro [12] and in vivo [13] models have been presented, in particular dietary supplementation studies in animal [14–16].

At the same time, specific studies on botanicals have been reported by Fredes et al. [17] and Ji et al. [18] focusing on the importance of these vegetal origin sources.

Nutraceuticals are a challenge for the future of prevention and therapy and a triggering tool in medicine area. The possibility to prevent and/or support a pharmacological therapy, which is nowadays mainly based on pharmaceuticals, can be a powerful tool to face pathological, chronic, long-term diseases in subjects who do not qualify for a pharmacological therapy. The big challenge is to improve nutraceuticals bioavailability and clear their mechanism of action adopting nanotechnologies as new delivery approach and clinical studies to assess and detail how they work in detail [19,20]. At the same time, the interest to new food sources and exploring novel nutraceuticals which beyond their nutritional value have also added value as contributing bioactive substances tailored to specific health conditions for a better results in term of efficacy and safety is stimulating interest and research worldwide for new sources and sustainable environmental friendly solutions [21–23].

This Special Issue end point has been to contribute to the growth of this area of research, trigger interest or research on food and add information scientifically substantiated by new data.

We would like to thank all the authors and the reviewers of the papers published in this Special Issue for their great contribution and effort. We are also grateful to the editorial board members and to the staff of the journal for their kind support during the preparation of this Special Issue.

Author Contributions: All authors listed have made a substantial, direct and intellectual contribution to the work, and approved it for publication. All authors have read and agreed to the published version of the manuscript.

Conflicts of Interest: The authors declare no conflict of interest.

References

1. Santini, A.; Novellino, E. Nutraceuticals: Beyond the Diet before the Drugs. *Curr. Bioact. Compd.* **2014**, *10*, 1–12. [CrossRef]
2. Durazzo, A.; Lucarini, M.; Souto, E.B.; Cicala, C.; Caiazzo, E.; Izzo, A.A.; Novellino, E.; Santini, A. Polyphenols: A concise overview on the chemistry, occurrence, and human health. *Phytother. Res.* **2019**, *33*, 2221–2243. [CrossRef] [PubMed]
3. Santini, A. Nutraceuticals: Redefining a Concept. *Ann. Pharmacol. Pharm.* **2018**, *3*, 1147.
4. Santini, A.; Novellino, E. To Nutraceuticals and Back: Rethinking a Concept. *Foods* **2017**, *6*, 74. [CrossRef] [PubMed]
5. Daliu, P.; Santini, A.; Novellino, E. A decade of nutraceutical patents: Where are we now in 2018? *Expert Opin. Ther. Pat.* **2018**, *28*, 875–882. [CrossRef] [PubMed]
6. Santini, A.; Novellino, E. Nutraceuticals-shedding light on the grey area between pharmaceuticals and food. *Expert Rev. Clin. Pharmacol.* **2018**, *11*, 545–547. [CrossRef] [PubMed]
7. Daliu, P.; Santini, A.; Novellino, E. From pharmaceuticals to nutraceuticals: Bridging disease prevention and management. *Expert Rev. Clin. Pharmacol.* **2019**, *12*, 1–7. [CrossRef]
8. Lu Martínez, A.A.; Báez González, J.G.; Bautista Villarreal, M.; García Alanis, K.G.; Galindo Rodríguez, S.A.; García Márquez, E. Studied of Defatted Flour and Protein Concentrate of *Prunus serotine* and Applications. *Foods* **2020**, *9*, 29. [CrossRef]
9. Ullah, S.; Khalil, A.A.; Shaukat, F.; Song, Y. Sources, Extraction and Biomedical Properties of Polysaccharides. *Foods* **2019**, *8*, 304. [CrossRef]
10. Swat, M.; Rybicka, I.; Gliszczyńska-Świgło, A. Characterization of Fulvic Acid Beverages by Mineral Profile and Antioxidant Capacity. *Foods* **2019**, *8*, 605. [CrossRef]
11. Lucarini, M.; Durazzo, A.; Kiefer, J.; Santini, A.; Lombardi-Boccia, G.; Souto, E.B.; Romani, A.; Lampe, A.; Ferrari Nicoli, S.; Gabrielli, P.; et al. Grape Seeds: Chromatographic Profile of Fatty Acids and Phenolic Compounds and Qualitative Analysis by FTIR-ATR Spectroscopy. *Foods* **2020**, *9*, 10. [CrossRef] [PubMed]
12. Liu, W.N.; Shi, J.; Fu, Y.; Zhao, X.H. The Stability and Activity Changes of Apigenin and Luteolin in Human Cervical Cancer Hela Cells in Response to Heat Treatment and Fe^{2+}/Cu^{2+} Addition. *Foods* **2019**, *8*, 346. [CrossRef] [PubMed]
13. Sayed, S.; Ahmed, M.; El-Shehawi, A.; Alkafafy, M.; Al-Otaibi, S.; El-Sawy, H.; Farouk, S.; El-Shazly, S. Ginger Water Reduces Body Weight Gain and Improves Energy Expenditure in Rats. *Foods* **2020**, *9*, 38. [CrossRef] [PubMed]

14. Omri, B.; Amraoui, M.; Tarek, A.; Lucarini, M.; Durazzo, A.; Cicero, N.; Santini, A.; Kamoun, M. *Arthrospira Platensis* (Spirulina) Supplementation on Laying Hens' Performance: Eggs Physical, Chemical, and Sensorial Qualities. *Foods* **2019**, *8*, 386. [CrossRef] [PubMed]
15. Omri, B.; Alloui, N.; Durazzo, A.; Lucarini, M.; Aiello, A.; Romano, R.; Santini, A.; Abdouli, H. Egg Yolk Antioxidants Profiles: Effect of Diet Supplementation with Linseeds and Tomato-Red Pepper Mixture before and after Storage. *Foods* **2019**, *8*, 320. [CrossRef] [PubMed]
16. Omri, B.; Larbi Manel, B.; Jihed, Z.; Durazzo, A.; Lucarini, M.; Romano, R.; Santini, A.; Abdouli, H. Effect of a Combination of Fenugreek Seeds, Linseeds, Garlic and Copper Sulfate on Laying Hens Performances, Egg Physical and Chemical Qualities. *Foods* **2019**, *8*, 311. [CrossRef]
17. Fredes, C.; Parada, A.; Salinas, J.; Robert, P. Phytochemicals and Traditional Use of Two Southernmost Chilean Berry Fruits: Murta (*Ugni molinae* Turcz) and Calafate (*Berberis buxifolia* Lam.). *Foods* **2020**, *9*, 54. [CrossRef]
18. Ji, M.Y.; Bo, A.; Yang, M.; Xu, J.F.; Jiang, L.L.; Zhou, B.-C.; Li, M.H. The Pharmacological Effects and Health Benefits of Platycodon grandifloras-A Medicine Food Homology Species. *Foods* **2020**, *9*, 142. [CrossRef]
19. Souto, E.B.; Silva, G.F.; Dias-Ferreira, J.; Zielinska, A.; Ventura, F.; Durazzo, A.; Lucarini, M.; Novellino, E.; Santini, A. Nanopharmaceutics: Part I-Clinical Trials Legislation and Good Manufacturing Practices (GMP) of Nanotherapeutics in the EU. *Pharmaceutics* **2020**, *12*, 146. [CrossRef]
20. Souto, E.B.; Silva, G.F.; Dias-Ferreira, J.; Zielinska, A.; Ventura, F.; Durazzo, A.; Lucarini, M.; Novellino, E.; Santini, A. Nanopharmaceutics: Part II-Production Scales and Clinically Compliant Production Methods. *Nanomaterials* **2020**, *10*, 455. [CrossRef]
21. Campos, J.R.; Severino, P.; Ferreira, C.S.; Zielinska, A.; Santini, A.; Souto, S.B.; Souto, E.B. Linseed Essential Oil—Source of Lipids as Active Ingredients for Pharmaceuticals and Nutraceuticals. *Curr. Med. Chem.* **2019**, *26*, 1–22. [CrossRef] [PubMed]
22. Salehi, B.; Venditti, A.; Sharifi-Rad, M.; Kregiel, D.; Sharifi-Rad, J.; Durazzo, A.; Lucarini, M.; Santini, A.; Souto, E.B.; Novellino, E.; et al. The Therapeutic Potential of Apigenin. *Int. J. Mol. Sci.* **2019**, *20*, 1305. [CrossRef] [PubMed]
23. Lucarini, M.; Durazzo, A.; Romani, A.; Campo, M.; Lombardi-Boccia, G.; Cecchini, F. Bio-Based Compounds from Grape Seeds: A Biorefinery Approach. *Molecules* **2018**, *23*, 1888. [CrossRef] [PubMed]

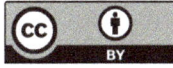

© 2020 by the authors. Licensee MDPI, Basel, Switzerland. This article is an open access article distributed under the terms and conditions of the Creative Commons Attribution (CC BY) license (http://creativecommons.org/licenses/by/4.0/).

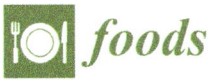

Article

Studied of Defatted Flour and Protein Concentrate of *Prunus serotine* and Applications

Analía A. Lu Martínez [1], Juan G. Báez González [1,*], Minerva Bautista Villarreal [1], Karla G. García Alanis [1], Sergio A. Galindo Rodríguez [2] and Eristeo García Márquez [3,*]

[1] Universidad Autónoma de Nuevo León, Facultad de Ciencias Biológicas, Departamento de Alimentos, Avenida Universidad s/n, Ciudad Universitaria, San Nicolás de los Garza, NL 66455, Mexico; liamtz18@hotmail.com (A.A.L.M.); minevillareal@hotmail.com (M.B.V.); karla_alanis23@hotmail.com (K.G.G.A.)
[2] Universidad Autónoma de Nuevo León, Facultad de Ciencias Biológicas, Laboratorio de Nanotecnología, Avenida Universidad s/n, Ciudad Universitaria, San Nicolás de los Garza, NL 66455, Mexico; sagrod@yahoo.com.mx
[3] Centro de Investigación y Asistencia en Tecnología y Diseño del Estado de Jalisco, Autopista Mty-Aeropuerto Km 10 Parque PIIT, Vía de Innovación 404, Apodaca, NL 66629, Mexico
* Correspondence: juan.baezgn@uanl.edu.mx (J.G.B.G.); egarcia@ciatej.mx (E.G.M.)

Received: 16 November 2019; Accepted: 23 December 2019; Published: 27 December 2019

Abstract: *Prunus serotine* seed, was processed to produce a defatted flour (71.07 ± 2.10% yield) without hydrocyanic acid. The total protein was 50.94 ± 0.64%. According to sensory evaluation of cookies with *P. serotine* flour, the highest score in overall impression (6.31) was at 50% flour substitution. Its nutritional composition stood out for its protein and fiber contents 12.50% and 0.93%, respectively. Protein concentrate (*Ps*PC) was elaborated (81.44 ± 7.74% protein) from defatted flour. Emulsifying properties of *Ps*PC were studied in emulsions at different mass fractions; ϕ = 0.002, 0.02, 0.1, 0.2, and 0.4 through physicochemical analysis and compared with whey protein concentrate (WPC). Particle size in emulsions increased, as did oil content, and results were reflected in microscope photographs. *Ps*PC at ϕ 0.02 showed positive results along the study, reflected in the microphotograph and emulsifying stability index (ESI) test (117.50 min). At ϕ 0.4, the lowest ESI (29.34 min), but the maximum emulsifying activity index (EAI) value (0.029 m^2/g) was reached. WPC had an EAI value higher than *Ps*PC at $\phi \geq 0.2$, but its ESI were always lower in all mass fraction values. *Ps*PC can compete with emulsifiers as WPC and help stabilize emulsions.

Keywords: *Prunus serotine*; defatted flour; soluble protein; protein concentrate; emulsifying properties; emulsion stability

1. Introduction

Nowadays, there is an increasing demand for products of high nutritional quality [1]. Proteins are one of the major components of the human diet because of their nutritional properties. They are also responsible for physicochemical properties such as solubility, water, and oil retention capacity, foaming and emulsifying capacity, viscosity, and gelation, among others. The proteins impact not only the quality of the products, but also acceptance by consumers [2].

Protein is available in a variety of dietary sources [3]. In recent years, the growing concern of consumers with respect to animal safety has forced the industry to use vegetable proteins [4–6]. This type of proteins has health benefits, e.g., reduction of blood cholesterol levels, prevention of obesity and lower risk of heart diseases and cancer [7]. Vegetable proteins, when mixed with cereals, provide an alternative source of amino acids [3], which is why enrichment of other protein sources such as oilseeds and legumes with cereal-based foods has received considerable attention [8].

Baked snacks, such as bread and cookies, are widely accepted and consumed throughout the world and have become an attractive target for feeding and nutritional status improvement programs. This is especially true for cookies, because they not only offer a good vehicle for protein enrichment for consumers, but also because of their wide-spread consumption (5.9 per capita in 2019) and long shelf life [9–11].

The implementation of wheat flour substitutes or mimicry are desirable alternatives to achieve not only a decrease in calories, but also, to obtain a healthier nutritional profile in their composition [12,13]. Legumes and oilseeds such as soy, sunflower, barley, melon seeds, peanuts, hazelnuts, walnuts, sesame seeds, cashews, and almonds, are some alternative sources of flour [9,10].

Also, food grade films, hydrogels, foams, and emulsifiers have been developed from vegetable proteins. Emulsions are capable of absorbing at the oil-in water interface or air-in water dispersion [7,14]. These are part of many processed food formulations. Proteins are widely used for encapsulation of active substances. The proteins are used as a wall material around the active principle droplet, manifesting advantages such as biocompatibility, biodegradability, amphiphilic and hydrophobic and functional properties [15]. Moreover, vegetable proteins can be combined with other polymers, forming a variety of complexes with different structures (e.g., double networks, mosaic textures and cross-linked structures) [7].

In emulsions, the emulsifying activity index, emulsifying stability index, droplet size, interfacial properties and viscosity parameters are used [1]. Other techniques that help to understand the structure of the emulsions and morphology of the particles, particle size, and colloid instabilities (e.g., flocculation, aggregation) are light microscopy, SEM, and dynamic or static light scattering [16]. Among the vegetable proteins emulsifiers options, we found mainly leguminous foodstuffs like soy, lupin, peas, and chickpeas, cereals like wheat, barley, corn, and rice and oil seed such as peanuts, sunflowers, canola, flaxseed, and sesame. [7,17].

In Mexico, the oilseed *Prunus serotine* is widely distributed, and can be found in 16 states of the Republic. Nowadays the production of the fruit goes to 467.96 tons per year [18,19]. However, only the fruit and leaves have been used since colonial times for nourishment and medicinal purposes [20]. While the seed is still of little economic value because of the waste of its nutritional benefits, since it is only consumed as a toasted snack, the main nutrients in its composition are unsaturated fatty acids (89.9%) such as oleic, linoleic, and α-eleostearic acid, crude fiber (10.73 ± 1.49%) and protein (37.95 ± 0.16%) with 88.12 ± 0.72% of digestibility [18,21]. A protein value higher than other oilseeds like *P. dulcis* (19.91%) and *Arachis hypogaea* (22.82%), having lysine as the limiting amino acid. It has also been reported that digestibility values higher than 80% are related to an efficient amino acid bioavailability [18].

Its oil composition is also considered unique because of the significant content of α-eleostearic acid [22]. This acid can be a nutraceutical ingredient because it is capable of providing beneficial health effects, including prevention and/or treatment of a disease [23]. Some studies report that it effectively suppresses growth of cancer cells, lowers serum lipid levels in mammals, and has been proposed as chemotherapeutic agent against breast cancer. *P. serotine* seed oil increase its potential as functional and nutraceutical ingredient [22].

Biotic and abiotic metabolites can contaminate crops and plant-based foods; therefore, toxins must be examined [24]. Cyanogenic glycosides occur in a wide range of food plant species, such as cassava root, apples, lima beans, passion fruit, and almonds [25]. Almonds contain amygdalin as a cyanogenic glycoside (a secondary metabolite) [26]. This metabolite produces hydrogen cyanide (HCN) when it is hydrolyzed. Its effects go from intoxication symptoms to neuropathic problems [27]. Nevertheless, the toasting process to which *P. serotine* seed is subjected as snack, helps to not produce amygdalin because of the temperature it is subjected to. The pericarp of *P. serotine* accumulates amygdalin, but it is acyanogenic because it lacks enzymes to release HCN [28]. In addition, it is devoid of oil content, as well as cyanide components [22]. All these circumstances, along with the fact that the seed has been used for human nutrition since ancient times, allow us to assume that it has little or no toxicity [28].

However, there are some treatments that can reduce or eliminate the risk of poisoning, whereby the focus in on removal of glycoside through washing and/or pressing the food, by enzymatic breakdown of the glycoside, destroying the enzyme or a combination of these methods [29].

From *P. serotine* seed, two valuable products can be obtained, namely α-eleostearic acid with nutraceutical potential applications and the defatted seed with high protein content, which can be used for the development of biscuit products and concentrate protein for the stabilization of emulsions.

We have previously evaluated the study of *P. serotine* oil, so we are focusing on the second product and its derivates. Therefore, the aim was to evaluate *P. serotine* defatted flour without hydrogen cyanide risk in cookies and protein concentrate in emulsion stability.

2. Materials and Methods

P. serotine seeds were obtained from Xochimilco's market in Mexico City, Mexico. Wheat flour (*Triticum* spp.) and canola oil were purchased from a local food store in Monterrey, Nuevo Leon, Mexico. Whey protein concentrate (WPC, MB Pro-mix, 80%) was food grade from Marquez Bros, International, Inc.-whey division, Hanford, CA. Solvents: hexane, *n*-propanol, boric acid, ethanol, phosphoric acid, and hydrochloric acid were of analytical grade (J.T. Baker reagents, Azcapotzalco, Mexico City, Mexico). The reagents sodium chloride, sodium hydroxide, sodium azide, sodium carbonate, sodium tartrate and copper sulphate were purchased from Development of Chemical Specialities in Monterrey, Nuevo Leon, Mexico. Picric acid was from Acce Microbiology in Guadalupe, Nuevo Leon, Mexico, and Coomassie brilliant blue G-250 from ThermoFisher Scientific, Mexico. Sucrose, Tris(hydroxymethyl)aminomethane, SDS, Folin & Ciocalteu's and bovine serum albumin (BSA) were from Sigma-Aldrich, Mexico.

2.1. P. serotine Defatted Flour

A defatted flour was elaborated from the seeds of *P. serotine* (Scheme 1). Seeds were cracked open with a sterilized metal squeezer, washed with 2.5% NaCl and distilled water (1:5, *w/v*) for 30 min with constant magnetic stirring, followed by scalding with hot water at 90 °C for 5 min, and drained for 7 min, followed by drying for 1 h at 60 °C in an oven with air circulation. Once dried, the oil was removed with a manual oil press (Kinetic, Henan Wecare Industry Co. Ltd., Jiaozuo, China) and the residue (ground seed) toasted to 100 °C for 25 min [29]. Subsequently, the remaining oil was removed by constant magnetic stirring with hexane (1: 5, *w/v*) to 25 ± 2 °C for 1 h. The ground seed was washed and filtered through Whatman paper No. 4 and dried in a hood extractor for 6 h. Finally, it was chopped in a blender and passed through a 70-mesh screen to obtain a *P. serotine* defatted flour [2].

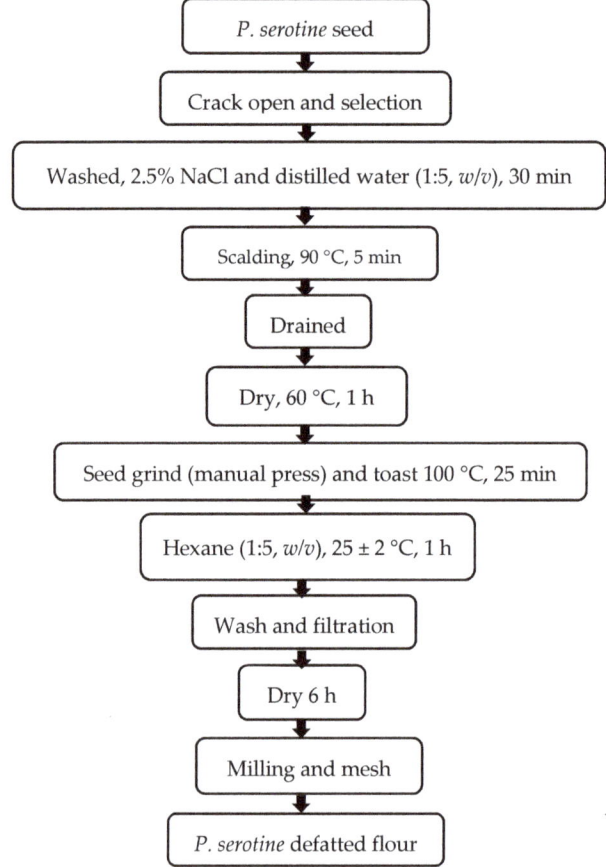

Scheme 1. Physical-chemistry process to obtain *P. serotine* defatted flour.

The flour yield was determined by the following formula:

$$\text{Flour yield (\%)} = \frac{\text{Flour weight (g)}}{\text{Seed weight (g)}} * 100 \tag{1}$$

2.2. Particle Size

In order to measure the particle size of the *P. serotine* defatted flour, the methodology of Khor et al. [30] was used with some modifications. The flour was measured in a Mastersizer 3000 Hydro LV (Malvern Instruments Ltd., Worcestershire, UK) using the liquid unit. The particle size was evaluated through the volume-weight mean diameter ($D_{4,3}$) at 25 ± 2 °C, as Belorio et al. [31] report. Optical properties of the sample were defined as refractive index 1.37, isopropyl alcohol as dispersant, and an absorption of 0.1. The results were expressed in μm as means ± standard deviation. Wheat flour (*Triticum* spp.) was used as control.

2.3. Chemical Composition

Analysis were performed on *P. serotine* defatted flour by using Association of Official Analytical Chemistry [32] and compared with wheat flour (control). Moisture, ash, and crude fiber were evaluated gravimetrically (AOAC 14.006, AOAC 925.15 and AOAC 962.09, respectively). The Goldfish method (AOAC 920.36C) was used to determine the fat content. The protein was measured using the Kjeldahl method (AOAC 930.29) and total carbohydrates were determined by the difference using the following equation:

$$HC\ (\%) = [100 - (protein + lipids + ash + crude\ fiber)] \qquad (2)$$

2.4. Grignard Test

To verify that during the process of making *P. serotine* defatted flour, hydrocyanic acid (HCN) was eliminated, a qualitative test was used according to Castro and Rodriguez [33]. Picrosodic papers were prepared and then circles of filter paper (Whatman No. 4) were soaked with 1% picric acid solution and allowed to dry in the dark until they changed color to deep yellow. Once dried, they were impregnated with 10% sodium carbonate and allowed to dry. Afterwards, they were fixed on the lid of amber bottles and two drops of 10% sodium carbonate were added, preventing it from dripping.

The *P. serotine* defatted flour was placed inside the jar to fill a third of it and covered quickly. The bottles were stored in the dark and after 24 h, a reading was taken. As a control, only fractionated *P. serotine* seeds were used (without any treatment). If the paper´s yellow color was maintained or it became light orange, there would be absolutely no problem in its consumption, but if it changed to intense orange or pink, it could only be consumed with caution and if the color became reddish or dark brown, it would not be safe to consume.

2.5. Cookie Preparation

Four variations of cookie recipe were made according to Jia et al. [34] with some modifications. The cookie dough formula is presented in Table 1. The control recipe was 100% commercial wheat flour (Fc) and the other four were 100, 75, 50, and 25%, respectively, with *P. serotine* defatted flour (F1 to F4, respectively). Butter and sugar were mixed, then creamed with a Kitchen Aid mixer at low speed for one min. Vanilla essence and egg were added and mixed for one minute. In another bowl, all dry ingredients (flour, baking powder, and salt) were sifted and gradually added to the previous mix at low speed for 1 min and then medium speed for one min. When all the ingredients were integrated and homogenized, the dough was wrapped in plastic and allowed to cool at 4 °C for 1 h.

Table 1. Cookie dough formula.

Ingredients	Weight (g)
Flour (Fc, F1, F2, F3, F4)	150
Baking powder	3
Salt	3.5
Butter without salt	73
Sugar	66.6
Egg	25
Vanilla essence	2.5

Fc corresponds to 150 g of wheat flour, F1 corresponds to 150 g of *P. serotine* defatted flour, F2 corresponds to 112.5 g of *P. serotine* defatted flour and 37.5 g of wheat flour, F3 corresponds to 75 g of *P. serotine* defatted flour and 75 g of wheat flour and F4 corresponds to 37.5 g of *P. serotine* defatted flour and 112.5 g of wheat flour.

Once the dough had rested, it was kneaded and spread with a rolling pin and 2 × 2 cm and 0.5 cm high square cookies were cut and, placed in an aluminum tray with waxed paper to prevent them from sticking. The oven was preheated at 160 °C for 15 min and the cookies were baked for 12 min at the same temperature. After removal from the oven, the cookies were left to cool at room temperature (25 ± 2 °C).

2.6. Sensory Evaluation and Chemical Composition

The evaluation was carried out in the Sensory Evaluation Laboratory of the Faculty of the College of Food Science at the Autonomous University of Nuevo Leon, Mexico. Fifty-five panelists (untrained) participated in the sensory test based on Jia et al. [34]. These individuals were seated at individual tables in different compartments. A 9-point hedonic scale was used (1 = extreme dislike, 5 = neither like nor dislike, 9 = extreme like) to evaluate the cookies texture, appearance, color, smell, taste, mouthfeel, aftertaste, and overall impression. Scores of five and higher for overall impressions were considered acceptable in this study. Cookies with 3-digit random number codes were randomly presented to the panelists, who were instructed to cleanse their palates with distilled water (25 °C) between sensory analyses. Chemical composition analysis (fat, protein, crude fiber and carbohydrate) involved quantification in the cookies with the highest score for the overall impression attribute, as specified in Section 2.3.

2.7. Extraction of Soluble Proteins

Proteins were extracted sequentially from *P. serotine* defatted flour according to the procedure described by Ramirez Pimentel et al. [35] and Raya Perez et al. [28], with the following solvents: distilled water (albumins), 0.5 M NaCl solution in 50 mM Tris pH 8 (globulins), 55% (*v/v*) 2-propanol (prolamins) and 0.1 M boric acid with 0.5% SDS pH 8 (glutelins).

The flour:solvent mixture (ratio 1:10, *w/v*) was stirred for 1 h at 25 ± 2 °C. The extracts were centrifuged (Hermle Z326, Labortechnik GmbH, Wehingen, Germany) at 13,000 g at 25 ± 2 °C for 20 min and the supernatants filtered (Whatman No. 4). The extraction with each solvent was repeated on the same sample sequentially and the supernatants of the three extractions were combined.

2.8. Soluble Protein Determination

Soluble proteins were quantified from the soluble protein extractions as reported by Lopez Dellamary Toral [36] based on the Bradford [37] technique, with some modifications. Bovine serum albumin (BSA) was used as a standard (0.05 to 0.5 mg/mL). The soluble protein fractions were diluted with 50 mM Tris-HCl buffer at pH 7, to obtain values within the standard range concentration. Albumin concentration was 0.49 mg/mL, globulin 0.26 mg/mL, prolamin 0.33 mg/mL, and glutelin 0.24 mg/mL. In microplates, 20 µL of each extract was added in triplicate, using wells consecutively with 200 µL of Bradford reagent (0.01% Coomassie Blue G-250, 4.75% ethanol, 85% H_3PO_4), allowing to stand for 2 min. The samples were evaluated (microplate reader-Anthos 2020 version 2.0.5) at 620 nm.

2.9. Electrophoresis

Protein patterns were analyzed according to Syros et al. [38] with some modifications based on Bio-Rad laboratories [39] using polyacrylamide gel electrophoresis (SDS-PAGE). Two glass plates were placed in the electrophoresis chamber, fixing them with plastic spacers and polyacrylamide gel (4–20%) with a 10-well comb (Mini-PROTEAN TGX, Precast protein gels, Bio-Rad Laboratories, Inc. Irvine, CA, USA).

In gel rails, 20 µL of each extraction of soluble protein fraction were placed (at the same previous concentrations) with distilled water. After electrophoresis, the gel was completely immersed in a fixing solution and washed three times for 10 min with distilled water. The gel was immersed and stirred in Coomassie blue dye solution (G-250) until bands were clearly evidenced.

2.10. Isoelectric Point (pI)

The isoelectric point of the *P. serotine* defatted flour was determined according to the theoretical determination of proteins and other macromolecules, through zeta potential (ζ-potential) which is the most direct characterization of the repulsion or attraction strength between their acid-base residues [40,41]. For this, a mixture of flour: deionized water in a 1:20 ratio (w/v) at different pH with 0.1 N NaOH and 0.1 N HCl was vortexed for two minutes. Zetasizer Nano ZS90 light scattering equipment (Malvern Instruments, Worcestershire, England, UK) was used. The measures were in automatic mode using a universal immersion cell (ZEN 1002, Malvern Instrument, Worcestershire, UK) at 25 °C. The results were reported as the average of three separate injections, with three measures per injection. The averages of triplicate values were used as the values for zeta potential reported.

2.11. Prunus serotine Protein Concentration (PsPC)

To obtain *PsPC* the results obtained from the p*I* were taken as a basis. Variations of the procedure were undertaken to determine the one that was repeatable and had protein concentrate values $\geq 80\%$ and $\leq 90\%$. All procedures were initiated by mixing the *P. serotine* defatted flour for 1 h in vortex with distilled water at pH 11 with 0.1 N NaOH (25 ± 2 °C), ratio 1:20 (w/v). Then the sample was isolated by centrifugation (Hermle Z326, Labortechnik GmbH, Wehingen, Germany) at 13,000 g for 30 min and filtered through No. 4 Whatman paper to obtain two fractions (residue and supernatant).

In the first variation, up to two extractions of the residue obtained in the first part of the process were carried out with 5% NaCl (1:20, w/v), at two extraction times (30 min and 1 h) in vortex at 25 °C, followed by centrifugation (Hermle Z326, Labortechnik GmbH, Wehingen, Germany) at 13,000 g for 30 min and filtered, again obtaining two fractions. The residue was analyzed utilizing the Kjeldhal method [32] to ensure the lowest protein loss in the process. The resulting supernatant was combined with the supernatant obtained in the first part, to subsequently acidify and solubilize the protein with HCl as shown in Scheme 1. The precipitate was stored until analysis at -20 °C. The pH for acidification were 3.0, 3.7, and 4.5.

In the second variation, the residue of the first part was automatically discarded and the supernatant was acidified with HCl and left to rest for 30 min. Finally, it was centrifuged and filtered under the previous conditions. The precipitate was collected and stored at -20 °C until use. Three acid pH values (3.0, 3.7, and 4.5) were tested (Scheme 2).

All final precipitates were analyzed according to proximal analysis via the Kjeldhal method based on AOAC 930.29 [32]. The yield was determined by the following equation:

$$Protein\ concentrate\ yield\ (\%) = \frac{Precipitate\ weight\ (g)}{Defatted\ flour\ weight\ (g)} * 100 \qquad (3)$$

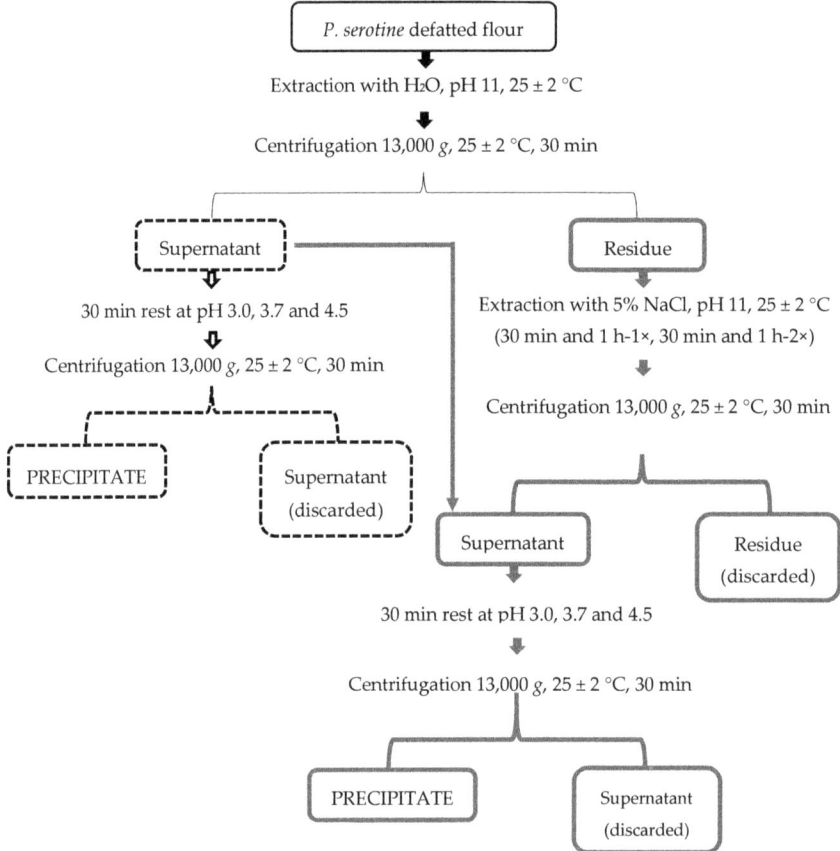

Scheme 2. The diagram in gray indicates the procedure for obtaining protein concentrate from the *P. serotine* defatted flour with NaCl treatment and acid pH. 1× indicating that the extraction was performed once, and 2×, that it was repeated twice. The black dots indicate the procedure for obtaining protein concentrate from the *P. serotine* defatted flour by direct acidification.

2.12. Preparation of Emulsions

The emulsifying agents (PsPC and whey protein concentrate) were prepared at 1% *w/v* in deionized water and solubilized with constant stirring. Then the sample was allowed to hydrate overnight at 4 °C. Afterwards, 0.05% sodium azide was mixed to prevent microbial growth. Different amounts of canola oil 0.1, 1, 5, 10, and 20 g were added, to obtain a variety of mass fractions (ϕ = 0.002, 0.02, 0.1, 0.2, and 0.4). The emulsions were mixed in a homogenizer (OMNI International GLH, Georgia, United States) at an initial speed of 1000 rpm for 2 min and subsequently at 3000 rpm for 3 min. All emulsions were made in triplicate and stored at 25 ± 2 °C for 18 days, and every three days, all the following analyzes were made. Whey protein concentrate (WPC) was used as a control [42,43].

2.13. Droplet Size Measurement

Particle size was determined by integrated light scattering using a Mastersizer 3000 Hydro LV (Malvern Instruments Ltd., Worcestershire, UK). The emulsions were analyzed immediately after preparation in quintuplicate. Laser diffraction measures the particle size distribution (diameter equivalent to the volume) from the angular variation of the intensity of scattered light when the laser beam passes through the particles dispersed in solution. The data are then integrated based on the angular dispersion intensity, calculating the particle size through the Mie theory of light scattering. The droplet size of emulsions was evaluated through volume-surface mean diameter ($D_{3,2}$) at 25 ± 2 °C as Guo and Mu reports [1]. Optical properties of the sample were defined as refractive index 1.43 for *PsPC* and 1.46 for WPC, water as dispersant and an absorption of 0.1. The results were expressed as means ± standard deviation [30].

2.14. Emulsifying Activity Index and Emulsifying Stability Index (EAI and ESI)

The EAI and ESI were assayed via the colorimetric method, previously reported by Guo and Mu [1]. Immediately after homogenizing each emulsion, 20 µL from the bottom was taken and diluted with 5 mL of 0.1% SDS solution. It was vortexed for 5 min and, the absorbance was measured in a spectrophotometer (UV-Visible-Genesys 10s, Thermo scientific, Cambridge, MA, USA) at 500 nm [1]. The *EAI* and *ESI* were calculated using the following equations:

$$EAI\left(\frac{m^2}{g}\right) = \frac{2 * 2.303 * A_0 * dilution\ factor}{c * 1 * (1 - \phi) * 10,000} \quad (4)$$

where *c* is the initial protein concentration which is 1% *w/v*, φ is the oil weight fraction, dilution factor was 250.

$$ESI\ (min) = \frac{A_0}{A_0 - A_{10}} * t \quad (5)$$

where A_0 and A_{10} are the absorbance of the diluted emulsions at 0 and 10 min, respectively and, *t* was 10 min.

2.15. Interfacial Protein Concentration

According to Eichberg and Mokrasch [44] and Guo and Mu [1], interfacial protein concentration was quantified. Two milliliters of freshly prepared emulsions were diluted with 2 mL of 50% sucrose solution (*w/v*) and vortexed for 5 min at 25 ± 2 °C. In a centrifuge tube, 2 mL of the solution were mixed with 7 mL of 5% sucrose solution (*w/v*) and all samples were centrifuged (Spectrafuge 6C, Labnet International, Inc., New York, NY, USA) at 3500*g* for 30 min at 25 ± 2 °C. Once centrifuged, three phases were observed: the oil drops in the upper phase, an intermediate phase corresponding to the 5% sucrose solution, and the aqueous phase in the lower part of the tube. The tubes were frozen at −40 °C for 24 h and then the upper layer of the oil was removed.

The proteins adsorbed from the oil phase were removed by adding 20 mL of 1% SDS (*w/v*) solution. To determine the concentration of adsorbed protein, 1 mL of the sample was mixed with 3 mL of an alkaline copper reagent (A: 2% Na_2CO_3, 0.4% NaOH, 0.16% sodium tartrate, and 1% SDS with B: 4% $CuSO_4 \cdot 5H_2O$, in a ratio of 100:1). The samples were vigorously stirred, and allowed to rest at 25 ± 2 °C for 10 min. Subsequently, 0.3 mL of 2 N Folin-Ciocaletu was added and allowed to stand for 45 min at 25 ± 2 °C. The absorbance was immediately measured at 660 nm in a spectrophotometer (UV-Visible-Genesys 10s, Thermo scientific, Cambridge, MA, USA) against a blank. Bovine serum albumin (BSA) was used as a standard. The interfacial protein concentration was calculated as:

$$T\left(\frac{mg}{m^2}\right) = C_{ad}/S_V \quad (6)$$

where C_{ad} (mg/mL) is the concentration of adsorbed protein and S_V is the specific interfacial area (m^2/mL emulsion) of the emulsion droplets.

2.16. Optical Microscopy

The optical microscopy photographs were taken based on Huang et al. [45] with small modifications. Emulsions were mixed in vortex for 1 min prior to analysis. A drop of the emulsion was placed between the coverslip and microscope slide. The globules of the emulsions were examined and observed under bright field illumination with 40× objective lens on a Leica microscope (Leica DM500, 9435 Heerbrugg, Switzerland) along with the software Leica LAS EZ 2.0.0, Ltd., Application Suite (Leica Microsystems, 9435 Heerbrugg, Switzerland).

2.17. Statistical Analysis

Data from the replicated experiments were analyzed to determine whether the variances were statistically homogeneous, and the results were expressed as the mean ± standard deviation (SD). Statistical comparisons were made by one-way variance analysis (ANOVA) followed by Tukey's test using Statgraphics centurion XVII Software. The difference between means was considered significant at $p < 0.05$.

3. Results and Discussion

3.1. Particle Size of Defatted Flour

P. serotine defatted flour had a yield of 71.07 ± 2.10%. Its particle size ($D_{4,3}$) was 5.10 ± 0.03 μm, which was minor for the commercial wheat flour (*Triticum* spp.) with 7.31 ± 0.01 μm, making *P. serotine* flour 1.4 times smaller.

The AOAC 965.22 [46] mentioned that wheat flour must be able to pass through a No. 70 mesh (212 μm) to be acceptable commercially, and *P. serotine* flour in the process of elaboration did pass through this mesh screen and its particle size was smaller than that of wheat flour (control).

It is already known that the particle size of wheat flour can influence cookie quality, but this can also be true for gluten-free flours. Belorio et al. [31] observed that cookies with smaller values of the elastic component (G') correspond to flours with higher values of $D_{4,3}$. Meanwhile, the biggest elastic values (G') were found in doughs elaborated from finer flours.

3.2. Chemical Composition

The moisture in both flours passed the test mentioned in Codex Standard 152-1985 [47]. *P. serotine* defatted flour was 4.6 times less moisture than wheat flour (Table 2). It was not possible to remove all the oil contained in the *P. serotine* seed. After the separation process, 3.4% was quantified. Possibly because of the oil being bound to proteins contained in *P. serotine*, it also contains 5 times more protein and 1.5 times as much total fiber than wheat flour and 2 times less carbohydrates [48].

Table 2. Nutritional components of two flours.

Component (%)	*P. serotine*	Wheat [1] (*Triticum* spp.)
Moisture	2.58 ± 0.09 [b]	11.92 [a]
Ash	5.36 ± 0.24 [a]	0.47 [b]
Fat	3.36 ± 0.31 [a]	0.98 [b]
Protein	50.94 ± 0.64 [a]	10.33 [b]
Crude Fiber	4.03 ± 0.27 [a]	2.7 [b]
Carbohydrates	36.31 ± 1.09 [b]	76.31 [a]

The values are the average of five assays ± standard deviations of the flours. Mean values labeled with a different letter in the same file are significantly different ($p < 0.005$). [1] Wheat nutritional values were consulted on https://fdc.nal.usda.gov/fdc-app.html#/food-details/168936/nutrients.

3.3. Grignard Test

Zumaeta Cordova and Gonzales Díaz [29] mentioned that the treatments that allow the release of hydrocyanic acid from glycosides and their subsequent elimination by drying or heating, are those that guarantee greater safety (100 °C for 25 min).

The experiment showed that in the control sample (fractionated seed without treatment), the paper impregnated with picric acid changed from yellow to deep orange, which indicated that the food could be consumed, but with caution. Meanwhile, the flour with treatment paper remained with the same yellow color. This indicated that there were no potential consumption problems (Figure 1).

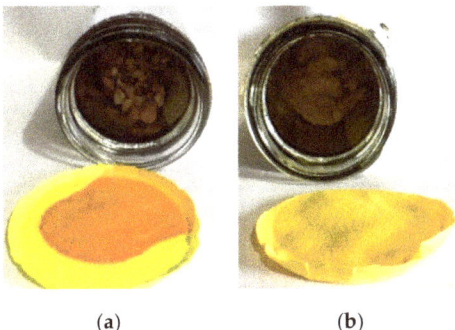

(a) (b)

Figure 1. (a) *P. serotine* seed without treatment. (b) *P. serotine* defatted flour with treatment.

We believe that due to the low concentration of cyanogenic compounds, the consumption of *P. serotine* seeds has not caused any poisoning problems. In addition, the seed has been toasted for a long period of time prior to consumption.

According to Alveano Aguerrebere [20], there is no significant difference between the protein content of the seed in its toasted version (37.95 ± 0.16%), compared to when it is raw (36.55 ± 0.22%). Also, Garcia Aguilar et al. [18] mentioned that there is no significant difference in the values of in vitro protein digestibility of raw (88.12 ± 0.72%) and toasted (89.40 ± 1.32%) *P. serotine* seeds.

3.4. Sensory Evaluation

The effects of the addition of *P. serotine* defatted flour are shown in Table 3. A decrease in the scores of all sensory attributes and the overall impression of the cookies was found with the addition of *P. serotine* defatted flour. However, the maximum amount of *P. serotine* defatted flour accepted by the untrained panelists in the cookies was 75% (F2) based on the value obtained in the overall acceptability category though the formulation with *P. serotine* defatted flour showing the highest acceptability level was F3 with a substitution of 50%.

Table 3. Effects of *P. serotine* defatted flour on sensory attributes of cookies.

Sensory Attributes	Fc	F1	F2	F3	F4
Color	7.38 ± 2.01 [a]	4.49 ± 2.01 [c]	5.93 ± 2.03 [b]	6.96 ± 1.49 [a, b]	6.91 ± 1.97 [a, b]
Smell	7.43 ± 1.78 [a]	4.81 ± 1.99 [c]	6.04 ± 2.03 [b]	6.59 ± 1.46 [a, b]	6.48 ± 1.77 [a, b]
Taste	7.38 ± 1.70 [a]	2.55 ± 1.55 [c]	5.73 ± 2.18 [b]	5.53 ± 1.74 [b]	6.07 ± 2.14 [b]
Texture	7.33 ±1.88 [a]	3.95 ± 1.96 [c]	5.73 ± 1.92 [b]	5.76 ± 1.73 [b]	6.65 ± 1.67 [a, b]
Appearance	7.49 ± 1.99 [a]	4.56 ± 2.08 [c]	5.78 ± 2.01 [b]	6.85 ± 1.42 [a]	6.78 ± 1.82 [a, b]
Mouthfeel	7.33 ± 1.76 [a]	3.16 ± 1.61 [c]	5.39 ± 2.34 [b]	5.69 ± 1.76 [b]	6.05 ± 2.04 [b]
Aftertaste	6.89 ± 1.72 [a]	2.89 ± 1.71 [c]	5.27 ± 2.16 [b]	5.60 ± 2.12 [b]	5.78 ± 2.15 [b]
Overall impression	7.45 ± 1.54 [a]	3.27 ± 1.72 [c]	5.84 ± 1.79 [b]	6.31 ± 1.60 [b]	6.18 ± 1.88 [b]

The values are the average of fifty-five assay ± standard deviations of the sensory attributes of cookies with *P. serotine* defatted flour and wheat flour. Mean values labeled with a different letter in the same file are significantly different ($p < 0.005$).

The results obtained in the evaluation show that the cookies that were made with 75 to 25% *P. serotine* defatted flour (F2 to F4) received a score greater than five in overall impression, making them acceptable. These cookies had greater acceptance compared to other cookies made with Californian almonds (*P. dulcis*), for which maximum acceptance was only 20% substitution, with a score of 5.25 in overall impression [34].

3.5. Cookie Chemical Composition

Based on the results obtained from the sensory test, a decision was made to carry out the chemical analysis on Fc cookies (100% wheat flour) because it was preferred by the evaluators. Of the cookies made with *P. serotine* defatted flour, those substituted by 50 and 25% (F3 and F4) were selected as a result of obtaining the highest score in overall impression (Table 4).

Table 4. Nutritional components in cookies with wheat and *P. serotine* defatted flour.

Component (%)	Fc	F3	F4
Fat	68.08 ± 0.29 [a]	61.94 ± 0.27 [a]	58.48 ± 0.27 [a]
Protein	0.71 ± 0.06 [c]	12.50 ± 0.03 [a]	11.79 ± 0.02 [b]
Crude Fiber	0.00 ± 0.00 [a]	0.93 ± 0.04 [a]	0.88 ± 0.03 [a]
Carbohydrates	31.20 ± 0.05 [a]	24.63 ± 0.05 [c]	28.85 ± 0.08 [b]

The values are the average of three assays ± standard deviations of cookies with wheat and *P. serotine* defatted flour. Mean values labeled with a different letter in the same file are significantly different ($p < 0.005$).

Cookies made with *P. serotine* defatted flour stood out for having fiber and for their protein content, up to 17 times higher than cookies with wheat flour (Fc), as well as, for presenting 6.57 and 2.35% lower carbohydrates, and 6.14 and 9.6% lower fat content (F3 and F4, respectively) than control cookies. In addition, it can be said that cookies made with 50 and 25% *P. serotine* defatted flour have a lower gluten content compared to control cookies, since almonds are the best vegetable sources of gluten-free protein and one of the most popular ingredients in the preparation of gluten-free foods, making them a healthy alternative for people suffering from celiac disease [49].

3.6. Soluble Protein Determination

From the *P. serotine* defatted flour 16.4 ± 2.54 g soluble protein was extracted/100 mL of solution, which is equivalent to 32.15 ± 0.49% of total protein content. The soluble protein profile was albumin 76.95 ± 2.29%, globulin 13.60 ± 2.56%, glutelin 6.16 ± 0.99%, and prolamin 3.29 ± 0.37%. The relative concentration of soluble protein with respect to insoluble proteins was 3.3:1 (Table 5). Raya Perez et al. [28], also quantified soluble protein in *P. serotine* and also reported albumin as the predominating fraction, followed by globulin, glutelin, and finally prolamin.

Table 5. Soluble protein content in *P. serotine* defatted flour.

Soluble Protein	Protein Content (mg/mL)	Fraction Content with Respect of Total Soluble Protein (%)
Albumin	126.09 ± 3.74 [a]	76.95 ± 2.29 [a]
Globulin	22.29 ± 4.20 [b]	13.60 ± 2.56 [b]
Prolamin	5.39 ± 0.60 [d]	3.29 ± 0.37 [d]
Glutelin	10.09 ± 1.61 [c]	6.16 ± 0.99 [c]

The values are the average of three assays ± standard deviations of the soluble proteins in *P. serotine* defatted flour. Mean values labeled with a different letter in the same column are significantly different ($p < 0.005$).

3.7. Electrophoresis

The SDS-PAGE patterns for *P. serotine* defatted flour is reported in Figure 2. The molecular weight of albumin varied in a range from 63 to 20 KDa (lane 2 and 6). In globulins, it varied between 63 and 20 KDa (lane 3 and 7), in prolamins, it ranged from 60 to 20 KDa (lane 4 and 8), and in glutelins from 60 to 12 KDa (lane 5 and 9).

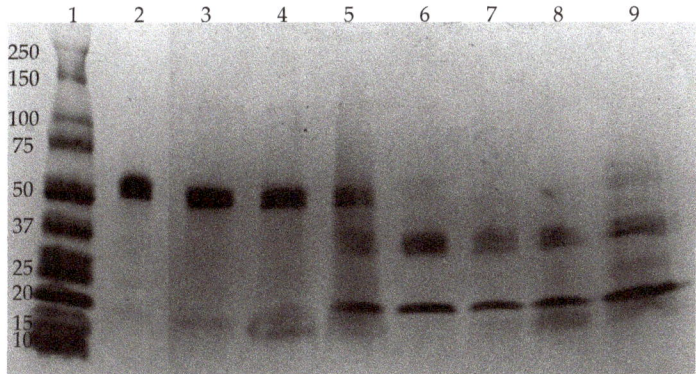

Figure 2. Soluble protein patterns of *P. serotine* defatted flour. 1. Molecular weight markers, lanes 2 to 5 (without 2-mercaptoethanol); 2. albumin; 3. globulin; 4. prolamin; 5. glutelin. Lanes 6 to 9, as lanes 2 to 5 but with 2-mercaptoethanol.

The molecular weights obtained were similar to the ones reported by Raya Perez et al. [28]. Albumin weight varied between 65 and 20 KDa, globulin between 65 and 14 KDa and prolamins and glutelins between 65 and 12 KDa, respectively.

Albumins and globulins are the main storage proteins of dicotyledonous plants (e.g., legumes and oilseeds), whereas prolamins and glutelins predominate in monocotyledonous plants (e.g., cereals). As expected of a nitrogen source, storage proteins are rich in asparagine (and aspartate), glutamine (and glutamate), and arginine [50], which is the case of *P. serotine* seed. According to Garcia Aguilar et al. [18] the seed contains 116.97 mg/g of asparagine, 273.73 mg/g of glutamine, and 87.42 mg/g of arginine (toasted version), the three amino acids showing the highest values.

Sze Tao and Sathe [2] have reported that pepsin is the most efficient protease hydrolyzing almond (*P. dulcis*) protein, especially for polypeptides with molecular weights from 15 to 42 KDa. Typically, pepsin hydrolysis produced polypeptides with 15 to 36 KDa, followed by 15 to 20 KDa and some with 20 to 40 KDa. Therefore, *P. serotine* defatted flour protein may be useful in production of food protein hydrolysate and did not necessarily involve an additional process.

3.8. Isoelectric Point (pI)

The isoelectric point of an amino acid is the pH value at which the amino acid is doubly ionized or in zwitterion concentration and is deduced from the Henderson–Hasselbach equation, as the average of the pK values of the stages that form and decompose the zwitterion. The point of intersection of calibration curve with the x-axis is pI value of protein [34,51].

As a result of the conductivity measurement at different pH of the *P. serotine* defatted flour, it was found that the specific pI for this oilseed was 3.7 (Figure 3). This value can be attributed to the high content of acidic amino acids present in the oilseed (aspartic acid 112.29 mg/g and glutamine 256.84 mg/g), which influenced the low value of pI [17]. In addition, this value is within the optimum range for the precipitation of oil proteins such as peanuts (4.0 ± 0.25), coinciding with what other researchers have reported [52].

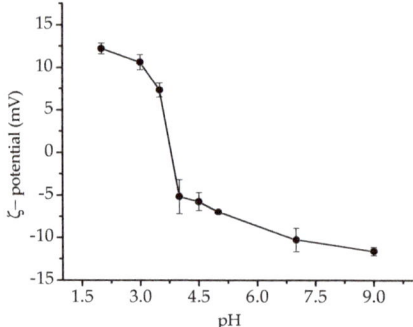

Figure 3. Isoelectric point (pI) of *P. serotine* defatted flour as a function change of concentration of hydrogen concentration.

3.9. Prunus serotine Protein Concentration (PsPC)

The *P. serotine* defatted flour was subjected to different treatments to obtain a process that is repeatable, standardized, and therefore reliable. The processes were adjusted and carried out as the results were obtained.

Usually to solubilize protein from oilseed meal, alkaline solutions are used. Solutions with a pH of 9 to 12 have higher protein yields. However, in values of pH 12 and higher, isolates with better quality are not always obtained [53].

The salts increase the solubility through the salting-in process, whereby the counter ions cover the ionic charges of protein molecules [54]. NaCl is a solubilizing agent, and the combination of alkali and salt is often used to improve protein solubility [53]. Table 6 shows the results of treating the flour with an alkaline pH followed by the interaction with a saline solution at different numbers of extractions in order to extract and recover the highest protein content of the first residue of flour.

Table 6. Treatments to obtain protein content in *P. serotine* defatted flour.

Sample	No. of Extractions	Time of Extraction (min)	Flour:NaCl Ratio (pH 11)	pH for Protein Precipitation	Protein Content (%)
P. serotine defatted flour	1	30	1:12	4.5	73.47 ± 0.92 [a, b]
	1	30	1:12	3.0	75.37 ± 2.86 [a]
	1	30	1:6	3.7	66.30 ± 7.80 [b]
	1	30	1:6	3.0	70.78 ± 4.50 [a, b]
	1	30	1:3	3.0	69.15 ± 3.07 [a, b]

Protein Content in Final Precipitate of *P. serotine* Defatted Flour with Direct Acidification.

Sample	No. of Extractions	Time of Extraction (min)	pH for Protein Precipitation	Protein Content (%)
P. serotine defatted flour	1	30	4.5	63.99 ± 6.63 [b]
	1	30	3.7	76.66 ± 7.36 [a, b]
	1	30	3.0	81.99 ± 6.96 [a]

The values are the average of three assays ± standard deviations of protein extractions from *P. serotine* defatted flour. Mean values labeled with a different letter in the same file are significantly different ($p < 0.005$).

The sample subjected to two extractions of one hour each with NaCl at a 1:20 (*w/v*) ratio at pH 11 had the lowest remaining protein in the residue (13.30 ± 0.39%), which would indicate that this process allows the collection of more protein in the supernatant of the treated sample.

The most common approach to recover solubilized proteins is by precipitating it with pH adjustment. In peanuts, some authors use pH 4.5 [53,54], while other researchers mention that the optimum pH can be within the isoelectric region between pH 3.0 and 5.0 [47]. Based on all these data, the following pH were used to precipitate the proteins of the supernatants: 4.5, 3.7, and 3.0.

The final protein content precipitated from the collected supernatant was not enough to reach the desired value of protein concentrate (whey protein concentrate ≥ 80%). The resulting values were: 56.77 ± 9.20 (pH 4.5), 66.96 ± 1.21 (pH 3.7), and 72.02 ± 5.01 (pH 3.0). This was attributed to the fact that at a high ionic strength, proteins can be almost completely precipitated from their solution because of dehydration in the protein molecules, thus reducing their solubility [53]. Therefore, the number and time of extraction was reduced in this, as well as in the flour:NaCl ratio (Table 6). At the same time, tests were carried out on the *P. serotine* defatted flour involving interaction only with an alkaline solution at pH 11 and then the supernatant was acidified to identify, in which acidic pH was the most effective.

The results obtained when precipitating the supernatants at pH 3.0 compared to other pH values (3.7 and 4.5) yielded a higher protein percentage. This was corroborated with the direct acidification process, which showed a concentrate value of 81.99 ± 6.96%.

The procedure was repeated two more times and results show that the treatment with direct acidification was the most effective. The average value of protein concentration in the final *P. serotine* defatted flour precipitate was 82.0%.

Researchers have identified and quantified the amino acids present in *P. serotine* seed, as well as its total and soluble protein [18,20,40]. However, there are still no reports on the uses or applications of *P. serotine* protein concentrate, making this work one of the first in its findings.

3.10. Droplet Size Measurement of Emulsions

In Figure 4, it can be seen that emulsions with more oil content had the largest droplet size. As the days passed, the particle size increased when $\phi \geq 0.2$. In every *PsPC* emulsion, the maximum droplet size value was reached at different days, but it could be considered as average on day 10. While in WPC emulsions, the range of days to reach the maximum droplet size was more stable (between days 6 and 12), the particle size was more dispersed compared to the *P. serotine* protein.

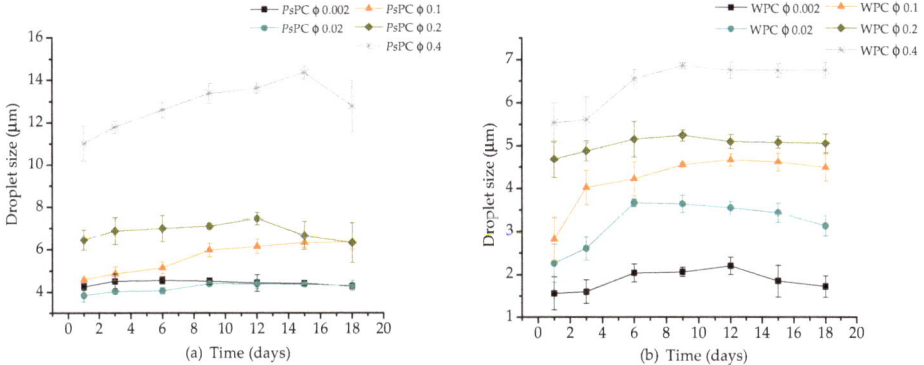

Figure 4. Droplet size ($D_{3,2}$) of emulsions with (**a**) protein concentrate (*PsPC*) (1% *w/v*) compared to (**b**) whey protein concentrate (WPC) (1% *w/v*) at different ϕ.

The *PsPC* emulsion at ϕ 0.02 presented a droplet size of 4.39 ± 0.08 µm as a maximum, becoming the smallest and more constant emulsion during the time of experiment, and for WPC, it was at ϕ 0.002, with a value of 2.20 ± 0.20 µm. In both the control (WPC) and *PsPC* emulsions, on the other hand, at ϕ 0.4, the droplet size had the highest value of 6.88 ± 0.11 µm (day 9) and 14.36 ± 0.31 µm (day 15), respectively, during storage time because of coalescence.

A small droplet size is of interest in emulsion studies, because they are strongly correlated with high emulsion stability [16]. Authors such as Pandolfe [55] and Floury et al. [56] have reported that the increase of oil in emulsions led to a gradual increase of oil droplet sizes. Part of the effect may be due to the limitation of surfactants in emulsions, since as the oil content increases, the available proteins decreases, limiting the stabilizing benefits of the protein, thus favoring the coalescence of the oil drops, and therefore, increasing the diameter. We suggest that emulsion stability is due to the hydrophobicity of the polypeptide chain. The mean diameter of the droplets in food emulsions can vary from less than 0.2 µm (for cream liqueurs) to greater than 100 µm (for salad dressings), depending on the product [57].

3.11. Emulsifying Activity Index and Emulsifying Stability Index (EAI and ESI)

Compared with other particles, the protein particles have emulsifying properties and great potential to form soft particles [42]. The ability of a protein to form an emulsion can be defined as an emulsifying activity index (EAI), which determines the approximate amount of interfacial area that can be stabilized per unit amount of protein. Additionally, the stability of the emulsion over a specific time period is referred to as the emulsifying stability index (ESI) [58]. The EAI increased as did the mass fraction in *Ps*PC emulsions (Figure 5). The effect was similar in the control emulsions.

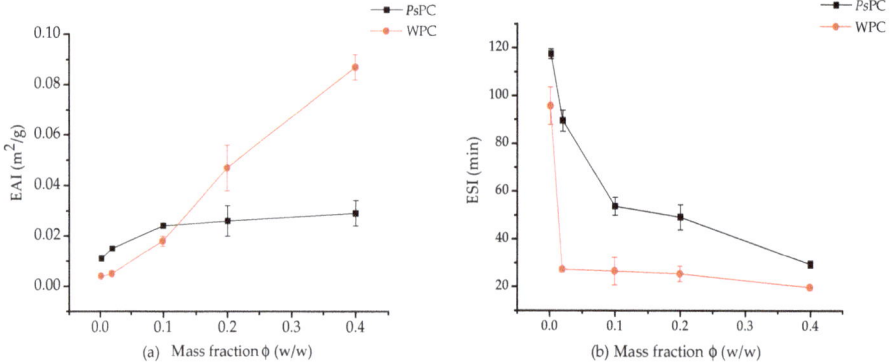

Figure 5. (**a**) Emulsifying activity index (EAI) and (**b**) emulsifying stability index (ESI) of *Ps*PC emulsions compared with WPC at different φ.

On the contrary, the stability time diminished as the mass fraction (φ) increased in ESI (Figure 5). In *Ps*PC emulsions, ESI went from 117.50 ± 2.17 (φ = 0.002) to 29.34 ± 1.48 min (φ = 0.4) and in WPC emulsions, from 95.83 ± 7.95 (φ = 0.002) to 19.87 ± 1.08 min (φ = 0.4). For the control emulsions, less stability time was always reported compared to those of *Ps*PC.

Different authors have mentioned similar characteristics in almond proteins, wheat gluten, and acidic subunits of soy (11S globulin) [2,59]. Guo and Mu [1] also got similar results when they studied emulsifying properties of sweet potato protein and found that at low protein concentrations (<1%, *w/v*), the EAI values are greater, because it facilitates the formation of new droplets, and with the increase of oil, ESI value decreases. Nevertheless, at oil volumes >35% *v/v*, there is a marked increase in ESI, a phenomenon that has been reported also by Sun and Gunasekaran [60] for whey protein isolates.

EAI can be related with interfacial effect and low interaction with aqueous solutions. Our previous droplet size results can be associated with the EAI; as these indexes increased, the droplet size also increased. This can be attributed to the proteins that are surface active molecules with the capacity to improve the stability of oil-in-water emulsions, creating a protective membrane that generate repulsive interactions between oil droplets [16].

3.12. Interfacial Protein Concentration

The effect of interfacial protein concentration shows the oil drops phase separation after being centrifuged. The values suggest that emulsions were stable. When values of φ < 0.2 were used, it was difficult to separate the phases and reported the values.

Table 7 shows the results of emulsions with ϕ 0.2 and 0.4. Control emulsions with WPC showed that as the volume of oil increases, the protein content at the interface is diminished.

Table 7. Interfacial protein concentration in PsPC and whey protein concentrate (WPC) emulsions.

Sample	Mass Fraction (ϕ)	Interfacial Protein Concentration (mg/m^2)
PsPC	0.2	0.009 ± 0.0
	0.4	0.023 ± 0.0
WPC	0.2	0.015 ± 0.0
	0.4	0.014 ± 0.0

The values are the average of three assay ± standard deviations of interfacial protein concentration in PsPC and WPC emulsions.

The interfacial protein concentration in control emulsions was more constant, in contrast with PsPC, which showed a higher value as oil volume increased, allowing more stability.

3.13. Optical Microscopy

The microphotographs in function of PsPC and WPC are shown in Figures 6 and 7, respectively. The images reflect the results of droplet size analysis. It shows that as the mass fraction of emulsions increased, the droplet size also decreased and began to show coalescence. Guo and Mu [1] report similar results. The maximum droplet size can be seen between day 9 and 12 in both emulsions.

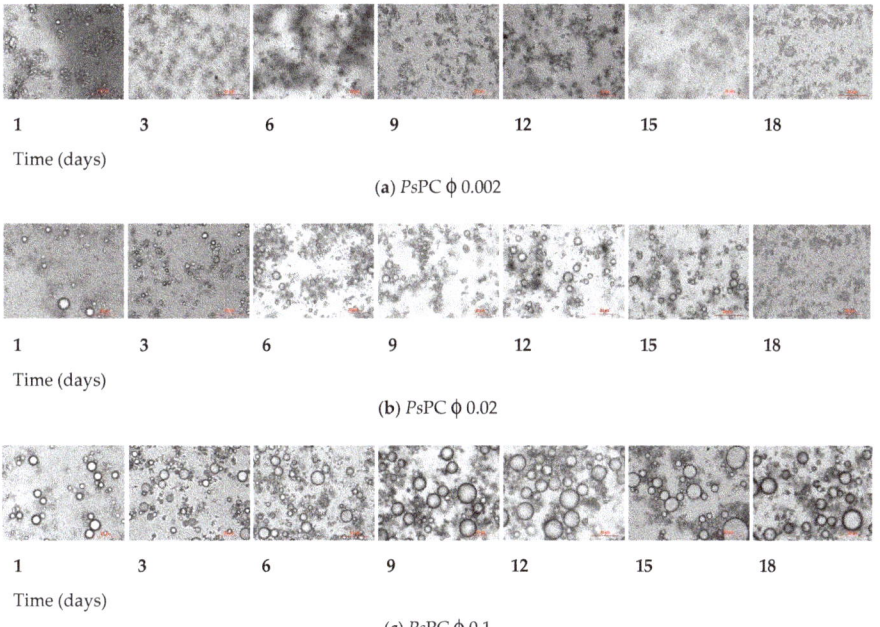

Figure 6. Cont.

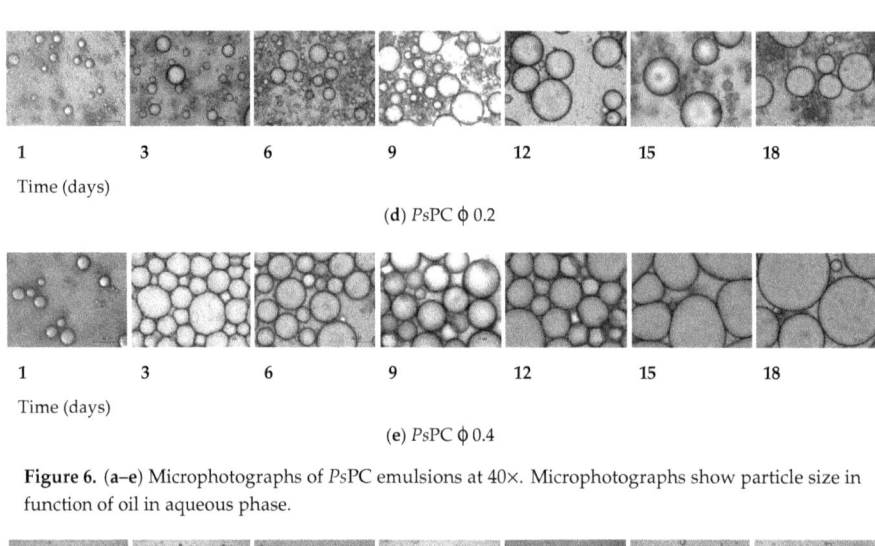

(d) *Ps*PC ɸ 0.2

(e) *Ps*PC ɸ 0.4

Figure 6. (**a**–**e**) Microphotographs of *Ps*PC emulsions at 40×. Microphotographs show particle size in function of oil in aqueous phase.

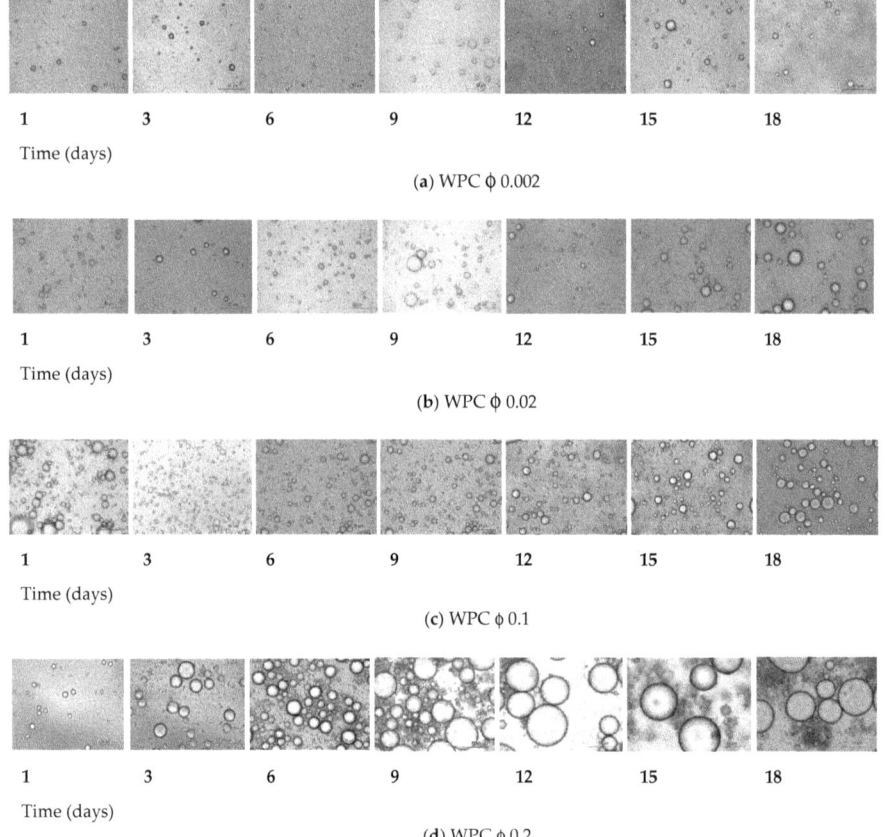

(a) WPC ɸ 0.002

(b) WPC ɸ 0.02

(c) WPC ɸ 0.1

(d) WPC ɸ 0.2

Figure 7. *Cont.*

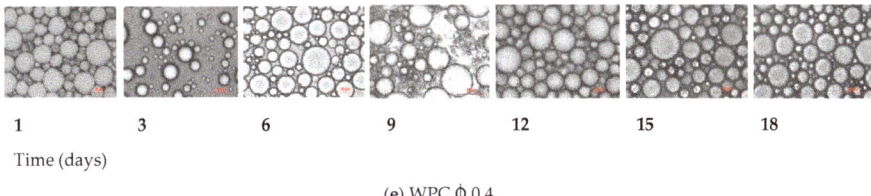

(e) WPC ϕ 0.4

Figure 7. (**a**–**e**) Microphotographs of WPC emulsions at 40×. The particle size changes depending on the oil phase increase.

WPC and *Ps*PC emulsions at their smallest mass fractions ($\phi = 0.002$ and $\phi = 0.02$) showed more homogenization.

4. Conclusions

The *P. serotine* seed is an important source of protein and mainly contains albumin. *P. serotine* defatted flour can be used to replace wheat flour at 50% in the preparation of cookies with acceptable sensory property. We believe that it is necessary to remove all cyanogenic compounds in flour of *P. serotine*. The Grignard test shows a positive reaction in flour without thermic treatment. The content of raw fiber in cookies was almost the same in all treatments. *P. serotine* flour purification can be a concentrated protein source with possible applications to stabilize emulsions.

The alkaline (pH 11) and acid (pH 3.0) process showed a higher concentration of protein than the ionic force process as a function of the sodium chloride concentration. The protein concentrate is comparable to WPC in that it forms stable emulsions with oil content of less than 20% by weight, without changing the particle size during 18 days of storage.

Author Contributions: A.A.L.M., J.G.B.G., E.G.M., K.G.G.A. conceived and designed the experiments; A.A.L.M. and M.B.V. performed the experiments; J.G.B.G., A.A.L.M., M.B.V., K.G.G.A., S.A.G.R., and E.G.M. analyzed the data; J.G.B.G., K.G.G.A., and E.G.M. helped with reagents/plant materials/analysis tools; and A.A.L.M., M.B.V., J.G.B.G. and E.G.M. were involved in drafting the manuscript and revising it. All authors have approved the final version. All authors have read and agreed to the published version of the manuscript.

Funding: We thank CONACyT for the financial support through the project PN-2015-01-1470 and UANL-PAICyT CT723-19.

Acknowledgments: We would like to thank Consejo Nacional de Ciencia y Tecnología (CONACyT) for financially supporting through the project Problemas Nacionales-2015-01-1470 and financially supporting A.A.L.M. to obtain her Ph.D. (scholarship 611290), and Universidad Autónoma de Nuevo León (UANL) for financially supporting through the project PAICyT CT723-19.

Conflicts of Interest: The authors declare no conflict of interest. The funders had no role in the design of the study; in the collection, analysis, or interpretation of data; in the writing of the manuscript, or in the decision to publish the results.

References

1. Guo, Q.; Mu, T.H. Emulsifying properties of sweet potato protein: Effect of protein concentration and oil volume fraction. *Food Hydrocoll.* **2011**, *25*, 98–106. [CrossRef]
2. Sze Tao, K.W.C.; Sathe, S.K. Functional properties and in vitro digestibility of almond (*Prunus dulcis* L.) protein isolate. *Food Chem.* **2000**, *69*, 153–160. [CrossRef]
3. Hoffman, J.R.; Falvo, M.J. Protein-Which is Best? *J. Sports Sci. Med.* **2004**, *3*, 118–130. [PubMed]
4. Jiménez Yan, L.; Brito, A.; Cuzon, G.; Gaxiola, G.; García, T.; Taboada, G.; Soto, L.A.; Brito, R. Energy balance of *Litopenaeus vannamei* postlarvae fed on animal or vegetable protein based compounded feeds. *Aquaculture* **2006**, *260*, 337–345. [CrossRef]
5. Sawashita, N.; Naemura, A.; Shimizu, M.; Morimatsu, F.; Ijiri, Y.; Yamamoto, J. Effect of dietary vegetable and animal proteins on atherothrombosis in mice. *Nutrition* **2006**, *22*, 661–667. [CrossRef]

6. Choi, Y.S.; Choi, J.H.; Han, D.J.; Kim, H.Y.; Lee, M.A.; Jeong, J.Y.; Chung, H.J.; Kim, C.J. Effects of replacing pork back fat with vegetable oils and rice bran fiber on the quality of reduced-fat frankfurters. *Meat Sci.* **2010**, *84*, 557–563. [CrossRef]
7. Lin, D.; Wei, L.; Alan, K.; Longtao, Z.; Baodong, Z.; Song, M. Interactions of vegetable proteins with other polymers: Structure-function relationships and applications in the food industry. *Trends Food Sci. Technol.* **2017**, *68*, 130–144. [CrossRef]
8. Alobo, A.P. Effect of sesame seed flour on millet biscuit characteristics. *Plant Food Hum. Nutr.* **2001**, *56*, 195–202. [CrossRef]
9. Ogunsina, B.S.; Radha, C.; Indrani, D. Quality characteristics of bread and cookies enriched with debittered *Moringa oleifera* seed flour. *Int. J. Food Sci. Nutr.* **2011**, *62*, 185–194. [CrossRef]
10. Wani, A.A.; Sogi, D.S.; Sing, P.; Khatkar, B.S. Influence of watermelon seed protein concentrates on dough handling, textural and sensory properties of cookies. *J. Food Sci. Technol.* **2013**, *52*, 2139–2147. [CrossRef]
11. Cookies and Crackers Europe Statista Market Forecast. Available online: https://www.statista.com/outlook/40100300/102/cookies-crackers/europe (accessed on 12 December 2019).
12. Giarnetti, M.; Paradiso, V.M.; Caponino, F.; Summo, C.; Pasqualone, A. Fat replacement in shortbread cookies using an emulsion filled gel based on inulin and extra virgin olive oil. *LWT Food Sci. Technol.* **2015**, *63*, 339–345. [CrossRef]
13. Swanson, R.B.; Perry, J.M. Modified oatmeal and chocolate chip cookies: Evaluation of the partial replacement of sugar and/or fat to reduce calories. *Int. J. Consum. Stud.* **2007**, *31*, 265–271. [CrossRef]
14. Berton Carabin, C.; Schroën, K. Towards new food emulsions: Designing the interface and beyond. *Curr. Opin. Food Sci.* **2019**, *27*, 74–81. [CrossRef]
15. Nesterenko, A.; Alric, I.; Silvestre, F.; Durrieu, V. Vegetable proteins in microencapsulation: A review of recent interventions and their effectiveness. *Ind. Crops Prod.* **2013**, *42*, 469–479. [CrossRef]
16. Tavernier, I.; Wijaya, W.; Van der Meeren, P.; Dewettinck, K.; Patel, A.R. Food-grade particles for emulsion stabilization. *Trends Food Sci. Technol.* **2016**, *50*, 159–174. [CrossRef]
17. Wang, R.; Tian, Z.; Chen, L. A novel process for microencapsulation of fish oil with barley protein. *Food Res. Int.* **2011**, *44*, 2735–2741. [CrossRef]
18. García Aguilar, L.; Rojas Molina, A.; Ibarra Alvarado, C.; Rojas Molina, J.I.; Vázquez Landaverde, P.A.; Luna Vázquez, F.J.; Zavala Sánchez, M.A. Nutritional value and volatile compounds of black cherry (*Prunus serotina*) seeds. *Molecules* **2015**, *20*, 3479–3495. [CrossRef]
19. Anuario Estadístico de la Producción Agrícola. Available online: http://infosiap.siap.gob.mx/aagricola_siap_gb/ientidad/index.jsp (accessed on 16 October 2019).
20. Alveano Aguerrebere, I. Estudio Químico y Farmacológico de la Semilla de *Prunus serotina*. Master's Thesis, Universidad Autonoma de Querétaro, Querétaro, Mexico, November 2010.
21. Páez Reyes, L.M.; Sánchez Olarte, J.; Velasco Torres, M.; Álvarez Gaxiola, J.F.; Argumedo Macías, A. Propuesta de estrategia para el mejoramiento del cultivo de capulín en los municipios de Domingo Arenas, Calpan y San Nicolás de los Ranchos. *Ra Ximhani* **2013**, *9*, 109–119. [CrossRef]
22. Alveano Aguerrebere, I.; Rojas Molina, A.; Dave Oomah, B.; Drover, J.C.G. Characteristics of *Prunus serotine* seed oil. *Food Chem.* **2011**, *124*, 983–990. [CrossRef]
23. Santini, A.; Novellino, E. Nutraceuticals-shedding light on the grey are between pharmaceuticals and foods. *Expert Rev. Clin. Pharmacol.* **2018**, *11*, 545–547. [CrossRef]
24. Cimmino, A.; Andolfi, A.; Zonno, M.C.; Troise, C.; Santini, A.; Tuzi, A.; Vurro, M.; Ash, G.; Evidente, A. Phomentrioloxin: A phytotoxic pentasubstituted geranylcycloxentriol produced by *Phomopsis* sp., a potential mycoherbicide for *Carthamus lanatus* biocontrol. *J. Nat. Prod.* **2012**, *75*, 1130–1137. [CrossRef] [PubMed]
25. Cressey, P.; Saunders, D.; Goodman, J. Cyanogenic glycosides in plant-based foods available in New Zealand. *Food Addit. Contam. Part A* **2013**, *30*, 1946–1953. [CrossRef] [PubMed]
26. Vetter, J. Plant cyanogenic glycosides. *Toxicon* **2000**, *38*, 11–36. [CrossRef]
27. Lee, J.; Zhang, G.; Wood, E.; Castillo, C.R.; Mitchell, A.E. Quantification of amygdalin in nonbitter, semibitter, and bitter almonds (*Prunus dulcis*) by UHPLC-(ESI) QqQ MS/MS. *J. Agric. Food Chem.* **2013**, *61*, 7754–7759. [CrossRef] [PubMed]
28. Raya Pérez, J.C.; Aguirre Mancilla, C.L.; Tapia Aparicio, R.; Ramírez Pimentel, J.G.; Covarrubias Prieto, J. Caracterización de las proteínas de reserva y composición mineral de la semilla de capulín (*Prunus serotina*). *Polibotánica* **2012**, *34*, 203–215.

29. Zumaeta Cordova, L.; Gonzales Díaz, G. Aceptabilidad y valor Nutricional de la Pasta de la hoja de yuca (*Manihot esculenta*) Utilizada en Distintos Productos Alimenticios. Bachelor's Thesis, Universidad Nacional de la Amazonia Peruana, Iquito, Peru, 11 August 2014.
30. Khor, Y.P.; Kosh, S.P.; Long, K.; Long, S.; Syed Ahmad, S.; Tan, C. A comparative study of the physicochemical properties of a virgin coconut oil emulsion and commercial food supplement emulsion. *Molecules* **2014**, *19*, 9187–9202. [CrossRef]
31. Belorio, M.; Sahagún, M.; Gómez, M. Influence of flour particle size distribution on the quality of maize gluten-free cookies. *Foods* **2019**, *8*, 83. [CrossRef]
32. Association of Official Analytical Chemist (AOAC). *Official Methods of Analysis of International*, 16th ed.; AOAC: Rockville, Maryland, MD, USA, 1998.
33. Reacción de Grignard para Detectar Compuestos del Ácido Cianhídrico en Sorgo. Available online: https://inta.gob.ar/documentos/reaccion-de-grignard-para-detectar-compuestos-del-acido-cianidrico-en-sorgo (accessed on 28 August 2018).
34. Jia, C.; Huang, W.; Abdel-Samie, M.A.-S.; Huang, G.; Huang, G. Dough rheological, mixolab mixing, and nutritional characteristics of almond cookies with and without xylanase. *J. Food Eng.* **2011**, *105*, 227–232. [CrossRef]
35. Ramírez Pimentel, J.G.; Herrera Herrera, A.; Aguirre Mancilla, C.L.; Covarrubias Prieto, J.; Iturriaga de la Fuente, G.; Raya Pérez, J.C. Caracterización de las proteínas de reserva y contenido mineral de semilla de melón (*Cucumis melo* L.). *Rev. Mex. Cienc. Agríc.* **2016**, *7*, 1667–1678. [CrossRef]
36. López Dellamary Toral, F.A. Aislamiento y Caracterización de Proteinas de las Semillas Maduras de *Enterolobium cyclocarpum* para su Aprovechamiento Alimenticio. Ph.D. Thesis, Universidad de Colima, Colima, México, November 2000.
37. Bradford, M.C. A rapid and sensitive method for the quantitation of microgram quantities of protein utilizing the principle of protein dye binding. *Anal. Biochem.* **1976**, *72*, 248–254. [CrossRef]
38. Syros, T.; Yupsanis, T.; Economou, A. Fractionation and electrophoretic patterns of storage proteins of *Ebenus cretica*. A preliminary survey as a tool in taxonomy. *Biol. Plant.* **2003**, *46*, 435–443. [CrossRef]
39. Mini-PROTEAN Tetra Cell. Available online: https://www.bio-rad.com/webroot/web/pdf/lsr/literature/10007296D.pdf (accessed on 5 September 2018).
40. Feng, X.; Dai, H.; Ma, L.; Yu, Y.; Tang, M.; Li, Y.; Hu, W.; Liu, T.; Zhang, Y. Food-grade gelatin nanoparticles: Preparation, characterization, and preliminary application for stabilizing pickering emulsions. *Foods* **2019**, *8*, 479. [CrossRef] [PubMed]
41. Xiong, T.; Ye, X.; Su, Y.T.; Chen, X.; Sun, H.; Li, B.; Chen, Y. Identification and quantification of proteins at adsorption layer of emulsion stabilized by pea protein isolates. *Colloids Surf. B* **2018**, *171*, 1–9. [CrossRef]
42. Sillero, A.; Maldonado, A. Isoelectric point determination of proteins and other macromolecules: Oscillating method. *Comput. Biol. Med.* **2006**, *36*, 157–166. [CrossRef] [PubMed]
43. Yesiltas, B.; Sorensen, A.M.; García Moreno, P.J.; Anankanbil, S.; Guo, Z.; Jacobsen, C. Combination of sodium caseinate and succinylated alginate improved stability of high fat fish oil-in-water emulsions. *Food Chem.* **2018**, *255*, 290–299. [CrossRef]
44. Eichberg, J.; Mokrasch, L.C. Interference by oxidized lipids in the determination of protein by the Lowry procedure. *Anal. Biochem.* **1969**, *30*, 386–390. [CrossRef]
45. Huang, X.; Kakuda, Y.; Cui, W. Hydrocolloids in emulsions: Particle size distribution and interfacial activity. *Food Hydrocoll.* **2011**, *15*, 533–542. [CrossRef]
46. Norma del Codex para la Harina del Trigo. Available online: file:///C:/Users/FAM%20TT/Downloads/CXS_152s%20(1).pdf (accessed on 12 March 2017).
47. CODEX-STAN-152-1985. Norma del Codex para la Harina de Trigo. (Rev.1 -1995). Available online: http://www.colpos.mx/bancodenormas/ninternacionales/CODEX-STAN-152-1985.pdf (accessed on 5 April 2017).
48. USDA. U.S. Department of Agriculture. Available online: https://fdc.nal.usda.gov/fdc-app.html#/food-details/168936/nutrients (accessed on 20 January 2019).
49. CINECA IRIS Institutional Research Information System. Available online: http://hdl.handle.net/11369/363087 (accessed on 15 May 2019).
50. González Pérez, S.; Arellano, J.B. Vegetable protein isolates. In *Handbook of Hydrocolloids*, 2nd ed.; Phillips, G.O., Williams, P.A., Eds.; Woodhead Publishing: Salamanca, Spain, 2009; pp. 383–419.

51. UNSA Investiga Repositorio Institucional. Available online: http://repositorio.unsa.edu.pe/handle/UNSA/6553 (accessed on 12 October 2017).
52. Ferreyra, J.C.; Kuskoski, E.M.; Bordignon Luiz, M.T.; Barrera Arellano, D.; Fett, R. Propiedades emulsificantes y espumantes de las proteínas de harina de cacahuate (*Arachis hypogaea* Lineau). *Grasas Aceites* **2007**, *58*, 264–269.
53. Arntfield, S.D. *Proteins from Oil-Producing Plants*, 2nd ed.; Woodhead Publishing: Winnipeg, MB, Canada, 2018; pp. 146–167.
54. Universidad Nacional de Quilmnes. Available online: http://ufq.unq.edu.ar/Docencia-Virtual/BQblog/Salting-in-Salting-out-precipitacion-solventes (accessed on 2 September 2018).
55. Pandolfe, W.D. Effect of premix condition, surfactant concentration, and oil level on the formation of oil-in-water emulsions by homogenization. *J. Disper. Sci. Techol.* **1995**, *16*, 633–650. [CrossRef]
56. Floury, J.; Desrumaux, A.; Lardieres, J. Effect of high-pressure homogeniztion on droplet size distributions and rheological properties of model oil-in-water emulsions. *Innov. Food Sci. Emerg. Technol.* **2000**, *1*, 127–134. [CrossRef]
57. McClements, D.; Decker, E. Lipid Oxidation in Oil-in-Water Emulsions: Impact of Molecular Environment on Chemical Reactions in Heterogeneous Food Systems. *J. Food Sci.* **2000**, *65*, 1270–1282. [CrossRef]
58. Tirgar, M.; Silcock, P.; Carne, A.; Birch, E.J. Effect of extraction method on functional properties of flaxseed protein concentrates. *Food Chem.* **2017**, *215*, 417–424. [CrossRef] [PubMed]
59. Liu, M.; Lee, D.S.; Damodaran, S. Emulsifying properties of acidic subunits of soy 11S globulin. *J. Agric. Food Chem.* **1999**, *47*, 4970–4975. [CrossRef] [PubMed]
60. Sun, C.H.; Gunasekaran, S. Effects of protein concentration and oil phase volume fraction on the stability and rheology of menhaden oil-in water emulsions stabilized by whey protein isolate with xanthan gum. *Food Hydrocoll.* **2009**, *23*, 165–170. [CrossRef]

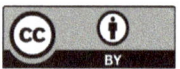

© 2019 by the authors. Licensee MDPI, Basel, Switzerland. This article is an open access article distributed under the terms and conditions of the Creative Commons Attribution (CC BY) license (http://creativecommons.org/licenses/by/4.0/).

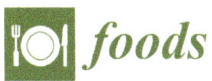

Review

Sources, Extraction and Biomedical Properties of Polysaccharides

Samee Ullah [1,2], Anees Ahmed Khalil [2], Faryal Shaukat [1] and Yuanda Song [1,*]

[1] Colin Ratledge Center for Microbial Lipids, Center for Functional Foods and Health, School of Agriculture Engineering and Food Science, Shandong University of Technology, Zibo 255049, China
[2] University Institute of Diet and Nutritional Sciences, Faculty of Allied Health Sciences, The University of Lahore, Lahore 54000, Pakistan
* Correspondence: ysong@sdut.edu.cn; Tel.: +86-139-0617-4047

Received: 16 July 2019; Accepted: 28 July 2019; Published: 1 August 2019

Abstract: In the recent era, bioactive compounds from plants have received great attention because of their vital health-related activities, such as antimicrobial activity, antioxidant activity, anticoagulant activity, anti-diabetic activity, UV protection, antiviral activity, hypoglycemia, etc. Previous studies have already shown that polysaccharides found in plants are not likely to be toxic. Based on these inspirational comments, most research focused on the isolation, identification, and bioactivities of polysaccharides. A large number of biologically active polysaccharides have been isolated with varying structural and biological activities. In this review, a comprehensive summary is provided of the recent developments in the physical and chemical properties as well as biological activities of polysaccharides from a number of important natural sources, such as wheat bran, orange peel, barely, fungi, algae, lichen, etc. This review also focused on biomedical applications of polysaccharides. The contents presented in this review will be useful as a reference for future research as well as for the extraction and application of these bioactive polysaccharides as a therapeutic agent.

Keywords: bioactive polysaccharides; extraction; biomedical applications

1. Introduction

Polysaccharides are considered as vital bio-macromolecules for all living organisms, which are structurally comprised of homo or hetero monosaccharides and uronic acids connected with glycosidic linkages [1–3]. They are predominantly found in various parts of plants, animals, fungi, bacteria, and seaweed, and play a critical role in numerous physiological functions of life [4]. Polysaccharides along with lipids, proteins, and polynucleotides are classified as the most pivotal four macromolecules in life sciences. Bioactive polysaccharides are known as polysaccharides produced from living organisms, and/or are functionalized from sugar-based materials possessing biological effects on organisms. Moreover, during the last decades, bioactive polysaccharides have been investigated as therapeutic agents against many chronic diseases due to their biodegradability, non-toxic nature, and biocompatibility [5]. Studies have shown that polysaccharides possess a wide range of pharmacological perspectives such as antioxidative, antitumor, antimicrobial, anti-obesity, hypolipidemic, antidiabetic, and hepato-protective properties [6–8]. They have been investigated extensively for the development of novel products in the field of cosmetics, food, medicine, petrochemicals, and paper [3,9,10]. Particularly, in the medicinal industry, polysaccharides are mostly used as pharmaceuticals and medical biomaterials (hypoglycemic, anti-osteoarthritic, and anticancer products) to curtail the effect of respective metabolic syndromes [9,11].

The potentiality of bioactive polysaccharides is strongly influenced depending upon their configuration and chemical structure. Nevertheless, the macromolecular configurations of plant cellular polysaccharides, particularly hetero polysaccharides (hemicelluloses), are very complex owing to the occurrence of various monosaccharides acting as isobaric stereoisomers [12,13]. Additionally, polysaccharides present in plants, microorganisms (bacteria, fungi, and yeasts), animals, and algae are chemically and/or physically bound with various other biomolecules like lignin, proteins, lipids, polynucleotides, and a few minerals [14]. Hence, to understand the importance of bioactive polysaccharides in the domain of life sciences resulted in the multi-disciplinary collaboration of scientists from the fields of microbiology, phytology, glycol-biology, nutrition, food sciences, and glycol-medicine [5]. Polysaccharides both in the simple and complex glycol-conjugated form are renowned for various bioactive functions, for instance, antivirus, antioxidant, antimicrobial, anticancer, antidiabetic, reno-protective, immunomodulatory, and anti-stress perspectives.

2. Sources of Bioactive Polysaccharides

Bioactive polysaccharides are categorized broadly depending upon their sources, structure, applications, solubility, and chemical composition. On the basis of chemical composition, they are characterized as homopolysaccharides (homoglycans) and heteropolysaccharides (heteroglycans). Homoglycans comprise of a single type of monosaccharide, such as glycogen and cellulose which consists of glucose molecules, whereas heteroglycans are made up of a different type of monosaccharides, for example, heparin and chondroitin sulfate (CS) [15].

According to the glycosides linked on to the glycan, polysaccharides can also be classified as proteoglycans and glycoproteins, glycolipids, and glycoconjugates [16,17]. According to grouping based on origins, bioactive polysaccharides are usually classified as those derived from animals (chondroitin sulfate, heparin, and hyaluronan), plants (pectin, inulin, Ginseng polysaccharides, xylans, and arabinans), bacteria (exopolysaccharides, capsular polysaccharides, and peptidoglycans), lichen, fungi, and algae. In the section below, bioactive properties associated with polysaccharides are reviewed depending upon their natural sources in order to understand their functionality.

2.1. Bioactive Polysaccharides in Dietary Fibers

The FAO (Food and Agriculture Organization) defined dietary fibers as a variety of indigestible plant polysaccharides including pectins, cellulose, gums, hemicelluloses, oligosaccharides, and various lignified compounds. Dietary fibers are the type of polysaccharides that are biologically active in their innate form and/or after enzymatic and chemical treatments. For instance, celluloses and hemicelluloses directly stimulate the bowel movement, whereas inulin is fermented by microflora with the intent to prevent various gastrointestinal disorders [18]. Dietary fibers play a vital role in prevention from various diseases especially hyperlipidemia, cardiovascular complications, and obesity. Gums, inulin, and pectin are capable of slowing down the passage of food in the digestive tract, reducing serum cholesterol concentrations, hindering the absorption of sugar from food to bloodstream and, therefore, avoiding sudden hyperglycemic conditions post food ingestion.

Among dietary fibers, lignin, cellulose, and hemicellulose are classified as insoluble fibers which help in the stimulation of the bowel movement, speeds up the removal of waste via the digestive tract, and helps in prevention of hemorrhoids, constipation, and diverticulosis [19,20]. Results of various epidemiological investigations and clinical trials have suggested that consumption of moderate or higher levels of dietary fiber efficiently reduces the risk of numerous metabolic syndromes like diabetes [21], strokes [22], hypertension [23,24], hyperlipidemia/hypercholesterolemia, [25,26], obesity, and cancer [27]. Usually, ingestion of dietary fiber has health modulating benefits, like increased stool bulk, reduced intestinal transit time, a decline in levels of total cholesterol (TC) and postprandial blood glucose, and/or insulin contents [27–29]. Keeping in view the significance of dietary fibers with special reference to human health and their associated mechanism of actions, these are considered as an abundant source of bioactive polysaccharides. Table 1 summarizes the types, names, sources, composition, and physiological effects of dietary fiber polysaccharides from various studies and trials.

2.2. Bioactive Polysaccharides in Herbs

Herbs have attained a significant position in traditional medicines (Indian Ayurveda, ancient Chinese medicine, phytomedicine in western countries, and Japanese Kamp medicine) of numerous countries owing to their associated curing benefits against numerous diseases. Outcomes of recent pharmacological studies have illuminated that the chief component of herbal medicines usually comprises of tannins, polysaccharides, high molar mass proteins, and low molar mass constituents like terpenoids (quassinoids, sesquiterpenes, and *Rabdosia* diterpenes), saponins, alkaloids (protoberberine alkaloid, phenanthridine, etc.), and flavonoids (*Scutellaria* flavones) [30]. Among the above-mentioned compounds in herbal medicines, polysaccharides are believed to be main bioactive compounds responsible for various pharmacological potentials like antitumor, antioxidant, hepato-protective, antiviral, radio-protective, immuno-stimulatory, and anti-fatigue activities [31–35]. Innate polysaccharides present in numerous herbs are known for stimulation of the human immune system, inhibition of viral replication, scavenging free radicals, and inhibition of lipid peroxidation [33,36,37]. Recent advancements regarding the application of polysaccharides present in herbal medicines for prevention and cure of diseases are documented in Table 1.

Table 1. Biological activities of bioactive polysaccharides.

Polysaccharides	Biological Activities	Mechanism of Action	References
β-glucan	Anti-obesity activity	• Reduced energy intake • Increase in fullness and satiety • Decreased hunger and increased satiety and fullness.	[38]
Pectin, Algal Fucoidan	Anti-microbial activity	• Inhibitory effects on the entry of enveloped viruses including herpes and HIV into cells • Inhibit the formation of syncytium formation	[39,40]
Fucoidan, Polygonum multiflorum Thunb Polysaccharides	Anti-oxidant activity	• Inhibited ERK and p38-MAPK signaling pathways scavenging free radicals (e.g., superoxide anion radical, hydroxyl radical, and hydroxyl peroxide), • Prevents lipid oxidation and protein glycation • Inhibits the formation of ROS and RNS	[40,41]
Red algae sulfated polysaccharides, Carrageenan, Fucoidan, Chondroitin sulfate	Anti-inflammatory activity	• Lowered the expression of inducible nitric oxide synthase (iNOS) • Inhibited the expressions of TNF-a, interleukin-1b (IL-1b) and interferon-c (IFN-c) • Repressed pro-inflammatory cytokines • Suppresses the activity of COX-2	[40,42,43]
β-glucan	Anti-diabetic activity	• Suppressed the formation of AGE • Reduced postprandial glucose and insulin responses • Increases the level of antioxidant enzymes in the body	[38]
Konjac glucomannan	Hypo-cholesterolemic activity	• Reduced the plasma cholesterol • Significantly lowered Serum total, HDL-C, and LDL-C • Reduces the concentration of serum MDA	[44]
Pectin, Ginseng polysaccharides, Heparan sulfate	Anti-tumour activity	• Constrains the production of prostaglandin E2 • Prevents from the oxidation of DNA • Stimulates macrophages to produce helper types 1 and 2 (Th1 and Th2) cytokines • Promotes the formation of ternary complexes • Displaces growth factors	[39,45,46]
Ginseng polysaccharides	Immune modulatory activity	• Downregulates the secretion of inflammation related mediator nitric oxide (NO) and cytokines (TNF-a, IL-6, and IL-1b) • Reduces the activation of neutrophils	[45]
β-glucan, Pectin, Gums, Konjac glucomannan	Gastro-protective activity	• Supplement increased faecal bulk • Alter postprandial lipid and lipoprotein composition	[19,44]
Acanthopanax polysaccharides	Neuro-protective activity	• Increase SOD and GSH-Px activities and IL-10 levels • Reduces the levels of MDA, IL-1, and TNF-α • Prevents the formation of inflammatory cytokines	[47]

2.3. Bioactive Polysaccharides in Algae and Lichens

Polysaccharides present in lichens and algae have been of great interest to the food scientists owing to their associated exceptional physical properties (stabilizing, gelling, and thickening capability) and biological potentials (immunomodulating, antiviral, anticoagulant, antitumor, antioxidative, anti-inflammatory, and anti-thrombotic activity) [48,49]. Basically, sulfated polysaccharides are the main group of the most attractive and interesting constituents in marine algae i.e., laminarans and fucoidans in the Phaeophyceae (brown algae), carrageenans in the Rhodophyceae (red algae), and ulvans in the Chlorophyceae (green algae) [40]. One of the most vital properties linked with sulfated polysaccharides is their anticoagulant characteristics. For instance, carrageenan (sulfated galactans) isolated from red algae and sulfated fucoidans extracted from brown algae are known to possess excellent anti-coagulant properties. Sulfated polysaccharides identified in algae have been stated to own equal or even stronger activities than those linked with heparin [32]. Various other biological properties of sulfated polysaccharides present in algae have been intensively investigated.

Experimentally, fucoidan has been reported to possess maximum antioxidative properties followed by alginate and laminaran, therefore protecting human health from the damage of ROS (reactive oxygen species). Likewise, the anticancer and anti-tumor characteristics of algae-based sulfated polysaccharides are found to be due to their antioxidative and free radical scavenging properties [50]. Moreover, inhibition of HIV and herpes viruses in cells owing to anti-viral potential of sulfated rhamnogalactans, carrageenans, and fucoidans have also been scientifically proven [40]. Immuno-modulating characteristics associated with algae-based sulfated polysaccharides were demonstrated by increasing the secreting and phagocytic activities of macrophages [51].

Polysaccharides derived from lichens (composite organism formed due to a symbiotic partnership among alga and fungus) are principally linear or rarely substituted α-glucans and/or β-glucans. This type of glucans isolated from lichens is reported to have a wide range of bioactive functions such as immunomodulatory perspectives, anti-tumor potential, and anti-viral characteristics [49,52,53]. The immuno-modulating activity of polysaccharides (β-glucans) derived from lichenin and lichens are linked to stimulation of a variety of immune responses like production of NO (nitric oxide) and ROS (reactive oxygen species) and release of cytokines and arachidonic acid metabolites [51]. Lichenin, also known as lichenan, consists of a galactoglucomannan (water-soluble hemicellulose) structure that is responsible for anti-thrombotic and anti-coagulant properties [54]. Bioactive properties related to sulfated polysaccharides from lichens and algae are highly dependent on their structural properties, for instance, sulfate concentration and distribution of sulfate groups on the main chain, stereochemistry, and molar masses. Hence, there is a need for the modification of innate sulfate polysaccharides to attain biologically active polysaccharides having desired molecular size and functionality for bioactive further application [40,55]. An overview of some recent advancements in this context are depicted in Table 2.

2.4. Bioactive Polysaccharides in Fungi

A wide range of bioactive saccharides is present in fungi ranging from monosaccharides to polysaccharides. They can be summarized as the intracellular or extracellular polysaccharides depending upon their presence in the fungi [56]. The bioactive polysaccharides derived from basidiomycetes are reported to have antitumor and anticancer activities and can prevent breast cancer in post-menopausal women. The compound which can inhibit tumors was first isolated from the basidiomycete *Boletus edulis* in 1957. In traditional medicine, several basidiomycete mushrooms are used as an immunosuppressant to treat cancer and even for treating AIDS [57]. Polysaccharopeptide (PSP) isolated from *Ganoderma lucidum* induces the inhibition of oncogenes and kill the tumor cells directly. Similarly, the bioactive polysaccharides schizophyllan, lentinan, and polysaccharide-K isolated from *Grifola frondosa* and *Trametes versicolor*, respectively, improve the immune function of the host and showed a synergistic effect with chemotherapy [58]. Just like mushrooms, another source of bioactive polysaccharides is *Cordyceps militaris*, and they possess a wide range of structurally different bioactive polysaccharides. Water-soluble polysaccharides from *C. militaris* contain a (1 → 4) galactose linkage and (1 → 3,6)-mannose linkage and branching usually arising from (1 → 4)-linked glucose. These polysaccharides were reported for their numerous biological activities including anti-tumor, immunomodulatory, antioxidant, and anti-inflammatory activities [56,59].

2.5. Bioactive Polysaccharides from Bacteria

Bacteria are a rich source of biologically active polysaccharides. On the base of structural properties, bacterial polysaccharides can be defined into five major classes: Exopolysaccharides (EPSs), capsular polysaccharides (CPSs), lipopolysaccharides (LPSs), peptidoglycans, and teichoic acids [60].

A lot of research has been done on hyperbranched bacterial polysaccharides (HBPSs). For example, highly branched dextran with a backbone of 75% (α-(1→6)-D-Glcp) with 19% of α-(1→3) and a few α-(1→2) branching [61], was separated from *Leuconostoc citreum* B-2 and studied extensively, and showed a water-holding capacity of up to 450% and an 80% water solubility index, consequently having potential applications in cosmetic, food, and pharmaceutical industries [62,63]. From an industrial point of view, EPSs producing Gram-negative prokaryotes (cyanobacteria) are important because of their ability to produce novel molecules. These EPSs usually linger as a sheath/capsule with the cells and when they are liberated from the cells they are termed as released polysaccharides. Some bacteria from the genus cyanobacterium, namely *Anabaena, Aphanocapsa, Cyanothece, Phormidium, Synechocystis,* and *Nostoc* are useful to produce sulfated EPSs, which also contain uronic acids [64]. Upon fermentation in the laboratory, polysaccharide yield from 0.5–4 g/L can be obtained from three known genera of marine bacteria, namely *Alteromonas* sp., *Pseudoalteromonas* sp. and *Vibrio* sp. [65]. Exopolysaccharide HE 800 is secreted by *Vibrio diabolicus* and it contains an equal amount of hexosamine and glucuronic acid, which can be depolymerized, N-deacetylated, and after chemical sulfurylation produce new derivatives of HE800. These derivatives are referred to as DRS HE800 and are structurally very close to heparan-sulfate [66]. Moreover, acidic and highly branched heteropolysaccharide (EPS GY785) is produced by the bacterium *Alteromonas infernus*. Non-saccharide units of EPS GY785 are composed of uronic acid and sugar (glucose and galactose) [67].

EPSs derived in the laboratory showed widespread biological activities like being an antioxidant, having cholesterol-lowering and inflammation-regulating properties, as well as anti-tumor, anti-coagulant, and antivirus activities [62,68]. Moreover, bacterial polysaccharides are used in Protein Glycan Coupling Technology (PGCT) to produce glycoconjugate vaccines against Gram-positive and Gram negative bacteria [69].

2.6. Bioactive Polysaccharides in Wood

Bioactive polysaccharides present in wood primarily consists of celluloses and some primary groups of hemicelluloses (glucans, arabinans, xylans, glucomannans, and galactans) [70,71]. Pectins and galacto-glucomannans derived from wood are stated to have radical scavenging properties and immune-stimulating activities [72,73]. Xylo-oligosaccharides (xylans) derived from dietary fibers, hard and/or softwood have been reported to be used efficiently as prebiotics by nutraceutical and medicinal industries [74]. Similarly, pentosane polysulfate—a xylan derivative being extracted from beech-wood—is also known as a biomedical agent for the treatment of interstitial cystitis, a bladder pain syndrome [75]. While most polysaccharides do not reveal biological properties unless they are subjected to some modification; derivatives of cellulose-like hydroxypropyl-cellulose (HPC), hydroxypropyl-methylcellulose (HPMC), hydroxyethyl-cellulose (HEC), and methyl-cellulose have evidently proven their functional roles in numerous fields (medicinal, cosmetics, food, and pharmaceutical) [76].

2.7. Bioactive Polysaccharides from other Sources

Sulfated glycosaminoglycans (GAGs) like keratin sulfate (KS), heparan sulfate (HS), dermatan sulfate (DS), and chondroitin sulfate (CS) belongs to a class known as animal-derived bioactive polysaccharides. Heparan sulfate comprises of repeated units of N-acetylated and sulfated disaccharides (glucosamine and glucuronic/iduronic acid) units [77–79]. Evidently, heparin is known to be the most effectual clinical anti-coagulant used in medical sciences. The anti-coagulation potential of heparin is mainly due to its particular structural arrangement, in which specifically the binding site of anti-thrombin III (ATIII, a non-vitamin K-dependent protease) is of central importance in the prevention of fibrin clot formation which is generated owing to the enzymatic activity of thrombin [80]. Better knowledge regarding the interlinkage among structural properties and activity of heparin creates an opportunity for the development of new drugs having more specificity and improved anti-coagulating properties. Furthermore, this structural-activity connection is also helpful in exploring various biomedical applications like anti-viral, anti-inflammatory, anti-cancer, and wound healing properties [78,79,81,82]. DS and CS chains comprise of sulfated N-acetylgalactosamine and iduronic acid (in case of DS)/glucuronic acid (in case of CS) disaccharide repeating units [83,84]. Both of these are functionally characterized as bioactive polysaccharides owing to their presence as a vital molecule in the extracellular matrix of the brain, which helps in regulation of cell migration, adhesion, and proliferation while healing of wounds, as well as proper signaling of growth factor in the skeleton [85–88].

On the other hand, HA (hyaluronic acid) primarily isolated form animal tissues comprise of the linear structure of non-sulfated glycosaminoglycan molecules with repeated units of β-(1-3)-N-acetyl-D-glucosamine, and β-(1-4)-D-glucuronic acid. It is also a vital constituent of the brain's extracellular matrix, which promotes mediation of cellular signaling, helps in healing of wounds, and morphogenesis. Owing to these properties, HA and their associated derivatives are predominantly being applied by the medical industry in eye surgery, viscosupplementation, and as a biomedical tool for drug delivery [89–91]. Chitin is known to be the most abundant polysaccharide present in the exoskeleton of shrimps and crabs, the cell walls of yeast and fungi, and the cuticles of insects. It is by far the second most copious polymer after cellulose and comprises of a random distribution of β-(1-4)-linked N-acetyl-glucosamine and N-glucosamine [92,93]. Industrially, chitosan is characterized as a vital derivative of chitin and is practically obtained due to partial deacetylation of chitin either by the action of enzyme chitin deacetylase or under alkaline conditions [94]. Bioactive properties (anti-cancer, anti-tumor, anti-bacterial, anti-inflammatory, etc.) associated with oligomers of chitosan and chitin, yielded owing to partial acidic hydrolysis, have earlier been documented [95].

3. Extraction and Quantification of Bioactive Polysaccharides

In general, bioactive potentials of naturally occurring polysaccharides are greatly dependent upon their molar mass and level and distribution of groups/side chains on the backbone. Therefore, isolation of polysaccharides from complex cellular plant matrices while keeping their bioactivity intact is of great significance. During the last decade, various innovative green extraction techniques (microwave-assisted, ultra-sonication, supercritical fluid extraction, and hot water extraction) are in practice for isolation of bioactive polysaccharides. These techniques have acquired great attention of scientists and researchers mainly due to their increased extraction rates, cost-effective nature, enviro-friendly characteristics, and structure preservative potentials [73,96,97].

Numerous scientific investigations have been implemented for the extraction and isolation of bioactive polysaccharides. The type of method adopted defines the physicochemical properties and antioxidant potential of isolated polysaccharides. For this purpose, a group of scientists compared the structural and antioxidant properties of bioactive polysaccharides extracted from Barrenwort (*Epimedium acuminatum*) through various extraction techniques (microwave-assisted, enzymatic, hot water extraction, and ultrasound-assisted extraction). They were of the view that bioactive polysaccharides isolated from hot water extraction had the highest antioxidant properties as compared to those extracted from other techniques, while their physicochemical properties were the same [98]. The hot water extraction method used in combination with various latest techniques (enzymatic pre-treatment, microwave, and ultrasound-assisted) are useful in increasing the yield and extraction productivity of polysaccharides. Likewise, enzymatic pre-treatment of raw material prior to extraction resulted in reduced extraction time, minimized the use of extraction solvents, preserved the bioactivities of the polysaccharides, and was energy efficient as compared to non-enzymatic pre-treated techniques [99]. In recent times, various ionic liquids have been formulated which aids in extraction of polysaccharides in a shorter time and at lower temperatures [100].

Table 2. Extraction techniques with reference to specific polysaccharides.

Type	Name	Sources	Extraction Techniques	Quantity/Yield	References
Dietary fibres	Cellulose	Coconut fibre	Acid Hydrolysis	32.8%	[101]
			Ammonium persulphate oxidation	49.6%	
			Ultrasound extraction	88.1%	
	Hemicelluloses	Wheat bran	Alkaline extraction	33.32%–64.1%	[102]
			Hydrothermal extraction	9% (14)	
	Pectins	Orange peels	Microwave-assisted extraction	24.2%	[103]
			Conventional extraction	18.32%	
			Ultrasound extraction	19.24%	
	B-glucan	Barley	Acidic extraction	4.6%	[104]
		Oats		6.97%	
		Barley bran	Alkaline extraction	5.6%–11.9%	
		Oat bran		3.9%–8.0%	
		Wheat bran		2.15%–2.51%	
		Barley		3.94%	
		Barley	Water extraction	2.5%–5.4%	
		Oat		2.1%–3.9%	
		Barley	Enzymatic extraction	5.22%	
		Oat		13.9%	
	Gums	Durian fruit	Aqueous extraction	59.7%	[105]
	Konjac glucomannan	*Amorphophallus konjac* plant	Water extraction using $Al_2(SO_4)_3$	59.02%	[106]
			Ethanol extraction	65.23%	
Herbs	Ginseng polysaccharides	*Panax ginseng* roots	Subcritical water extraction	63.1%	[107]
			Water extraction	14.71%	
			Ethanol extraction	17.96%	
	Astragalus polysaccharides	*Astragalus* roots	Water extraction	11.6% (20)	[108]
			Microwave-assisted extraction	16.07%	
			Ultrasound-assisted extraction	24.12%	
			Enzymatic hydrolysis extraction	9.78%	
	Polygonum multiflorum Thunb Polysaccharides	*Polygonum multiflorum* Thunb root	Ultrasound-assisted extraction	2.90%–4.72% (21)	[109]
			Ethanolic extraction	4.9% (22)	[110]
Algae and lichens	Green algae sulfated polysaccharides	Green algae, *Caulerpa racemosa*	Soxhlet extraction	10%–20% (23)	[111]
			Ultrasound assisted extraction	8.3% (24)	[112]
	Red algae sulfated polysaccharides (porphyran)	Red algae, *Porphyra haitanensis*	Ultrasound-assisted extraction	6.24% (25)	[113]
	Green algae sulfated Rhamnan	Green algae, *Monostroma latissimum*	Hot water extraction	15.9%	[114]
			Microwave-assisted extraction	53.1% (26)	
	Algal Fucoidan	Brown algae, *Ecklonia cava*	Aqueous extraction	53.33%	[115]
			Enzymatic extraction	57.00% (27)	
			Microwave assisted extraction	18.22% (30)	[116]
β-Glucans lichenan	Lichenan	*Cetraria islandica*	Hot water extraction	50.9%	[117]
	Pustulan	*Lasallia pustulata*	Hot water extraction	38%	
Fungi	Monosaccharides and polysaccharides	*Cordyceps militaris*, *Dictyophora* spp.	Hot water, alkali, and acidic solutions	6.36%–24.30%	[56,118]

In addition, this purification of polysaccharides from the crude extract is really of great importance as the linkage among structure and safety of products formed for food, pharmaceutical, and biomedical application depends on this. Purification could be achieved by using various techniques (gel filtration, ion exchange and affinity chromatography, ethanolic precipitation, and fractional precipitation), individually or in combination [32].

4. Biomedical Applications

Polysaccharides and their derived compounds are medicinally more preferred as compared to synthetic polymers owing to their biodegradability, non-toxic nature, biocompatibility, and low processing expenses. Mentioned benefits related to polysaccharides isolated from natural sources make them a valuable ingredient in the fields of pharmaceuticals, nutraceuticals, food, and cosmetic industries. At the present time, polysaccharides are been used in healthcare and disease control, while various novel areas have also been discovered like in cancer diagnosis, inhibition, and treatment; in drug delivery; in anti-bacterial and anti-viral perspectives; and in tissue engineering [92,119]. Therefore, this segment highlights the use of bioactive polysaccharides against various metabolic syndromes and in the above-mentioned novel areas.

4.1. Anti-Microbial and Antiviral

Various clinical investigations have authenticated that oral administration of pectin to infants and children significantly reduced diarrhea and other intestinal infections. This may be because of the decreased concentration of pathogenic bacteria like *Citrobacter*, *Salmonella*, *Enterobacter*, *Shigella*, *Proteus*, and *Klebsiella* [120]. A linear relationship has been documented among the concentration of probiotics and intestinal health [28].

The bioactive potential of fucoidans—a sulphated polysaccharide derived from marine brown seaweeds—have demonstrated noteworthy anti-viral potential against the cytomegalovirus, HIV, and HSV (herpes simplex virus) [121]. Additionally, few other seaweed-extracted polysaccharides like sulphated rhamnogalactans, carrageenans, and fucoidans have shown an inhibitory effect on viruses (HSV and HIV). Fucoidan comprises of a large quantity of L-fucose and sulphate groups along with fractions of galaturonic acid, xylose, mannose, and galactose. *Undaria pinnatifida* (marine brown alga) contains fucoidans and have been used in bone health supplementation mainly due to stimulation of osteoblastic cell differentiation. This sulphated polysaccharide has also been known to possess preventing action on UV-B-induced matrix metalloproteinase-1 (MMP-1) expression by inhibiting the ERK (extra-cellular signal regulated kinases) pathways. Therefore, it could be utilized as a functional ingredient in dermal ointments to prevent from skin photo-aging [40].

Some of the other fractions of algae have properties of virucidal and enzyme inhibitory activity inhibiting the formation of the syncytium. Besides, the sulfate group present is necessary for the anti-HIV activity and potency increases with the degree of sulfation.

4.2. Anti-Tumor/Cancer

Numerous scientists have explored dietary fibers as possessing potent anti-cancer properties. Amongst all, pectin has been investigated to reduce cancerous cell migration and tumor growth in a rat model that were administrated with modified citrus pectin [122]. This may be due to binding of pectin to galectin-3, which results in inhibitory action on some of its functional activities [123]. Anti-tumor mode of actions associated with dietary pectin are related to their immune-potentiation, probiotic properties, tumor growth inhibition, anti-mutagenic potential, and regulatory action of transformation-related oncogenes [124,125]. Anti-tumor mechanisms associated with pectin could be due to cellular immunological potential [126].

According to a study, ginseng polysaccharides were found to have a stimulating effect on DCs (dendritic cells) causing an elevated formation of IFN-g (interferon-g) [127]. It has also been documented that acidic ginseng polysaccharides (GPs) enhanced the production of cytotoxic cells against tumors and promoted macrophages for the production of Th1 and Th2 (helper type 1 and 2) cytokines [128,129]. Depending upon disease environment or timing of treatments, ginseng polysaccharides extracted from *Panax ginseng* demonstrated immuno-modulating perspectives mainly in an immunosuppressing or immuno-stimulating manner [130]. Acidic GP also revealed modulating action on the concentrations of antioxidative enzymes like GPx (glutathione peroxidase) and SOD (superoxide dismutase) probably due to induction of regulating cytokines [131,132]. Likewise, Lemmon et al. [132] found that the immuno-stimulating potential of acidic GPs isolated from American ginseng (*Panax quinquefolius*) was actually mediated by polysaccharides having molecular weight more than 100 kDa [34].

Furthermore, scientists have proven the fact that heparin administration may also have a beneficial impact on cancer and inflammation. Anti-cancerous, anti-inflammatory, and anti-tumor properties associated with heparin and its low molecular weight species are owing to the pathological functions of heparan sulfate (HS) chains of proteoglycan structure (HSPGs). Outcomes of an investigation validated that heparin transfers GRs (growth factors) stored by HS chains of HSPGs in the ECM (extracellular matrix) and on cell surfaces. Full-size heparin has potent pro-angiogenic properties as it increases the production of ternary complexes of heparin bound FGF2 and VEGF with GF receptors [45].

4.3. Anti-Obesity and Hypocholesterolemia

Numerous trials have shown a direct relationship between consumption of dietary fiber, rich diet/dietary fiber supplementation, and weight loss [133–137]. According to a meta-analysis comprising of 22 clinical trials, it was documented that a 12 g increase in the content of daily fiber intake resulted in a 10% decrease in energy intake along with a 1900 g decline in body weight [138]. More precisely, the administration of glucomannan (1.24 g/day) along with energy-restricted diet for five consecutive weeks caused a significant decrease in body weight as compared to the placebo group [139].

In a clinical trial on healthy volunteers, a drink containing oat β-glucan (10.5 g/400 g and 2.5 and 5 g/300 g) enhanced fullness sensation as compared to fiber-free drink [140,141]. Likewise, in healthy adolescents subjected to biscuits enriched with barley β-glucan (5.2%) helped in suppressing appetite ratings as compared to control biscuits [142]. Similarly, administration of bread formulated by barley β-glucan (3%) to volunteers resulted in decrease of hunger and increased satiety and fullness. This also resulted in a noteworthy decrease in energy intake at successive lunches [143]. On the other hand, a bar prepared from barley β-glucan (1.2 g) subjected to healthy volunteers did not change scores for energy intake and appetite scores as compared to control bars [144]. Effects of β-glucan on satiety depends upon the concentration, molecular weight (31–3100 kDa), solubility, and food carrying it [38].

Furthermore, a group of scientists investigated the hypocholesterolemic perspectives of a dietary supplement comprising equal content of konjac glucomannan (KGM) and chitosan [145]. The concentration of serum total cholesterol and low-density lipoprotein cholesterol (LDL-c) significantly reduced at the end of the trial (28th day). Fecal excretion of bile acids and neutral sterol were observed more at the commencement of the study as compared to the initiation of the study. Similarly, Chen et al. [146] investigated the impact of KGM supplementation (3.6 g/day) on levels of glucose and lipid biomarkers in hypercholesterolemic type-2 diabetic patients. Twenty-two diabetic patients having increased serum cholesterol content were selected for this study. As compared to the placebo group, KGM supplemented group showed decreased levels of LDL-c (20.7%), fasting glucose (23.2%), serum cholesterol (11.1%), and Apo-B (12.9%). Fecal bile acid and neutral sterol content were elevated significantly by 75.4% and 18.0%, respectively. Results of all the mentioned trials revealed that KGM supplementation could assist in the treatment of hypercholesterolemic diabetic patients [44].

4.4. Anti-Diabetic

Scientific evidences have shown that β-glucan can contribute to control glycemic responses. Numerous factors are found to affect such interactions like the nature of the food, concentration, and molecular weight of β-glucan. Among all these, the dose of β-glucan is considered to be the most important factor in regulating the impact of fiber on glycemic responses. As compared to other fibers, a small dose of β-glucan is sufficient to reduce the insulin and postprandial glucose responses in type 2 diabetic [147,148], healthy [149,150], and hyperlipidemic subjects [151]. Studies have revealed that consumption of breakfasts comprising of 4, 6, and 8.6 g of β-glucan momentously reduced the mean concentration of serum insulin and glucose as compared to control non-insulin-dependent diabetic mellitus subjects [147]. The content of exogenous glucose was noticed as 18% less in a polenta meal containing oat β-glucan (5 g) as compared to a control polenta meal without oat β-glucan-subjected individuals [152]. Likewise, consumption of a meal consisting of 13C-labelled glucose and β-glucan (8.9 g), for a period of three days, reduced (21%) the levels of exogenous 13C-glucose in plasma as compared to control meal having no β-glucan [38,153].

4.5. Gastro-Protective

An experimental trial conducted by means of two diverse types of resistant starches (one a high amylose granular resistant corn starch and the other was high amylose non-granular, dispersed, and retrograded resistant corn starch) to evaluate the influence on blood lipid concentration, fecal SCFA and bulking, and glycemic indexes. This study also comprised of supplements containing low fiber control and high fiber control. Outcomes of this trial revealed that high fiber control (wheat bran) and both resistance starches subjected groups showed an elevation in the fecal bulk as compared to the low fiber control group. Likewise, the average ratio of fecal SCFAs and butyrate had progressive effects on colon health. Xanthan gum may also be used in milk as a prebiotic for lactic acid bacteria. Similar trials regarding prebiotics have demonstrated protective implications on the sustainability of cultures under the presence of bile salts and refrigeration and low pH conditions. According to a study, guar gum has the capability to change lipoprotein and postprandial lipid compositions. Supplementation of guar gum has an influence on lipoprotein composition, lipemia, and postprandial glycaemia [19].

Chen et al. [154] explored the effect of KGM supplementation on the gastrointestinal response in volunteer subjects. They were of the view that KGM supplementation significantly elevated the dry and wet stool weight and defecation frequency to 21.7%, 30.2%, and 27.0%, correspondingly. The improved dry fecal mass may be due to the existence of plant soluble materials. Nevertheless, the bacterial biomass of total bacteria, bifido-bacteria, and lactobacilli increased in fecal mass in KGM supplemented groups. Furthermore, reduction in fecal pH and elevation in fecal short chain fatty acids (SCFAs) resulted in increased colonic fermentation owing to KGM supplementation [44].

4.6. Immune Modulatory

Ginseng polysaccharides (GPs) have not only been known to possess immune-stimulating perspectives but also are found to suppress the proinflammatory responses. According to a recent study, novel neutral polysaccharide (PPQN) derived from an American ginseng root was documented to have a suppressing effect against inflammation. This activity was reported due to the inhibitory effect of isolated polysaccharide on inflammatory-related mediators such as cytokines (IL-1b, IL-6, TNF-a) and NO (nitric oxide) in comparison with LPS (lipopolysaccharide) treatment. Owing to this mode of action, novel neutral polysaccharide isolated from an American ginseng root could be used in modulating numerous inflammatory-related health implications (tumor, cancer, etc.) [155]. Similarly, another study reported the inhibitory influence of ginseng polysaccharides on immunological responses noticed in collagen-induced arthritic subject [156]. *P. quinquefolius* (American ginseng) is extensively used for the preparation of numerous herbal products. Extracts of *P. quinquefolius* were found to suppress the immune-inflammatory response, reduced the activity of neutrophils, induced the formation of cytokines in the spleen, and elevated the production of splenic-B lymphocytes and bone marrow [157–160].

Platycodon grandifloras is an herbaceous plant which is used as folk medicines since ancient times to curb various diseases like asthma, bronchitis, and pulmonary tuberculosis. Proximate composition of *P. grandifloras* reveals that it is a rich source of carbohydrates (90%), protein (2.4%), ash (1.5%), and fat (0.1%). Polysaccharides extracted from roots of *P. grandifloras* have been reported to possess antidiabetic, hypolipidemic and hypocholesterolemic properties [161]. Furthermore, the inulin-type polysaccharides isolated from *P. grandifloras* (PGs) roots validated the immune-modulating impact on macrophages and B-cells, but had no effect on T-cells [162].

4.7. Anti-Inflammatory

Astragalus polysaccharides (APS) are known to possess anti-inflammatory effects on cytokines of $CD4^+$ T_h (T-helper) cells. In in-vitro antidiabetic models, an *Astragalus* polysaccharide has potentiated the lowering effect on the expression of T-helper 1 (Th1) and regulated the imbalance of Th1 and Th2. APS has reported to significantly enhance the gene expression of peroxisome-proliferator-activated receptor gamma (PPAR-γ) in a concentration-time dependent manner [163] and stimulated superoxide dismutase (SOD) anti-oxidative mechanism in type-1 diabetes mellitus (DM) models [164,165]. Moreover, APS reduced the expression of iNOS (inducible nitric oxide synthase) [122]. These inflammatory markers (NO, PPAR-γ, SOD, and iNOS) amongst diverse roles also perform numerous functions in regulating and stimulating inflammatory response [42].

Water-soluble sulfated polysaccharides (WSSPs) isolated from marine algae are also classified as anti-inflammatory compounds. On the other hand, very few pieces of evidence are present regarding anti-inflammatory perspectives of seaweed based sulfated polysaccharides. In vitro and in vivo studies have revealed that *Gracilaria verrucose-* and *Porphyra yezoensis*-derived sulfated polysaccharides stimulated the respiratory burst and phagocytosis in experimented mouse macrophages [40]. Orally administered chondroitin sulfate (CS) isolated from cartilage of Skate (*Raja kenojei*) affected arthritic conditions in a dose-dependent manner in chondroitin sulfate-treated groups. Pre- and post-treated groups that were subjected to CS (1000 mg kg^{-1}) revealed momentously decreased clinical scores as compared to vehicle treated groups. CS administration decreased the infiltration of inflammatory cells and prohibited from paw and knee joint destruction. Moreover, the results of RT-PCR showed that CS ingestion significantly repressed the expression of IL-1b (interleukin-1b), IFN-c (interferon-c), and TNF-α as compared to vehicle administered group. The CS-treated group reduced the formation of rheumatoid arthritis responses (IgG and IgM) in collagen-induced arthritic mice (CIA) model. Outcomes of this study authenticate the shielding potential of chondroitin sulfate in CIA mice mainly due to the inhibitory effect of pro-inflammatory cytokines formation [43].

4.8. Neuro-Protective

Acanthopanax senticosus derived polysaccharides comprised of uronic acid (22.5%), proteins (18.7%), and carbohydrates (58.3%). It could be established that *Acanthopanax*-based polysaccharides may not only help in improving symptoms regarding nervous defects but also reduced the infarct volume and water content of the brain in rats having cerebral ischemia–reperfusion injury. Additionally, polysaccharides isolated from *A. senticosus* elevated SOD, IL-10, and GSH-Px concentration and reduces the levels of TNF-α, IL-1, and MDA in brains tissues of experimented rats. Conclusively, bioactive polysaccharides extracted from *A. senticosus* protected brain damage due to antioxidative potential and inhibitory action on stimulation of inflammatory cytokines [47].

4.9. Anti-Oxidant

Bioactive acidic polysaccharides extracted from *Polygonum multiflorum* showed significant antioxidative properties (hydroxyl peroxide, superoxide anion radical, and hydroxyl radical), protein glycation and lipid oxidation. In addition to this, the intraperitoneal (i.p.) administration of *P. multiflorium*-based polysaccharides may increase the serum concentration of antioxidative characteristics in cyclophosphamide-induced anemic mice. Results of this study validate the use of *P. multiflorium* as a novel antioxidant tool to prevent oxidation [41]. Sulfated polysaccharides not only act as dietary fiber but also act as a natural antioxidant agent. They are responsible for the antioxidant properties possessed by marine algae. Various studies have recognized the use of numerous classes of SPs (alginic acid, Fucoidan, and laminaran) as potent antioxidative agents.

Antioxidative potential of SPs has classified by multiple in-vitro methods such as DPPH, FRAP, NO, ABTS radical scavenging, superoxide radical scavenging assay, and the hydroxyl radical scavenging assay. Additionally, Xue et al. [166] stated that many marine-based sulfated polysaccharides have shown antioxidant potential in organic solvents and a phosphatidylcholine-liposomal suspension [40].

4.10. Tissue Engineering

Application of bioactive polysaccharides and their derivatives in the field of tissue engineering (cell differentiation, cell adhesion, cell remodeling, cell proliferation, and cell responsive degradation) has opened new horizons in medical research, and therefore impelled the researchers to regenerate new tissues and define the structure of cellular growth [92]. Various bioactive polysaccharides including starch, chitosan, chondroitin sulfate, alginate, cellulose, chitin, hyaluronic acid, and their derivatives are being used as biomaterials in applications for tissue engineering [167]. Application of these bioactive polysaccharides as scaffolds in tissue engineering are required to accomplish some requirements such as non-toxicity, biodegradability having controlled the rate of degradation, biocompatibility, structural integrity, and suitable porosity [92].

Chitosan and chitin have all the required potential to act as scaffolds for tissue engineering mainly due to their mechanical strength, degradability, and immunogenicity. Hence, for tissue engineering they are being developed as 3D-hydrogels, free standing films, porous sponges, and fibrous scaffolds, inside which for in-vitro/in-vivo cultures the most suitable cell types are needed [168]. Designing of 3D-chitin/chitosan-based hydrogels and sponge scaffolds, and 2D-scaffolds for the purpose of cartilage and tendon regenerations, for encapsulation of stem cells ensuring their therapeutic application, and for utilizing these as a tool for regenerative medicine have been reported in numerous researches [169,170]. Furthermore, for bone regeneration purpose, the tissue engineering industry has formulated combinations of chitosan and hydroxyapatite and grafted chitosan and carbon nanotubes [171]. Along with this, numerous other bioactive polysaccharides like cellulose, hyaluronic acid, and starch have also been studied in detail to validate their use as a biomaterial for skin, bone, and cartilage tissue engineering [95].

4.11. Wound Healing and Wound Dressing

Numerous bioactive polysaccharides (alginate, chitin, hyaluronan, chitosan, and cellulose) are used for the preparation of wound healing materials owing to their intrinsic bio-compatible, less toxic, and pharmaceutical activities [172,173]. For instance, hyaluronan is a vital extracellular component possessing distinctive viscoelastic, hygroscopic, and rheological characteristics are well known for its tissue repairing properties owing to their physicochemical potentials and specific interaction with cells and extracellular matrices. It is documented earlier that hyaluronan has a multidimensional role regarding the repairing process of cell or wound healing specifically inflammation, granulation, formation of tissues, re-epithelialization, and remodeling. Various hyaluronan-derived products like esterified, cross-linked, or chemically modified products are medicinally used for wound healing and tissue repairing purposes [174]. While designing bioactive material for tissue engineering their wound healing properties is of great interest.

Naturally available wound dressing films either prepared by encapsulation or simply dispersion of the sodium alginate matrix in essential oils from cinnamon, lemon, tea, lemongrass, lavender, elicriso italic, peppermint, chamomile blue, and eucalyptus have demonstrated exceptional anti-fungal and anti-microbial activities, and therefore their application in disposable dressings for wounds could also be found [175]. Development of wound dressings obtained from cross-linkage between chitosan/silk fibroin blending membranes and di-aldehyde alginate have found to enhance cellular proliferative properties, suggesting their applications as wound healing agents [176]. Preparation of freestanding sodium alginate films or Ca^{2+} cross-linked alginate beads was achieved by mixing aqueous dispersions of PVPI (povidone iodine) and Na-Alg. These films/beads showed anti-fungal/anti-bacterial properties along with control release of povidone iodine into wounds as these products came into direct contact with the moist environment [175]. These applications validate the use of these products therapeutically in wound dressings. Some innovative wound dressings were prepared for external treatment of wounds by in situ injection of nanocomposite hydrogels that actually comprised of oxidized alginate, curcumin, and N, O-carboxymethyl chitosan. Results of various in vitro, in vivo, and histological investigations have proven the use of nanocurcumin, N, O-carboxymethyl chitosan, and oxidized alginate-based hydrogels as novel tools in wound dressings for their application as wound repairing agents. Furthermore, gamma radiations were successfully employed for the synthesis of silver nanoparticles comprising of alginate and polyvinyl pyrrolidone (PvP)-based hydrogels. These products have scientifically shown their capability regarding the prevention of fluid accumulations in exudate wounds [177]. The amalgamation of nano-silver particles provides a promising anti-microbial property and hence made these PvP-alginate hydrogels most appropriate for wound healing and dressing. Other than alginate and their associated derivatives, numerous other naturally occurring polysaccharides like hyaluronic acid, cellulose, chitosan, and chitin have been investigated by researchers to assess their wound healing applications [178].

4.12. Drug Delivery and Controlled Release

Application of bioactive polysaccharides as a novel agent in drug delivery and controlled release has also been studied by scientists owing to their least toxicity, minimum immunogenicity, and biocompatibility. Various naturally occurring polysaccharide-based drug delivery systems are in practice due to their targeted delivery/controlled release, shielding effect against premature degradation of drugs, improvement of intracellular transportation, enhancement of bioavailability of drugs, as well as delivery of small interfering RNA, antigens, and genes [179]. Delivery systems mentioned here usually possess covalent/ionic cross-linkages, poly-electrolyte complexes, conjugates of polysaccharides and drugs, and self-assembly [179]. Release of 3-D cross-linked drugs could be triggered by varying redox potential, pH, light, ions, temperature, and application of magnetic and/or electric fields [180]. Mainly the three most abundantly used polysaccharides i.e., alginate, chitin, cellulose, and chitosan are overviewed in detail as under in this portion.

Pharmaceutic application of cellulose and their associated derivatives could be classified either as pharmaceutical excipients for protecting purposes or as bioactive molecules themselves. Application of bioactive polysaccharides as pharmaceutical excipients in orally administrated drug delivery systems have been explored to enhance the solubility and bioavailability of drugs, to increase the final product (drug) stability, and to attain release profile from final formulations [181]. These days, microcrystalline cellulose, rice, and corn starches have been broadly engaged in formulations of capsule diluents, tablet dis-integrants, and glidants. Various cellulose derivatives like HPMC (hydroxypropyl methyl cellulose), MC (methyl cellulose), HPC (hydroxypropyl cellulose), and HEC (hydroxyethyl cellulose) possessing better physiochemical properties as compared to cellulose are evidently being used in pharmaceutical industries [182]. For instance, HPMC phthalate has significant pH depending solubility, specifically, stability under acidic conditions of the stomach while soluble in mild acidic to slight alkaline solutions and, hence, are being applied for controlled release of intestinal targeted drugs. In recent times, nanocellulose-based drug delivery systems comprising of CNCs (cellulose nanocrystals), NFC (nanofibrillated cellulose), and BC (bacterial cellulose) have been investigated comprehensively [183]. For example, the binding and release of the hydrochloride salt of doxorubicin and tetracycline have been explored extensively due to ionic cross-linked systems, in which sulfate groups on cellulose nanocrystals possessing negative charge are reversibly cross-linked ionically to counterpart positively charged drugs. Likewise, nanofibrillated cellulose-based films have also been investigated for entrapment of drugs and are being used in pharmaceutical industries for the production of long-lasting drug release systems [184].

Reconnoitering the application of chitin/chitosan as bio-molecular delivery vectors have impelled the scientists for the development of therapeutic drug delivery systems like siRNA (small interfering RNA) carriers, antigens, and genes [185]. In vivo, therapeutic application of chitosan-based siRNA carries has shown great potential as a tool for gene expression associated diseases. Inhibitory influence on human colorectal cancer gene expression due to the application of chitosan-siRNA nanoparticles have been studied in an earlier study [186]. It was noticed that chitosan-siRNA nanoparticles developed by ionic gelation with Na-tri-polyphosphate demonstrated a more targeted dene inhibiting impact owing to increased binding and loading effectiveness. Long-lasting delivery of encapsulated antigens or intra-dermal vaccines administered through chitosan microneedles transdermal delivery systems are documented to deliver more sustainable immune stimulation [187]. Though, the sensitivity of pH could also affect the stability issues of the drug delivery systems [179]. Various other bioactive polysaccharides like chondroitin, pectin, xanthan gum, dextran, chitin, gellan gum, chitosan, and dextran are also being used for controlled drug delivery [1,181].

5. Conclusions

Bioactive polysaccharides have acquired significant attention from scientists as functional biomolecules for the development of innovative and value-added products in the fields of pharmaceutics, food, cosmetics, and the biomedical industry. Their therapeutic application is mainly due to their bio-degradable, non-toxic, and bio-compatible nature. Extraction and isolation of naturally occurring bioactive polysaccharides possessing high purity with maximum extraction yield, meanwhile keeping in view that the native structure remains intact, are of great future concern and remains a field for further exploration. Momentous results to authenticate the use of these polysaccharides as a novel tool in the pharmaceutical and medicinal industry will require a multidimensional approach from scientists of various fields like healthcare, food science, organic chemistry, material science and engineering, as well as plant biology.

Author Contributions: S.U. and A.A.K. drafted this manuscript; Y.S. edited and reviewed the whole manuscript and provided suggestions to main authors with critical input and corrections; F.S. assisted in locating and interpreting the literature sources whenever or/and wherever was necessary; and all authors read and approved the final manuscript.

Funding: This work was supported by the National Natural Science Foundation of China (Grant Nos. 31670064 and 31271812), and TaiShan Industrial Experts Program.

Conflicts of Interest: Authors declare no conflict of interest.

References

1. Zhang, Y.; Wang, F. Carbohydrate drugs: Current status and development prospect. *Drug Discov. Ther.* **2015**, *9*, 79–87. [CrossRef] [PubMed]
2. Li, P.; Wang, F. Polysaccharides: Candidates of promising vaccine adjuvants. *Drug Discov. Ther.* **2015**, *9*, 88–93. [CrossRef] [PubMed]
3. Do Amaral, A.E.; Petkowicz, C.L.O.; Mercê, A.L.R.; Iacomini, M.; Martinez, G.R.; Rocha, M.E.M.; Cadena, S.M.S.C.; Noleto, G.R. Leishmanicidal activity of polysaccharides and their oxovanadium (iv/v) complexes. *Eur. J. Med. Chem.* **2015**, *90*, 732–741. [CrossRef] [PubMed]
4. Zong, A.; Cao, H.; Wang, F. Anticancer polysaccharides from natural resources: A review of recent research. *Carbohydr. Polym.* **2012**, *90*, 1395–1410. [CrossRef] [PubMed]
5. Colegate, S.M.; Molyneux, R.J. *Bioactive Natural Products: Detection, Isolation, and Structural Determination*; CRC Press: Boca Raton, FL, USA, 2007.
6. Zhang, C.; Gao, Z.; Hu, C.; Zhang, J.; Sun, X.; Rong, C.; Jia, L. Antioxidant, antibacterial and anti-aging activities of intracellular zinc polysaccharides from grifola frondosa sh-05. *Int. J. Biol. Macromol.* **2017**, *95*, 778–787. [CrossRef] [PubMed]
7. Sinha, V.; Kumria, R. Polysaccharides in colon-specific drug delivery. *Int. J. Pharm.* **2001**, *224*, 19–38. [CrossRef]
8. Dong, B.; Hadinoto, K. Direct comparison between millifluidic and bulk-mixing platform in the synthesis of amorphous drug-polysaccharide nanoparticle complex. *Int. J. Pharm.* **2017**, *523*, 42–51. [CrossRef]

9. Jung, B.; Shim, M.-K.; Park, M.-J.; Jang, E.H.; Yoon, H.Y.; Kim, K.; Kim, J.-H. Hydrophobically modified polysaccharide-based on polysialic acid nanoparticles as carriers for anticancer drugs. *Int. J. Pharm.* **2017**, *520*, 111–118. [CrossRef]
10. Nuti, E.; Santamaria, S.; Casalini, F.; Yamamoto, K.; Marinelli, L.; La Pietra, V.; Novellino, E.; Orlandini, E.; Nencetti, S.; Marini, A.M. Arylsulfonamide inhibitors of aggrecanases as potential therapeutic agents for osteoarthritis: Synthesis and biological evaluation. *Eur. J. Med. Chem.* **2013**, *62*, 379–394. [CrossRef]
11. Chen, Q.; Mei, X.; Han, G.; Ling, P.; Guo, B.; Guo, Y.; Shao, H.; Wang, G.; Cui, Z.; Bai, Y. Xanthan gum protects rabbit articular chondrocytes against sodium nitroprusside-induced apoptosis in vitro. *Carbohydr. Polym.* **2015**, *131*, 363–369. [CrossRef]
12. An, H.J.; Lebrilla, C.B. Structure elucidation of native n-and o-linked glycans by tandem mass spectrometry (tutorial). *Mass Spectrom. Rev.* **2011**, *30*, 560–578. [CrossRef]
13. MaKi-Arvela, P.I.; Salmi, T.; Holmbom, B.; Willfor, S.; Murzin, D.Y. Synthesis of sugars by hydrolysis of hemicelluloses-a review. *Chem. Rev.* **2011**, *111*, 5638–5666. [CrossRef] [PubMed]
14. Yang, L.; Zhang, L.-M. Chemical structural and chain conformational characterization of some bioactive polysaccharides isolated from natural sources. *Carbohydr. Polym.* **2009**, *76*, 349–361. [CrossRef]
15. Xiao, Z.; Tappen, B.R.; Ly, M.; Zhao, W.; Canova, L.P.; Guan, H.; Linhardt, R.J. Heparin mapping using heparin lyases and the generation of a novel low molecular weight heparin. *J. Med. Chem.* **2010**, *54*, 603–610. [CrossRef]
16. Gatti, G.; Casu, B.; Hamer, G.; Perlin, A. Studies on the conformation of heparin by 1h and 13c nmr spectroscopy. *Macromolecules* **1979**, *12*, 1001–1007. [CrossRef]
17. Varki, A.; Cummings, R.; Esko, J.; Stanley, P.; Hart, G.; Aebi, M.; Darvill, A.; Kinoshita, T.; Packer, N.; Prestegard, J. *Oligosaccharides and Polysaccharides—Essentials of Glycobiology*, 3rd ed.; Cold Spring Harbor Laboratory Press: Cold Spring Harbor, NY, USA, 2017.
18. Pool-Zobel, B.L. Inulin-type fructans and reduction in colon cancer risk: Review of experimental and human data. *Br. J. Nutr.* **2005**, *93*, S73–S90. [CrossRef]
19. Chawla, R.; Patil, G. Soluble dietary fiber. *Compr. Rev. Food Sci. Food Saf.* **2010**, *9*, 178–196. [CrossRef]
20. Tungland, B.; Meyer, D. Nondigestible oligo-and polysaccharides (dietary fiber): Their physiology and role in human health and food. *Compr. Rev. Food Sci. Food Saf.* **2002**, *1*, 90–109. [CrossRef]
21. Weng, L.-C.; Lee, N.-J.; Yeh, W.-T.; Ho, L.-T.; Pan, W.-H. Lower intake of magnesium and dietary fiber increases the incidence of type 2 diabetes in taiwanese. *J. Formos. Med. Assoc.* **2012**, *111*, 651–659. [CrossRef]
22. Casiglia, E.; Tikhonoff, V.; Caffi, S.; Boschetti, G.; Grasselli, C.; Saugo, M.; Giordano, N.; Rapisarda, V.; Spinella, P.; Palatini, P. High dietary fiber intake prevents stroke at a population level. *Clin. Nutr.* **2013**, *32*, 811–818. [CrossRef]
23. Viuda-Martos, M.; López-Marcos, M.; Fernández-López, J.; Sendra, E.; López-Vargas, J.; Pérez-Álvarez, J. Role of fiber in cardiovascular diseases: A review. *Food Sci. Food Saf.* **2010**, *9*, 240–258. [CrossRef]
24. Whelton, S.P.; Hyre, A.D.; Pedersen, B.; Yi, Y.; Whelton, P.K.; He, J. Effect of dietary fiber intake on blood pressure: A meta-analysis of randomized, controlled clinical trials. *LWW* **2005**, *23*, 475–481. [CrossRef]
25. Chau, C.-F.; Huang, Y.-L.; Lin, C.-Y. Investigation of the cholesterol-lowering action of insoluble fibre derived from the peel of citrus sinensis l. Cv. Liucheng. *Food Chem.* **2004**, *87*, 361–366. [CrossRef]
26. Kendall, C.W.; Esfahani, A.; Jenkins, D.J. The link between dietary fibre and human health. *Food Hydrocoll.* **2010**, *24*, 42–48. [CrossRef]
27. Lunn, J.; Buttriss, J. Carbohydrates and dietary fibre. *Nutr. Bull.* **2007**, *32*, 21–64. [CrossRef]
28. Anderson, J.W.; Baird, P.; Davis, R.H.; Ferreri, S.; Knudtson, M.; Koraym, A.; Waters, V.; Williams, C.L. Health benefits of dietary fiber. *Nutr. Rev.* **2009**, *67*, 188–205. [CrossRef]
29. Brown, L.; Rosner, B.; Willett, W.W.; Sacks, F.M. Cholesterol-lowering effects of dietary fiber: A meta-analysis. *Am. J. Clin. Nutr.* **1999**, *69*, 30–42. [CrossRef]
30. Tang, W.; Hemm, I.; Bertram, B. Recent development of antitumor agents from chinese herbal medicines. Part ii. High molecular compounds. *Planta Med.* **2003**, *69*, 193–201. [CrossRef]
31. Harlev, E.; Nevo, E.; Lansky, E.P.; Ofir, R.; Bishayee, A. Anticancer potential of aloes: Antioxidant, antiproliferative, and immunostimulatory attributes. *Planta Med.* **2012**, *78*, 843–852. [CrossRef]
32. Thakur, M.; Weng, A.; Fuchs, H.; Sharma, V.; Bhargava, C.S.; Chauhan, N.S.; Dixit, V.K.; Bhargava, S. Rasayana properties of ayurvedic herbs: Are polysaccharides a major contributor? *Carbohydr. Polym.* **2012**, *87*, 3–15. [CrossRef]

33. Tian, L.; Zhao, Y.; Guo, C.; Yang, X. A comparative study on the antioxidant activities of an acidic polysaccharide and various solvent extracts derived from herbal houttuynia cordata. *Carbohydr. Polym.* **2011**, *83*, 537–544. [CrossRef]
34. Jin, M.; Huang, Q.; Zhao, K.; Shang, P. Biological activities and potential health benefit effects of polysaccharides isolated from lycium barbarum l. *Int. J. Biol. Macromol.* **2013**, *54*, 16–23. [CrossRef]
35. Li, T.; Peng, T. Traditional chinese herbal medicine as a source of molecules with antiviral activity. *Antivir. Res.* **2013**, *97*, 1–9. [CrossRef]
36. Harhaji, T.L.M.; Mijatović, S.A.; Maksimović-Ivanić, D.D.; Stojanović, I.D.; Momčilović, M.B.; Tufegdžić, S.J.; Maksimović, V.M.; Marjanovi, Ž.S.; Stošić-Grujičić, S.D. Anticancer properties of ganoderma lucidum methanol extracts in vitro and in vivo. *Nutr. Cancer* **2009**, *61*, 696–707. [CrossRef]
37. Ke, M.; Zhang, X.-J.; Han, Z.-H.; Yu, H.-Y.; Lin, Y.; Zhang, W.-G.; Sun, F.-H.; Wang, T.-J. Extraction, purification of lycium barbarum polysaccharides and bioactivity of purified fraction. *Carbohydr. Polym.* **2011**, *86*, 136–141. [CrossRef]
38. El Khoury, D.; Cuda, C.; Luhovyy, B.; Anderson, G. Beta glucan: Health benefits in obesity and metabolic syndrome. *J. Nutr. Metab.* **2011**, *2012*. [CrossRef]
39. Zhang, W.; Xu, P.; Zhang, H. Pectin in cancer therapy: A review. *Trends Food Sci. Technol.* **2015**, *44*, 258–271. [CrossRef]
40. Wijesekara, I.; Pangestuti, R.; Kim, S.-K. Biological activities and potential health benefits of sulfated polysaccharides derived from marine algae. *Carbohydr. Polym.* **2011**, *84*, 14–21. [CrossRef]
41. Zhu, W.; Xue, X.; Zhang, Z. Structural, physicochemical, antioxidant and antitumor property of an acidic polysaccharide from polygonum multiflorum. *Int. J. Biol. Macromol.* **2017**, *96*, 494–500. [CrossRef]
42. Agyemang, K.; Han, L.; Liu, E.; Zhang, Y.; Wang, T.; Gao, X. Recent advances in astragalus membranaceus anti-diabetic research: Pharmacological effects of its phytochemical constituents. *Evid.-Based Complement. Altern. Med.* **2013**, *2013*. [CrossRef]
43. Volpi, N. Anti-inflammatory activity of chondroitin sulphate: New functions from an old natural macromolecule. *Inflammopharmacology* **2011**, *19*, 299–306. [CrossRef] [PubMed]
44. Behera, S.S.; Ray, R.C. Konjac glucomannan, a promising polysaccharide of amorphophallus konjac k. Koch in health care. *Int. J. Biol. Macromol.* **2016**, *92*, 942–956. [CrossRef] [PubMed]
45. Loh, S.H.; Park, J.-Y.; Cho, E.H.; Nah, S.-Y.; Kang, Y.-S. Animal lectins: Potential receptors for ginseng polysaccharides. *J. Ginseng Res.* **2017**, *41*, 1–9. [CrossRef] [PubMed]
46. Casu, B.; Naggi, A.; Torri, G. Heparin-derived heparan sulfate mimics to modulate heparan sulfate-protein interaction in inflammation and cancer. *Matrix Biol.* **2010**, *29*, 442–452. [CrossRef] [PubMed]
47. Xie, Y.; Zhang, B.; Zhang, Y. Protective effects of acanthopanax polysaccharides on cerebral ischemia–reperfusion injury and its mechanisms. *Int. J. Biol. Macromol.* **2015**, *72*, 946–950. [CrossRef] [PubMed]
48. Kim, S.-K.; Li, Y.-X. Medicinal benefits of sulfated polysaccharides from sea vegetables. *Adv. Food Nutr. Res.* **2011**, *64*, 391–402. [PubMed]
49. Olafsdottir, E.S.; Ingólfsdottir, K. Polysaccharides from lichens: Structural characteristics and biological activity. *Planta Medica* **2001**, *67*, 199–208. [CrossRef] [PubMed]
50. Chattopadhyay, N.; Ghosh, T.; Sinha, S.; Chattopadhyay, K.; Karmakar, P.; Ray, B. Polysaccharides from turbinaria conoides: Structural features and antioxidant capacity. *Food Chem.* **2010**, *118*, 823–829. [CrossRef]
51. Schepetkin, I.A.; Quinn, M.T. Botanical polysaccharides: Macrophage immunomodulation and therapeutic potential. *Int. Immunopharmacol.* **2006**, *6*, 317–333. [CrossRef] [PubMed]
52. Omarsdottir, S.; Freysdottir, J.; Olafsdottir, E.S. Immunomodulating polysaccharides from the lichen thamnolia vermicularis var. Subuliformis. *Phytomedicine* **2007**, *14*, 179–184. [CrossRef]
53. Zambare, V.P.; Christopher, L.P. Biopharmaceutical potential of lichens. *Pharm. Biol.* **2012**, *50*, 778–798. [CrossRef] [PubMed]
54. Martinichen-Herrero, J.; Carbonero, E.; Sassaki, G.; Gorin, P.; Iacomini, M. Anticoagulant and antithrombotic activities of a chemically sulfated galactoglucomannan obtained from the lichen cladoniaibitipocae. *Int. J. Biol. Macromol.* **2005**, *35*, 97–102. [CrossRef] [PubMed]
55. Ngo, D.-H.; Kim, S.-K. Sulfated polysaccharides as bioactive agents from marine algae. *Int. J. Biol. Macromol.* **2013**, *62*, 70–75. [CrossRef] [PubMed]

56. Zhang, J.; Wen, C.; Duan, Y.; Zhang, H.; Ma, H. Advance in cordyceps militaris (linn) link polysaccharides: Isolation, structure, and bioactivities: A review. *Int. J. Biol. Macromol.* **2019**, *132*, 906–914. [CrossRef] [PubMed]
57. Meng, X.; Liang, H.; Luo, L. Antitumor polysaccharides from mushrooms: A review on the structural characteristics, antitumor mechanisms and immunomodulating activities. *Carbohydr. Res.* **2016**, *424*, 30–41. [CrossRef] [PubMed]
58. Yu, Y.; Shen, M.; Song, Q.; Xie, J. Biological activities and pharmaceutical applications of polysaccharide from natural resources: A review. *Carbohydr. Polym.* **2018**, *183*, 91–101. [CrossRef] [PubMed]
59. Negre-Salvayre, A.; Coatrieux, C.; Ingueneau, C.; Salvayre, R. Advanced lipid peroxidation end products in oxidative damage to proteins. Potential role in diseases and therapeutic prospects for the inhibitors. *Br. J. Pharmacol.* **2008**, *153*, 6–20. [CrossRef] [PubMed]
60. Kamerling, J.P.; Gerwig, G.J. Strategies for the structural analysis of carbohydrates. *Compr. Glycosci.* **2007**, 1–68. [CrossRef]
61. Feng, F.; Zhou, Q.; Yang, Y.; Zhao, F.; Du, R.; Han, Y.; Xiao, H.; Zhou, Z. Characterization of highly branched dextran produced by leuconostoc citreum b-2 from pineapple fermented product. *Int. J. Biol. Macromol.* **2018**, *113*, 45–50. [CrossRef]
62. Chen, L.; Ge, M.-D.; Zhu, Y.-J.; Song, Y.; Cheung, P.C.K.; Zhang, B.-B.; Liu, L.-M. Structure, bioactivity and applications of natural hyperbranched polysaccharides. *Carbohydr. Polym.* **2019**, *223*, 115076. [CrossRef]
63. Cerning, J. Exocellular polysaccharides produced by lactic acid bacteria. *FEMS Microbiol. Rev.* **1990**, *7*, 113–130. [CrossRef] [PubMed]
64. Pereira, S.; Micheletti, E.; Zille, A.; Santos, A.; Moradas-Ferreira, P.; Tamagnini, P.; De Philippis, R. Using extracellular polymeric substances (eps)-producing cyanobacteria for the bioremediation of heavy metals: Do cations compete for the eps functional groups and also accumulate inside the cell? *Microbiology* **2011**, *157*, 451–458. [CrossRef] [PubMed]
65. Guezennec, J. Deep-sea hydrothermal vents: A new source of innovative bacterial exopolysaccharides of biotechnological interest? *J. Ind. Microbiol. Biotechnol.* **2002**, *29*, 204–208. [CrossRef] [PubMed]
66. Senni, K.; Pereira, J.; Gueniche, F.; Delbarre-Ladrat, C.; Sinquin, C.; Ratiskol, J.; Godeau, G.; Fischer, A.-M.; Helley, D.; Colliec-Jouault, S. Marine polysaccharides: A source of bioactive molecules for cell therapy and tissue engineering. *Mar. Drugs* **2011**, *9*, 1664–1681. [CrossRef] [PubMed]
67. Roger, O.; Kervarec, N.; Ratiskol, J.; Colliec-Jouault, S.; Chevolot, L. Structural studies of the main exopolysaccharide produced by the deep-sea bacterium alteromonas infernus. *Carbohydr. Res.* **2004**, *339*, 2371–2380. [CrossRef] [PubMed]
68. Zhou, Y.; Cui, Y.; Qu, X. Exopolysaccharides of lactic acid bacteria: Structure, bioactivity and associations: A review. *Carbohydr. Polym.* **2019**, *207*, 317–332. [CrossRef] [PubMed]
69. Kay, E.; Cuccui, J.; Wren, B.W. Recent advances in the production of recombinant glycoconjugate vaccines. *NPJ Vaccines* **2019**, *4*, 16. [CrossRef]
70. Gatenholm, P.; Tenkanen, M. *Industrially Isolated Hemicellulose*; ACS Symposium Series: Washington, DC, USA, 2004; pp. 1–2.
71. Barsett, H.; Ebringerová, A.; Harding, S.; Heinze, T.; Hromádková, Z.; Muzzarelli, C.; Muzzraelli, R.; Paulsen, B.; Elseoud, O. *Polysaccharides I: Structure, Characterisation and Use*; Springer Science & Business Media: Berlin, Germany, 2005; Volume 186.
72. Ebringerová, A.; Hromádková, Z.; Hříbalová, V.; Xu, C.; Holmbom, B.; Sundberg, A.; Willför, S. Norway spruce galactoglucomannans exhibiting immunomodulating and radical-scavenging activities. *Int. J. Biol. Macromol.* **2008**, *42*, 1–5. [CrossRef]
73. Le Normand, M.; Mélida, H.; Holmbom, B.; Michaelsen, T.E.; Inngjerdingen, M.; Bulone, V.; Paulsen, B.S.; Ek, M. Hot-water extracts from the inner bark of norway spruce with immunomodulating activities. *Carbohydr. Polym.* **2014**, *101*, 699–704. [CrossRef]
74. Aachary, A.A.; Prapulla, S.G. Xylooligosaccharides (xos) as an emerging prebiotic: Microbial synthesis, utilization, structural characterization, bioactive properties, and applications. *Food Sci. Food Saf.* **2011**, *10*, 2–16. [CrossRef]
75. Van Ophoven, A.; Vonde, K.; Koch, W.; Auerbach, G.; Maag, K.P. Efficacy of pentosan polysulfate for the treatment of interstitial cystitis/bladder pain syndrome: Results of a systematic review of randomized controlled trials. *Curr. Med. Res. Opin.* **2019**, 1–9. [CrossRef] [PubMed]

76. Li, J.; Mei, X. *Applications of Cellulose and Cellulose Derivatives in Immediate Release Solid Dosage*; ACS Publications: Washington, DC, USA, 2006.
77. Chappell, E.P.; Liu, J. Use of biosynthetic enzymes in heparin and heparan sulfate synthesis. *Bioorg. Med. Chem.* **2013**, *21*, 4786–4792. [CrossRef] [PubMed]
78. Linhardt, R.J. 2003 Claude S. Hudson award address in carbohydrate chemistry. Heparin: Structure and activity. *J. Med. Chem.* **2003**, *46*, 2551–2564. [CrossRef] [PubMed]
79. Sakiyama-Elbert, S.E. Incorporation of heparin into biomaterials. *Acta Biomater.* **2014**, *10*, 1581–1587. [CrossRef] [PubMed]
80. Schedin-Weiss, S.; Richard, B.; Hjelm, R.; Olson, S.T. Antiangiogenic forms of antithrombin specifically bind to the anticoagulant heparin sequence. *Biochemistry* **2008**, *47*, 13610–13619. [CrossRef] [PubMed]
81. Rajangam, K.; Behanna, H.A.; Hui, M.J.; Han, X.; Hulvat, J.F.; Lomasney, J.W.; Stupp, S.I. Heparin binding nanostructures to promote growth of blood vessels. *Nano Lett.* **2006**, *6*, 2086–2090. [CrossRef] [PubMed]
82. Zhang, F.; Walcott, B.; Zhou, D.; Gustchina, A.; Lasanajak, Y.; Smith, D.F.; Ferreira, R.S.; Correia, M.T.S.; Paiva, P.M.; Bovin, N.V. Structural studies of the interaction of crataeva tapia bark protein with heparin and other glycosaminoglycans. *Biochemistry* **2013**, *52*, 2148–2156. [CrossRef] [PubMed]
83. Silbert, J.E.; Sugumaran, G. Biosynthesis of chondroitin/dermatan sulfate. *IUBMB Life* **2002**, *54*, 177–186. [CrossRef]
84. Takegawa, Y.; Araki, K.; Fujitani, N.; Furukawa, J.-I.; Sugiyama, H.; Sakai, H.; Shinohara, Y. Simultaneous analysis of heparan sulfate, chondroitin/dermatan sulfates, and hyaluronan disaccharides by glycoblotting-assisted sample preparation followed by single-step zwitter-ionic-hydrophilic interaction chromatography. *Anayticall Chem.* **2011**, *83*, 9443–9449. [CrossRef]
85. Sugahara, K.; Mikami, T.; Uyama, T.; Mizuguchi, S.; Nomura, K.; Kitagawa, H. Recent advances in the structural biology of chondroitin sulfate and dermatan sulfate. *Curr. Opin. Struct. Biol.* **2003**, *13*, 612–620. [CrossRef]
86. Kwok, J.; Warren, P.; Fawcett, J. Chondroitin sulfate: A key molecule in the brain matrix. *Int. J. Biochem. Cell Biol.* **2012**, *44*, 582–586. [CrossRef]
87. Zou, X.; Foong, W.; Cao, T.; Bay, B.; Ouyang, H.; Yip, G. Chondroitin sulfate in palatal wound healing. *J. Dent. Res.* **2004**, *83*, 880–885. [CrossRef]
88. Alliston, T. Chondroitin sulfate and growth factor signaling in the skeleton: Possible links to mps vi. *J. Pediatr. Rehabil. Med.* **2010**, *3*, 129–138.
89. Balazs, E.A. Therapeutic use of hyaluronan. *Struct. Chem.* **2009**, *20*, 341–349. [CrossRef]
90. Gaffney, J.; Matou-Nasri, S.; Grau-Olivares, M.; Slevin, M. Therapeutic applications of hyaluronan. *Mol. BioSyst.* **2010**, *6*, 437–443. [CrossRef]
91. Prestwich, G.D. Hyaluronic acid-based clinical biomaterials derived for cell and molecule delivery in regenerative medicine. *J. Control. Release* **2011**, *155*, 193–199. [CrossRef]
92. Khan, F.; Ahmad, S.R. Polysaccharides and their derivatives for versatile tissue engineering application. *Macromol. Biosci.* **2013**, *13*, 395–421. [CrossRef]
93. Logesh, A.; Thillaimaharani, K.; Sharmila, K.; Kalaiselvam, M.; Raffi, S. Production of chitosan from endolichenic fungi isolated from mangrove environment and its antagonistic activity. *Asian Pac. J. Trop. Biomed.* **2012**, *2*, 140–143. [CrossRef]
94. Khor, E.; Lim, L.Y. Implantable applications of chitin and chitosan. *Biomaterials* **2003**, *24*, 2339–2349. [CrossRef]
95. Rinaudo, M. Main properties and current applications of some polysaccharides as biomaterials. *Polym. Int.* **2008**, *57*, 397–430. [CrossRef]
96. Chao, Z.; Ri-Fu, Y.; Tai-Qiu, Q. Ultrasound-enhanced subcritical water extraction of polysaccharides from lycium barbarum l. *Sep. Purif. Technol.* **2013**, *120*, 141–147. [CrossRef]
97. Song, T.; Pranovich, A.; Holmbom, B. Separation of polymeric galactoglucomannans from hot-water extract of spruce wood. *Bioresour. Technol.* **2013**, *130*, 198–203. [CrossRef]
98. Cheng, H.; Feng, S.; Jia, X.; Li, Q.; Zhou, Y.; Ding, C. Structural characterization and antioxidant activities of polysaccharides extracted from epimedium acuminatum. *Carbohydr. Polym.* **2013**, *92*, 63–68. [CrossRef]
99. Chen, S.; Chen, H.; Tian, J.; Wang, J.; Wang, Y.; Xing, L. Enzymolysis-ultrasonic assisted extraction, chemical characteristics and bioactivities of polysaccharides from corn silk. *Carbohydr. Polym.* **2014**, *101*, 332–341. [CrossRef]

100. Abe, M.; Fukaya, Y.; Ohno, H. Extraction of polysaccharides from bran with phosphonate or phosphinate-derived ionic liquids under short mixing time and low temperature. *Green Chem.* **2010**, *12*, 1274–1280. [CrossRef]
101. Do Nascimento, D.M.; Dias, A.F.; De Araújo Junior, C.P.; De Freitas Rosa, M.; Morais, J.P.S.; De Figueirêdo, M.C.B. A comprehensive approach for obtaining cellulose nanocrystal from coconut fiber. Part II: Environmental assessment of technological pathways. *Ind. Crops Prod.* **2016**, *93*, 58–65. [CrossRef]
102. Matavire, T.O. Extraction and Modification of Hemicellulose from Wheat Bran to Produce Entrapment Materials for the Controlled Release of Chemicals and Bioactive Substances. Master's Thesis, Stellenbosch University, Stellenbosch, South Africa, March 2018.
103. Boukroufa, M.; Boutekedjiret, C.; Petigny, L.; Rakotomanomana, N.; Chemat, F. Bio-refinery of orange peels waste: A new concept based on integrated green and solvent free extraction processes using ultrasound and microwave techniques to obtain essential oil, polyphenols and pectin. *Ultrason. Sonochem.* **2015**, *24*, 72–79. [CrossRef]
104. Maheshwari, G.; Sowrirajan, S.; Joseph, B. Extraction and isolation of β-glucan from grain sources—A review. *J. Food Sci.* **2017**, *82*, 1535–1545. [CrossRef]
105. Amid, B.T.; Mirhosseini, H. Optimisation of aqueous extraction of gum from durian (durio zibethinus) seed: A potential, low cost source of hydrocolloid. *Food Chem.* **2012**, *132*, 1258–1268. [CrossRef]
106. Yanuriati, A.; Marseno, D.W.; Harmayani, E. Characteristics of glucomannan isolated from fresh tuber of porang (amorphophallus muelleri blume). *Carbohydr. Polym.* **2017**, *156*, 56–63. [CrossRef]
107. Zhang, Y.; Zhang, Y.; Taha, A.A.; Ying, Y.; Li, X.; Chen, X.; Ma, C. Subcritical water extraction of bioactive components from ginseng roots (panax ginseng ca mey). *Ind. Crops Prod.* **2018**, *117*, 118–127. [CrossRef]
108. Guo, Z.; Lou, Y.; Kong, M.; Luo, Q.; Liu, Z.; Wu, J. A systematic review of phytochemistry, pharmacology and pharmacokinetics on astragali radix: Implications for astragali radix as a personalized medicine. *Int. J. Mol. Sci.* **2019**, *20*, 1463. [CrossRef]
109. Zhu, W.; Xue, X.; Zhang, Z. Ultrasonic-assisted extraction, structure and antitumor activity of polysaccharide from polygonum multiflorum. *Int. J. Biol. Macromol.* **2016**, *91*, 132–142. [CrossRef]
110. Lv, L.; Cheng, Y.; Zheng, T.; Li, X.; Zhai, R. Purification, antioxidant activity and antiglycation of polysaccharides from polygonum multiflorum thunb. *Carbohydr. Polym.* **2014**, *99*, 765–773. [CrossRef]
111. Alves, A.; Caridade, S.G.; Mano, J.F.; Sousa, R.A.; Reis, R.L. Extraction and physico-chemical characterization of a versatile biodegradable polysaccharide obtained from green algae. *Carbohydr. Res.* **2010**, *345*, 2194–2200. [CrossRef]
112. Xu, S.-Y.; Huang, X.; Cheong, K.-L. Recent advances in marine algae polysaccharides: Isolation, structure, and activities. *Mar. Drugs* **2017**, *15*, 388. [CrossRef]
113. Yu, X.; Zhou, C.; Yang, H.; Huang, X.; Ma, H.; Qin, X.; Hu, J. Effect of ultrasonic treatment on the degradation and inhibition cancer cell lines of polysaccharides from porphyra yezoensis. *Carbohydr. Polym.* **2015**, *117*, 650–656. [CrossRef]
114. Tsubaki, S.; Oono, K.; Hiraoka, M.; Onda, A.; Mitani, T. Microwave-assisted hydrothermal extraction of sulfated polysaccharides from ulva spp. and monostroma latissimum. *Food Chem.* **2016**, *210*, 311–316. [CrossRef]
115. Lee, W.-W.; Ahn, G.; Wijesinghe, W.; Yang, X.; Ko, C.-I.; Kang, M.-C.; Lee, B.-J.; Jeon, Y.-J. Enzyme-assisted extraction of ecklonia cava fermented with lactobacillus brevis and isolation of an anti-inflammatory polysaccharide. *Algae* **2011**, *26*, 343–350. [CrossRef]
116. Rodriguez-Jasso, R.M.; Mussatto, S.I.; Pastrana, L.; Aguilar, C.N.; Teixeira, J.A. Microwave-assisted extraction of sulfated polysaccharides (fucoidan) from brown seaweed. *Carbohydr. Polym.* **2011**, *86*, 1137–1144. [CrossRef]
117. Murray, P.G.; Grassick, A.; Laffey, C.D.; Cuffe, M.M.; Higgins, T.; Savage, A.V.; Planas, A.; Tuohy, M.G. Isolation and characterization of a thermostable endo-β-glucanase active on 1, 3-1, 4-β-d-glucans from the aerobic fungus talaromyces emersonii cbs 814.70. *Enzym. Microb. Technol.* **2001**, *29*, 90–98. [CrossRef]
118. Nie, S.; Cui, S.W.; Xie, M.; Phillips, A.O.; Phillips, G.O. Bioactive polysaccharides from cordyceps sinensis: Isolation, structure features and bioactivities. *Bioact. Carbohydr. Diet. Fibre* **2013**, *1*, 38–52. [CrossRef]
119. Klein, S. *Polysaccharides in Oral Drug Delivery: Recent Applications and Future Perspectives*; ACS Symposium Series: Washington, DC, USA, 2009; pp. 13–30.

120. Olano-Martin, E.; Gibson, G.R.; Rastall, R. Comparison of the in vitro bifidogenic properties of pectins and pectic-oligosaccharides. *J. Appl. Microbiol.* **2002**, *93*, 505–511. [CrossRef]
121. Witvrouw, M.; De Clercq, E. Sulfated polysaccharides extracted from sea algae as potential antiviral drugs. *Gen. Pharmacol. Vasc. Syst.* **1997**, *29*, 497–511. [CrossRef]
122. Nangia-Makker, P.; Hogan, V.; Honjo, Y.; Baccarini, S.; Tait, L.; Bresalier, R.; Raz, A. Inhibition of human cancer cell growth and metastasis in nude mice by oral intake of modified citrus pectin. *J.Natl. Cancer Inst.* **2002**, *94*, 1854–1862. [CrossRef]
123. Lattimer, J.M.; Haub, M.D. Effects of dietary fiber and its components on metabolic health. *Nutrients* **2010**, *2*, 1266–1289. [CrossRef]
124. Georgiev, Y.; Ognyanov, M.; Yanakieva, I.; Kussovski, V.; Kratchanova, M. Isolation, characterization and modification of citrus pectins. *J. BioSci. Biotechnol.* **2012**, *1*, 223–233.
125. Cheng, H.; Li, S.; Fan, Y.; Gao, X.; Hao, M.; Wang, J.; Zhang, X.; Tai, G.; Zhou, Y. Comparative studies of the antiproliferative effects of ginseng polysaccharides on ht-29 human colon cancer cells. *Med. Oncol.* **2011**, *28*, 175–181. [CrossRef]
126. Jeon, C.; Kang, S.; Park, S.; Lim, K.; Hwang, K.W.; Min, H. T cell stimulatory effects of korean red ginseng through modulation of myeloid-derived suppressor cells. *J. Ginseng Res.* **2011**, *35*, 462. [CrossRef]
127. Kim, M.-H.; Byon, Y.-Y.; Ko, E.-J.; Song, J.-Y.; Yun, Y.-S.; Shin, T.; Joo, H.-G. Immunomodulatory activity of ginsan, a polysaccharide of panax ginseng, on dendritic cells. *Korean J. Physiol. Pharmacol.* **2009**, *13*, 169–173. [CrossRef]
128. Kim, K.-H.; Lee, Y.-S.; Jung, I.-S.; Park, S.-Y.; Chung, H.-Y.; Lee, I.-R.; Yun, Y.-S. Acidic polysaccharide from panax ginseng, ginsan, induces th1 cell and macrophage cytokines and generates lak cells in synergy with ril-2. *Planta Medica* **1998**, *64*, 110–115. [CrossRef]
129. Lee, Y.; Chung, I.; Lee, I.; Kim, K.; Hong, W.; Yun, Y. Activation of multiple effector pathways of immune system by the antineoplastic immunostimulator acidic polysaccharide ginsan isolated from panax ginseng. *Anticancer Res.* **1997**, *17*, 323–331.
130. Yoo, D.-G.; Kim, M.-C.; Park, M.-K.; Park, K.-M.; Quan, F.-S.; Song, J.-M.; Wee, J.J.; Wang, B.-Z.; Cho, Y.-K.; Compans, R.W. Protective effect of ginseng polysaccharides on influenza viral infection. *PLoS ONE* **2012**, *7*, e33678. [CrossRef]
131. Sun, Y. Structure and biological activities of the polysaccharides from the leaves, roots and fruits of panax ginseng ca meyer: An overview. *Carbohydr. Polym.* **2011**, *85*, 490–499. [CrossRef]
132. Lemmon, H.R.; Sham, J.; Chau, L.A.; Madrenas, J. High molecular weight polysaccharides are key immunomodulators in north american ginseng extracts: Characterization of the ginseng genetic signature in primary human immune cells. *J. Ethnopharmacol.* **2012**, *142*, 1–13. [CrossRef]
133. Rigaud, D.; Ryttig, K.; Angel, L.; Apfelbaum, M. Overweight treated with energy restriction and a dietary fibre supplement: A 6-month randomized, double-blind, placebo-controlled trial. *Int. J. Obes.* **1990**, *14*, 763–769.
134. Birketvedt, G.; Aaseth, J.; Florholmen, J.; Ryttig, K. Long-term effect of fibre supplement and reduced energy intake on body weight and blood lipids in overweight subjects. *Acta Medica (Hradec Kralove)* **2000**, *43*, 129–132.
135. Pittler, M.H.; Ernst, E. Guar gum for body weight reduction: Meta-analysis of randomized trials. *Am. J. Med.* **2001**, *110*, 724–730. [CrossRef]
136. Mueller-Cunningham, W.M.; Quintana, R.; Kasim-Karakas, S.E. An ad libitum, very low-fat diet results in weight loss and changes in nutrient intakes in postmenopausal women. *J. Am. Diet. Assoc.* **2003**, *103*, 1600–1606. [CrossRef]
137. Hays, N.P.; Starling, R.D.; Liu, X.; Sullivan, D.H.; Trappe, T.A.; Fluckey, J.D.; Evans, W.J. Effects of an ad libitum low-fat, high-carbohydrate diet on body weight, body composition, and fat distribution in older men and women: A randomized controlled trial. *Arch. Int. Med.* **2004**, *164*, 210–217. [CrossRef]
138. Howarth, N.C.; Saltzman, E.; Roberts, S.B. Dietary fiber and weight regulation. *Nutr. Rev.* **2001**, *59*, 129–139. [CrossRef]
139. Birketvedt, G.S.; Shimshi, M.; Thom, E.; Florholmen, J. Experiences with three different fiber supplements in weight reduction. *Med. Sci. Monit.* **2005**, *11*, PI5–PI8.
140. Lyly, M.; Liukkonen, K.-H.; Salmenkallio-Marttila, M.; Karhunen, L.; Poutanen, K.; Lähteenmäki, L. Fibre in beverages can enhance perceived satiety. *Eur. J. Nutr.* **2009**, *48*, 251–258. [CrossRef]

141. Lyly, M.; Ohls, N.; Lähteenmäki, L.; Salmenkallio-Marttila, M.; Liukkonen, K.-H.; Karhunen, L.; Poutanen, K. The effect of fibre amount, energy level and viscosity of beverages containing oat fibre supplement on perceived satiety. *Food Nutr. Res.* **2010**, *54*, 2149. [CrossRef]
142. Vitaglione, P.; Lumaga, R.B.; Montagnese, C.; Messia, M.C.; Marconi, E.; Scalfi, L. Satiating effect of a barley beta-glucan–enriched snack. *J. Am. Coll. Nutr.* **2010**, *29*, 113–121. [CrossRef]
143. Vitaglione, P.; Lumaga, R.B.; Stanzione, A.; Scalfi, L.; Fogliano, V. B-glucan-enriched bread reduces energy intake and modifies plasma ghrelin and peptide yy concentrations in the short term. *Appetite* **2009**, *53*, 338–344. [CrossRef]
144. Peters, H.P.; Boers, H.M.; Haddeman, E.; Melnikov, S.M.; Qvyjt, F. No effect of added β-glucan or of fructooligosaccharide on appetite or energy intake. *Am. J. Clin. Nutr.* **2008**, *89*, 58–63. [CrossRef]
145. Gallaher, D.D.; Gallaher, C.M.; Mahrt, G.J.; Carr, T.P.; Hollingshead, C.H.; Hesslink, R., Jr.; Wise, J. A glucomannan and chitosan fiber supplement decreases plasma cholesterol and increases cholesterol excretion in overweight normocholesterolemic humans. *J. Am. Col. Nutr.* **2002**, *21*, 428–433. [CrossRef]
146. Chen, H.-L.; Sheu, W.H.-H.; Tai, T.-S.; Liaw, Y.-P.; Chen, Y.-C. Konjac supplement alleviated hypercholesterolemia and hyperglycemia in type 2 diabetic subjects—A randomized double-blind trial. *J. Am. Col. Nutr.* **2003**, *22*, 36–42. [CrossRef]
147. Tappy, L.; Gügolz, E.; Würsch, P. Effects of breakfast cereals containing various amounts of β-glucan fibers on plasma glucose and insulin responses in niddm subjects. *Diabetes Care* **1996**, *19*, 831–834. [CrossRef]
148. Tapola, N.; Karvonen, H.; Niskanen, L.; Mikola, M.; Sarkkinen, E. Glycemic responses of oat bran products in type 2 diabetic patients. *Nutr. Metab. Cardiovasc. Dis.* **2005**, *15*, 255–261. [CrossRef]
149. Mäkeläinen, H.; Anttila, H.; Sihvonen, J.; Hietanen, R.; Tahvonen, R.; Salminen, E.; Mikola, M.; Sontag-Strohm, T. The effect of β-glucan on the glycemic and insulin index. *Eur. J. Clin. Nutr.* **2007**, *61*, 779. [CrossRef]
150. Maki, K.; Galant, R.; Samuel, P.; Tesser, J.; Witchger, M.; Ribaya-Mercado, J.; Blumberg, J.; Geohas, J. Effects of consuming foods containing oat β-glucan on blood pressure, carbohydrate metabolism and biomarkers of oxidative stress in men and women with elevated blood pressure. *Eur. J. Clin. Nutr.* **2007**, *61*, 786. [CrossRef]
151. Hallfrisch, J.; Scholfield, D.J.; Behall, K.M. Diets containing soluble oat extracts improve glucose and insulin responses of moderately hypercholesterolemic men and women. *Am. J. Clin. Nutr.* **1995**, *61*, 379–384. [CrossRef]
152. Nazare, J.A.; Normand, S.; Oste Triantafyllou, A.; Brac De La Perrière, A.; Desage, M.; Laville, M. Modulation of the postprandial phase by β-glucan in overweight subjects: Effects on glucose and insulin kinetics. *Mol. Nutr. Food Res.* **2009**, *53*, 361–369. [CrossRef]
153. Battilana, P.; Ornstein, K.; Minehira, K.; Schwarz, J.; Acheson, K.; Schneiter, P.; Burri, J.; Jequier, E.; Tappy, L. Mechanisms of action of β-glucan in postprandial glucose metabolism in healthy men. *Eur. J. Clin. Nutr.* **2001**, *55*, 327. [CrossRef]
154. Chen, H.-L.; Cheng, H.-C.; Liu, Y.-J.; Liu, S.-Y.; Wu, W.-T. Konjac acts as a natural laxative by increasing stool bulk and improving colonic ecology in healthy adults. *Nutrition* **2006**, *22*, 1112–1119. [CrossRef]
155. Wang, L.; Yu, X.; Yang, X.; Li, Y.; Yao, Y.; Lui, F.M.K.; Ren, G. Structural and anti-inflammatory characterization of a novel neutral polysaccharide from north american ginseng (panax quinquefolius). *Int. J. Biol. Macromol.* **2015**, *74*, 12–17. [CrossRef]
156. Zhao, H.; Zhang, W.; Xiao, C.; Lu, C.; Xu, S.; He, X.; Li, X.; Chen, S.; Yang, D.; Chan, A. Effect of ginseng polysaccharide on tnf-alpha and ifn-gamma produced by enteric mucosal lymphocytes in collagen induced arthritic rats. *J. Med. Plant Res.* **2011**, *5*, 1536–1542.
157. Pillai, R.; Lacy, P. Inhibition of neutrophil respiratory burst and degranulation responses by cvt-e002, the main active ingredient in cold-fx. *Allergy Asthma Clin. Immunol.* **2011**, *7*, A31. [CrossRef]
158. Biondo, P.D.; Goruk, S.; Ruth, M.R.; O'connell, E.; Field, C.J. Effect of cvt-e002™(cold-fx®) versus a ginsenoside extract on systemic and gut-associated immune function. *Int. Immunopharmacol.* **2008**, *8*, 1134–1142. [CrossRef]
159. Wang, M.; Guilbert, L.J.; Li, J.; Wu, Y.; Pang, P.; Basu, T.K.; Shan, J.J. A proprietary extract from north american ginseng (panax quinquefolium) enhances il-2 and ifn-γ productions in murine spleen cells induced by con-a. *Int. Immunopharmacol.* **2004**, *4*, 311–315. [CrossRef]

160. Wang, M.; Guilbert, L.J.; Ling, L.; Li, J.; Wu, Y.; Xu, S.; Pang, P.; Shan, J.J. Immunomodulating activity of cvt-e002, a proprietary extract from north american ginseng (panax quinquefolium). *J. Pharm. Pharmacol.* **2001**, *53*, 1515–1523. [CrossRef]
161. Kim, K.-S.; Seo, E.-K.; Lee, Y.-C.; Lee, T.-K.; Cho, Y.-W.; Ezaki, O.; Kim, C.-H. Effect of dietary platycodon grandiflorum on the improvement of insulin resistance in obese zucker rats. *J. Nutr. Biochem.* **2000**, *11*, 420–424. [CrossRef]
162. Han, S.B.; Park, S.H.; Lee, K.H.; Lee, C.W.; Lee, S.H.; Kim, H.C.; Kim, Y.S.; Lee, H.S.; Kim, H.M. Polysaccharide isolated from the radix of platycodon grandiflorum selectively activates b cells and macrophages but not t cells. *Int. Immunopharmacol.* **2001**, *1*, 1969–1978. [CrossRef]
163. Li, R.; Qiu, S.; Chen, H.; Wang, L. Immunomodulatory effects of astragalus polysaccharide in diabetic mice. *J. Chin. Integr. Med.* **2008**, *6*, 166–170. [CrossRef]
164. Chen, W.; Li, Y.-M.; Yu, M.-H. Astragalus polysaccharides: An effective treatment for diabetes prevention in nod mice. *Exp. Clin. Endocrinol. Diabetes* **2008**, *116*, 468–474. [CrossRef]
165. Chen, W.; Yu, M.; Li, Y. Effects of astragalus polysaccharides on ultrastructure and oxidation/apoptosis related cytokines' gene expression of non-obese diabetic mice's islets. Available online: https://europepmc.org/abstract/cba/636484 (accessed on 15 June 2019).
166. Xue, C.; Yu, G.; Hirata, T.; Terao, J.; Lin, H. Antioxidative activities of several marine polysaccharides evaluated in a phosphatidylcholine-liposomal suspension and organic solvents. *Biosci. Biotechnol. Biochem.* **1998**, *62*, 206–209. [CrossRef]
167. Oliveira, J.T.; Reis, R. Polysaccharide-based materials for cartilage tissue engineering applications. *J. Tissue Eng. Regen. Med.* **2011**, *5*, 421–436. [CrossRef]
168. Wan, A.C.; Tai, B.C. Chitin—a promising biomaterial for tissue engineering and stem cell technologies. *Biotechnol. Adv.* **2013**, *31*, 1776–1785. [CrossRef]
169. Croisier, F.; Jérôme, C. Chitosan-based biomaterials for tissue engineering. *Eur. Polymer J.* **2013**, *49*, 780–792. [CrossRef]
170. Lu, H.F.; Lim, S.-X.; Leong, M.F.; Narayanan, K.; Toh, R.P.; Gao, S.; Wan, A.C. Efficient neuronal differentiation and maturation of human pluripotent stem cells encapsulated in 3d microfibrous scaffolds. *Biomaterials* **2012**, *33*, 9179–9187. [CrossRef]
171. Venkatesan, J.; Kim, S.-K. Chitosan composites for bone tissue engineering—An overview. *Mar. Drugs* **2010**, *8*, 2252–2266. [CrossRef]
172. Barud, H.d.S.; De Araújo Júnior, A.M.; Saska, S.; Mestieri, L.B.; Campos, J.A.D.B.; De Freitas, R.M.; Ferreira, N.U.; Nascimento, A.P.; Miguel, F.G.; Vaz, M.M.d.O.L.L. Antimicrobial brazilian propolis (epp-af) containing biocellulose membranes as promising biomaterial for skin wound healing. *Evid.-Based Complement. Altern. Med.* **2013**, *2013*. [CrossRef]
173. Hrynyk, M.; Martins-Green, M.; Barron, A.E.; Neufeld, R.J. Alginate-peg sponge architecture and role in the design of insulin release dressings. *Biomacromolecules* **2012**, *13*, 1478–1485. [CrossRef]
174. Anilkumar, T.; Muhamed, J.; Jose, A.; Jyothi, A.; Mohanan, P.; Krishnan, L.K. Advantages of hyaluronic acid as a component of fibrin sheet for care of acute wound. *Biologicals* **2011**, *39*, 81–88. [CrossRef]
175. Liakos, I.; Rizzello, L.; Scurr, D.J.; Pompa, P.P.; Bayer, I.S.; Athanassiou, A. All-natural composite wound dressing films of essential oils encapsulated in sodium alginate with antimicrobial properties. *Int. J. Pharm.* **2014**, *463*, 137–145. [CrossRef]
176. Gu, Z.; Xie, H.; Huang, C.; Li, L.; Yu, X. Preparation of chitosan/silk fibroin blending membrane fixed with alginate dialdehyde for wound dressing. *Int. J. Biol. Macromol.* **2013**, *58*, 121–126. [CrossRef]
177. Singh, R.; Singh, D. Radiation synthesis of pvp/alginate hydrogel containing nanosilver as wound dressing. *J. Mate. Sci. Mater. Med.* **2012**, *23*, 2649–2658. [CrossRef]
178. Anisha, B.; Biswas, R.; Chennazhi, K.; Jayakumar, R. Chitosan–hyaluronic acid/nano silver composite sponges for drug resistant bacteria infected diabetic wounds. *Int. J. Biol. Macromol.* **2013**, *62*, 310–320. [CrossRef]
179. Mizrahy, S.; Peer, D. Polysaccharides as building blocks for nanotherapeutics. *Chem. Soc. Rev.* **2012**, *41*, 2623–2640. [CrossRef]
180. Alvarez-Lorenzo, C.; Blanco-Fernandez, B.; Puga, A.M.; Concheiro, A. Crosslinked ionic polysaccharides for stimuli-sensitive drug delivery. *Adv. Drug Deliv. Rev.* **2013**, *65*, 1148–1171. [CrossRef]
181. Reddy, K.; Krishna Mohan, G.; Satla, S.; Gaikwad, S. Natural polysaccharides: Versatile excipients for controlled drug delivery systems. *Asian J. Pharm. Sci.* **2011**, *6*, 275–286.

182. Jain, A.K.; Söderlind, E.; Viridén, A.; Schug, B.; Abrahamsson, B.; Knopke, C.; Tajarobi, F.; Blume, H.; Anschütz, M.; Welinder, A. The influence of hydroxypropyl methylcellulose (hpmc) molecular weight, concentration and effect of food on in vivo erosion behavior of hpmc matrix tablets. *J. Control. Release* **2014**, *187*, 50–58. [CrossRef]
183. Plackett, D.V.; Letchford, K.; Jackson, J.K.; Burt, H.M. A review of nanocellulose as a novel vehicle for drug delivery. *Nord. Pulp. Pap. Res. J.* **2014**, *29*, 105–118. [CrossRef]
184. Kolakovic, R.; Peltonen, L.; Laukkanen, A.; Hirvonen, J.; Laaksonen, T. Nanofibrillar cellulose films for controlled drug delivery. *Eur. J. Pharm. Biopharm.* **2012**, *82*, 308–315. [CrossRef]
185. Shelke, N.B.; James, R.; Laurencin, C.T.; Kumbar, S.G. Polysaccharide biomaterials for drug delivery and regenerative engineering. *Polym. Adv. Technol.* **2014**, *25*, 448–460. [CrossRef]
186. Ji, A.; Su, D.; Che, O.; Li, W.; Sun, L.; Zhang, Z.; Yang, B.; Xu, F. Functional gene silencing mediated by chitosan/sirna nanocomplexes. *Nanotechnology* **2009**, *20*, 405103. [CrossRef]
187. Chen, M.-C.; Huang, S.-F.; Lai, K.-Y.; Ling, M.-H. Fully embeddable chitosan microneedles as a sustained release depot for intradermal vaccination. *Biomaterials* **2013**, *34*, 3077–3086. [CrossRef]

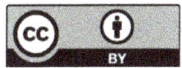

© 2019 by the authors. Licensee MDPI, Basel, Switzerland. This article is an open access article distributed under the terms and conditions of the Creative Commons Attribution (CC BY) license (http://creativecommons.org/licenses/by/4.0/).

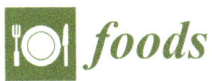

Article

Characterization of Fulvic Acid Beverages by Mineral Profile and Antioxidant Capacity

Monika Swat, Iga Rybicka * and Anna Gliszczyńska-Świgło

Institute of Quality Science, Poznań University of Economics and Business, al. Niepodległości 10, 61-875 Poznań, Poland; monika.swat@wp.pl (M.S.); anna.gliszczynska-swiglo@ue.poznan.pl (A.G.-Ś.)
* Correspondence: iga.rybicka@ue.poznan.pl; Tel.: +48-61-8-56-93-68

Received: 1 October 2019; Accepted: 18 November 2019; Published: 22 November 2019

Abstract: The main purpose of the study was to investigate the quality of fulvic acid-based food products. The concentrations of Ca, K, Mg, Na, Cu, Fe, Mn, and Zn, and antioxidant capacities of fulvic acid concentrates and ready-to drink beverages available on the global market were determined. The concentrations of minerals were determined using microwave plasma-atomic emission spectrometry. Antioxidant capacity was expressed as total polyphenol (TP) and flavonoid (TF) contents, the trolox equivalent antioxidant capacity (TEAC) and ferric reducing ability of plasma (FRAP) values. The daily portion of eight out of 14 products realized 45–135% of recommended daily allowance (RDA) for Fe. One of ready-to-drink beverages was also a good source of Mg (about 40% of RDA), and another one of Mn (about 70% of RDA). The concentrations of TP and TF in ready-to-drink beverages varied from 6.5 to 187 µg/mL, whereas in concentrates, from 5886 to 19,844 µg/mL. Dietary supplements or food products with fulvic acids may be a good source of antioxidant polyphenolic compounds and some minerals.

Keywords: antioxidant capacity; fulvic acids; functional beverage; iron; mineral

1. Introduction

Fulvic acids are natural, water-soluble polymers, which are the ingredients of humic substances defined as "a series of high molecular weight substances, yellow to black in colour, formed as a result of secondary synthesis reactions" [1,2]. They are complex substances without standard chemical formulae, which are present in soil and plants in trace amounts [3,4]. They are formed during the decomposition of decaying plants by microorganisms and they play essential functions in plants; e.g., are responsible for the absorption of nutrients and trace substances. Naturally, fulvic acids contain minerals (more than 70), amino acids, sugars, peptides, nucleic acids, phytochemical compounds, vitamins, and fragments of plant DNA [3]. Most of them occur in ionic form. This means that fulvic acids conduct electricity excellently and improve the absorption of other compounds interacting with them. Moreover, because of ionic minerals, fulvic acids help to increase their bioavailability in plants [5]. Fulvic acids are also chemically reactive because of the presence of many carboxyl and hydroxyl groups [3]. Due to their low molecular weights, they can transport minerals to plant cells in the root, stem, and leaves [6]. They also participate in the carbon cycle, because they are constantly recycled among plants, soil, and water [7].

The results of the studies on fulvic acid properties conducted with plants and plant cells indicate the positive effect of these substances on animal organisms. Kishor et al. [8] suggested that humic substances, consisting of 60–80% fulvic acids, have anticarcinogenic properties. They may be beneficial in cancer therapy due to their heavy metal chelating properties, binding of proteins delivering anticancer drugs, and inhibition of cancer cell proliferation [9–11]. Fulvic acids are also good free radical scavengers. They may scavenge superoxide ($O_2^{\bullet-}$), hypochlorous acid (HOCl), hydrogen peroxide (H_2O_2), hydroxyl radicals ($^{\bullet}OH$), peroxynitrite ($ONOO^-$), and singlet oxygen ($^1O_2$) [12,13].

Carrasco-Gallardo et al. [14] analysed the results of various clinical studies confirming the effect of fulvic acid consumption on the reduction the symptoms of Alzheimer's disease. Their studies suggested that fulvic acids can be potentially used to prevent this brain disorder, mainly due to their antioxidant properties. Many studies have provided the evidence that accumulation of oxidative stress products in brain tissue is closely associated with the development of Alzheimer's disease and antioxidant therapies are one of the promising therapeutic strategies for this disease [15]. It is thought that fulvic acids improve the absorption of iron, making it more bioavailable to bone marrow stem cells for formation of blood [16]. Van Rensburg [17] and Winkler and Gosh [18], in their reviews, listed few studies conducted with both animals and humans over several years on the safety of fulvic acids and their effects on human diseases. In these studies, fulvic acids were applied orally and topically. The studies were carried out using various doses and forms of fulvic acids, and with various durations. The results obtained suggested that fulvic acids are safe for humans; nevertheless, further studies to ensure their safety are still required. The recommended daily dose of fulvic acids for people is not established. Therefore, it is important to determine the optimal dosage of fulvic acids for different age groups to prevent them from overdosing.

Fulvic acids have been primarily used as products supporting the growth of plants and maintaining soil moisture. Currently, the food market has also become interested in them. Considering all the properties of fulvic acids, there is a potential to use them as a new, natural, and valuable food additives or supplements [19]. Due to the structure of fulvic acids and their chelating properties they can help to transport some nutrients, mainly minerals, to cells and remove deeply embedded toxins from the body [16]. Substances constituted up to 20% by fulvic acids have been used in traditional Indian medicine, "Ayurveda," for medicinal purposes for about 3000 years [20,21]. Fulvic acids intended for human consumption are currently available in concentrated form, ready-to-drink beverages and pills, but their variety on the food market is still small. These products are a potential source of minerals and antioxidant compounds. As far as is known, there are no data characterizing fulvic acid products in the aspects of either mineral profile or antioxidant capacity. Therefore, the objective of this study was to determine the content of selected macroelements and microelements and the antioxidant properties of fulvic acid beverages available on the global market.

2. Materials and Methods

2.1. Materials

The products were bought in 2015 in on-line stores. The analyses were performed for most of fulvic acid beverages available at that time on the global market. The experiments were repeated for the same products bought in 2018. The total of 14 beverages were included in the study—6 concentrates and 8 ready-to-drink beverages. According to the label description, fulvic acids in concentrated form originated from the Great Salt Lake in Utah (North America) and England. Fulvic acids in ready-to-drink beverages were obtained mainly from an aquatic source and/or soils of North America and South Africa.

2.2. Sample Preparation

For determination of minerals, the products tested were diluted with demineralized water (Hydrolab System, Wiślina, Poland). The dilution of ready-to-drink beverages was 10-fold and that of concentrates was 100-fold.

For determination of total phenolics (TP), total flavonoids (TF), and the antioxidant capacities, the products were centrifuged at $14{,}000\times g$ for 5 min (MiniSpin plus centrifuge, Eppendorf, Hamburg, Germany) and diluted with demineralized water if necessary.

2.3. Determination of Minerals

The concentrations of Ca, K, Mg, Na, Cu, Fe, Mn, and Zn were determined using microwave plasma-atomic emission spectrometry (Agilent MP-AES 4210) (Agilent Technologies, Melbourne, Australia) according to the method described in detail by Ozbek and Akman [22]. The analytical wavelengths and standard curves for minerals we analysed were: 616.217 nm and 0–50 µg/mL for Ca, 404.414 nm and 0–500 µg/mL for K, 383.829 nm and 0–20 µg/mL for Mg, 330.237 nm and 0–100 µg/mL for Na, 324.754 nm and 0–0.1 µg/mL for Cu, 371.993 nm and 0–10 µg/mL plus 259.940 nm and 10–100 µg/mL for Fe, 403.076 nm and 0–10 µg/mL for Mn, and 213.857 nm and 0–5 µg/mL for Zn. For each determination, at least two calibration curves were prepared, each adjusted to the expected concentration in the sample being analysed. Six determinations were performed for each sample.

2.4. Determination of Total Phenolics

The concentration of TP was determined according to Singleton and Rossi [23]. The method was adapted to 48-well microplates. In brief, 0.01 mL of each sample was mixed with 0.05 mL of the Folin–Ciocalteu reagent. After 3 min, 0.15 mL of 20% sodium carbonate and 0.79 mL of demineralized water were added and the solution was mixed. The plate was incubated for 2 h in the dark at room temperature. The absorbance was measured at 765 nm. At least six determinations were performed for each sample. The total content of phenolics was expressed in µg of gallic acid per millilitre of product.

2.5. Determination of Total Flavonoids

The concentration of TF was determined according to Karadeniz et al. [24]. The method was adapted to 48-well microplate and (±)-catechin was used as the standard. In brief, 0.10 mL of each sample was mixed with 0.50 mL of demineralized water and 0.03 mL of 5% $NaNO_2$. After 5 min, 0.06 mL of 10% $AlCl_3$ and 0.2 mL of 1M NaOH were added. After 5 min, 0.11 mL of demineralized water was added and the solution was mixed. The absorbance was measured at 510 nm and corrected for the absorbance of product sample and the absorbance of blank sample. At least six determinations were performed for each sample. The total content of flavonoids was expressed in µg of (±)-catechin per millilitre of the product.

2.6. Determination of the Antioxidant Capacity

The antioxidant capacity of fulvic acid products was determined using the TEAC method with $ABTS^{\bullet+}$ radical cation as described by Re et al. [25]. Moreover, the FRAP assay was carried out by the method of Benzie and Strain [26] with modifications previously described [27].

Briefly, the $ABTS^{\bullet+}$ radical cation was generated by reaction of 0.0077 g of ABTS dissolved in 1.8 mL of demineralized water with 0.2 mL of 0.0066 g/mL potassium persulphate. The reaction mixture was incubated in the dark at room temperature for 16 h [25]. The $ABTS^{\bullet+}$ radical cation working solution was obtained by dilution with methanol to an absorbance about 0.80 at 734 nm. The absorbance was measured 6 min after mixing 0.008 mL of sample with 0.792 mL of the $ABTS^{\bullet+}$ radical cation working solution. The TEAC value was calculated as the ratio of the linear regression coefficient of the calibration curve for five dilutions of the sample and the linear regression coefficient of the trolox standard curve. Three independent determinations were performed for each sample. The activity of each product was expressed as the TEAC value (in µmol of trolox/mL of product).

The FRAP assay is based on the reduction of a ferric 2,4,6-tripyridyl-s-triazine complex (Fe^{3+}-TPTZ) to the ferrous form (Fe^{2+}-TPTZ) in the presence of antioxidant. A volume of 0.008 mL of sample was added to 0.792 mL of the 10 mM ferric-TPTZ reagent and the increase in absorbance at 593 nm was measured after 8 min. The FRAP value was calculated as the ratio of the linear regression coefficient of the calibration curve for five dilutions of the sample and the linear regression coefficient of the $FeSO_4 \times 7 H_2O$ standard curve [27]. Three independent determinations were performed for each sample. Activity of each product was expressed as the FRAP value (µmol of Fe^{2+}/mL).

2.7. Statistical Analysis

Statistical analyses were carried out using Statistica 12.0 software (2013; StatSoft, Inc., Tulsa, OK, USA). All data were submitted to one-way analysis of variance (ANOVA). The significances of differences between mean values obtained for products were determined by the least significant differences tests at $\alpha = 0.05$. The comparison of data in Tables 1–3 is category-separated for clarity of data presentation.

Table 1. The content of macroelements in fulvic acid beverages.

Category of Product		Ca		K		Mg		Na	
		I [1]	II [1]	I	II	I	II	I	II
CONCENTRATE									
1	mg/mL	0.99 ± 0.01 [c]	2.09 ± 0.11 [b]	24.0 ± 0.2 [a]	24.1 ± 0.6 [a]	1.09 ± 0.02 [c]	1.05 ± 0.02 [c]	3.76 ± 0.14 [a]	3.62 ± 0.15 [a,b]
	mg/daily portion [2]	1.4	3.0	34	35	1.6	1.5	5.5	5.3
	%RDA/AI [3]	0.1%	0.3%	0.7%	0.7%	0.5%	0.5%	0.4%	0.4%
2	mg/mL	0.92 ± 0.05 [c,d]	0.91 ± 0.03 [d]	23.0 ± 0.4 [b]	23.0 ± 0.4 [b]	1.46 ± 0.02 [b]	1.46 ± 0.03 [b]	3.50 ± 0.21 [a,b]	3.32 ± 0.16 [b]
	mg/daily portion	0.6	0.6	16	16	1.0	1.0	2.5	2.3
	%RDA/AI	<0.1%	<0.1%	0.3%	0.3%	0.3%	0.3%	0.2%	0.2%
3	mg/mL	2.57 ± 0.17 [a]	2.62 ± 0.09 [a]	1.82 ± 0.17 [c]	1.98 ± 0.07 [c]	50 ± 2.3 [a]	48 ± 2.2 [a]	2.12 ± 0.06 [c]	2.05 ± 0.05 [c]
	mg/daily portion	7.2	7.3	5.1	5.5	139	135	5.9	5.7
	%RDA/AI	0.7%	0.7%	0.1%	0.1%	43%	42%	0.4%	0.4%
READY-TO-DRINK									
4	mg/mL	0.20 ± 0.01 [c]	0.33 ± 0.01 [b]	0.28 ± 0.01 [b]	0.18 ± 0.00 [c]	0.06 ± 0.01 [b]	0.07 ± 0.01 [a]	0.58 ± 0.02 [a]	0.57 ± 0.05 [a,b]
	mg/daily portion	5.6	9.2	7.8	5.0	1.7	2.0	16	16
	%RDA/AI	0.6%	0.9%	0.2%	0.1%	0.5%	0.6%	1.1%	1.1%
5	mg/mL	0.12 ± 0.01 [d]	0.20 ± 0.00 [c]	<0.01	<0.01	<0.01	<0.01	0.53 ± 0.04 [a,b]	0.52 ± 0.03 [b]
	mg/daily portion	3.4	5.6	0	0	0.3	0.3	15	15
	%RDA/AI	0.3%	0.6%	0	0	0.1%	0.1%	1%	1%
6	mg/mL	0.38 ± 0.03 [a]	0.37 ± 0.01 [a]	2.46 ± 0.06 [a]	2.56 ± 0.07 [a]	0.10 ± 0.00 [a]	0.10 ± 0.00 [a]	0.58 ± 0.04 [a]	0.62 ± 0.06 [a]
	mg/daily portion	6.1	5.9	40	41	1.6	1.6	9.3	9.9
	%RDA/AI	0.6%	0.6%	0.8%	0.9%	0.5%	0.5%	0.6%	0.7%
7	mg/mL	0.02 ± 0.00 [e]	0.02 ± 0.00 [e]	0.04 ± 0.00 [d]	0.04 ± 0.00 [d]	<0.01	<0.01	0.53 ± 0.01 [b]	0.54 ± 0.01 [b]
	mg/daily portion	10	10	20	20	0	0	265	270
	%RDA/AI	1%	1%	0.4%	0.4%	0	0	18%	18%

[1]—Production years: 2015 and 2018; [2]—the maximum daily intake; [3]—the percentage of recommended daily allowance (RDA)/adequate intake (AI) realized by maximum daily portion; a–e: significant differences ($p < 0.05$) between mean values for each mineral within the product categories are indicated by different letters.

Table 2. The content of microelements in fulvic acid beverages.

Category of Product		Cu		Fe		Mn		Zn	
		I [1]	II [1]	I	II	I	II	I	II
CONCENTRATE									
1	mg/mL	<0.01	<0.01	16.0 ± 1.5 [a]	14.0 ± 1.0 [a,b]	0.16 ± 0.00 [b]	0.16 ± 0.00 [b]	0.06 ± 0.00 [a]	0.05 ± 0.00 [a,b]
	mg/daily portion [2]	0	0	23	20	0.23	0.23	0.09	0.07
	%RDA [3]	0	0	129%	113%	13%	13%	1.1%	1.0%
2	mg/mL	<0.01	<0.01	13.0 ± 1.1 [b]	12.0 ± 1.1 [b]	0.20 ± 0.01 [a]	0.21 ± 0.00 [a]	0.04 ± 0.00 [b]	0.04 ± 0.00 [b]
	mg/daily portion	0	0	9.0	8.1	0.14	0.15	0.03	0.03
	%RDA	0	0	50%	45%	7.8%	8.2%	0.4%	0.4%
3	mg/mL	<0.01	<0.01	0.04 ± 0.00 [c]	0.04 ± 0.00 [c]	<0.01	<0.01	0.02 ± 0.00 [c]	0.02 ± 0.00 [c]
	mg/daily portion	0	0	0.11	0.11	0	0	0.06	0.06
	%RDA	0	0	0.6%	0.6%	0	0	0.7%	0.7%
READY-TO-DRINK									
4	mg/mL	<0.01	<0.01	0.83 ± 0.04 [b]	0.87 ± 0.04 [b]	<0.01	<0.01	0.01 ± 0.00 [b]	0.01 ± 0.00 [b]
	mg/daily portion	0	0	23	24	0	0	0.28	0.28
	%RDA	0	0	129%	135%	0	0	3.5%	3.5%
5	mg/mL	<0.01	<0.01	<0.01	<0.01	<0.01	<0.01	0.02 ± 0.00 [a]	0.01 ± 0.00 [b]
	mg/daily portion	0	0	0	0	0	0	0.56	0.28
	%RDA	0	0	0	0	0	0	7%	3.5%
6	mg/mL	<0.01	<0.01	1.19 ± 0.01 [a]	1.20 ± 0.01 [a]	0.08 ± 0.00	0.08 ± 0.00	0.01 ± 0.00 [b]	0.01 ± 0.00 [b]
	mg/daily portion	0	0	19	19	1.28	1.28	0.16	0.16
	%RDA	0	0	106%	107%	71%	71%	2%	2%
7	mg/mL	<0.01	<0.01	<0.01	<0.01	<0.01	<0.01	<0.01	<0.01
	mg/daily portion	0	0	0	0	0	0	0	0
	%RDA	0	0	0	0	0	0	0	0

[1]—Production years: 2015 and 2018; [2]—the maximum daily intake. [3]—the percentage of RDA realized by maximum daily portion; a-c: significant differences ($p < 0.05$) between mean values for each mineral within product categories are indicated by different letters.

Table 3. The antioxidant capacities expressed as the total polyphenol (TP) and total flavonoid (TF) (µg/mL), ferric reducing ability of plasma (FRAP) and trolox equivalent antioxidant capacity (TEAC) (µmol/mL) of fulvic acid beverages.

Category of Product		TP		TF		FRAP		TEAC	
		I[1]	II[1]	I	II	I	II	I	II
CONCENTRATE									
1	µg/mL	15,762 ± 140 [c]	16,457 ± 442 [b]	7321 ± 152 [a]	5886 ± 228 [b]	309 ± 15 [a]	235 ± 6 [b]	141 ± 5 [b]	117 ± 13 [c]
	µg/daily portion[2]	22,855	23,863	10,615	8535	448	341	204	170
2	µg/mL	12,814 ± 175 [d]	19,844 ± 231 [a]	6167 ± 163 [b]	7113 ± 270 [a]	309 ± 16 [a]	338 ± 18 [a]	150 ± 10 [b]	172 ± 9 [a]
	µg/daily portion[2]	8970	15,891	4317	4979	216	237	105	120
3		n.d.	n.d.	n.d.	n.d.	n.d.	n.d.	n.d.	n.d.
		n.d.	n.d.	n.d.	n.d.	n.d.	n.d.	n.d.	n.d.
READY-TO-DRINK									
4	µg/mL	44.7 ± 1.3 [b]	67.3 ± 2.8 [a]	17.1 ± 0.4 [e]	24.4 ± 0.6 [d]	n.d.	n.d.	n.d.	n.d.
	µg/daily portion	1252	1884	479	683	n.d.	n.d.	n.d.	n.d.
5	µg/mL	12.0 ± 2.6 [e]	12.0 ± 0.5 [e]	6.5 ± 0.5 [g]	8.1 ± 0.3 [f]	n.d.	n.d.	n.d.	n.d.
	µg/daily portion	336	336	182	227	n.d.	n.d.	n.d.	n.d.
6	µg/mL	22.0 ± 1.7 [c]	16.0 ± 0.5 [d]	187 ± 10 [a]	135 ± 20 [b]	4.8 ± 0.7	4.5 ± 0.1	n.d.	n.d.
	µg/daily portion	352	256	2992	2160	77	72	n.d.	n.d.
7	µg/mL	22.2 ± 0.8 [c]	21.4 ± 1.0 [c]	28.4 ± 0.6 [c]	29.3 ± 0.8 [c]	n.d.	n.d.	n.d.	n.d.
	µg/daily portion	11,100	10,700	14,200	14,650	n.d.	n.d.	n.d.	n.d.

[1]—production years: 2015 and 2018; [2]—the maximum daily intake, n.d.—not detected; a–g: significant differences ($p < 0.05$) between mean values for TP/TF/FRAP/TEAC within a product category were indicated by different letters.

3. Results and Discussion

Each producer of a fulvic acid beverage declared that they used a standard, repeatable, and controlled process to manufacture each batch of their product(s). On the other hand, they usually stated that some differences in the concentration of fulvic acids and individual trace substances may be observed because the starting material is a completely natural material, not subjected to any laboratory treatment. Because of this, products from different years (2015 and 2018) were regarded as independent samples. As products selected were from different categories (concentrates and ready-to-drink beverages); all results were expressed both per millilitre of the product and in regard to daily intake calculated for the maximum portion suggested by producers.

Tables 1 and 2 present the concentrations of macroelements and microelements in fulvic acid beverages. The percentages of the realization of recommended daily allowances (RDAs for Ca, Mg, Cu, Fe, Mn, and Zn) and adequate intakes (AIs for K and Na) were calculated for the maximum daily portions suggested by the producers. The maximum portions were: 1.45 mL, 0.7 mL, and 2.8 mL for concentrates 1, 2, and 3, respectively. For ready-to-drink beverages 4, 5, 6, and 7 they were 28 mL, 28 mL, 16 mL, and 500 mL, respectively. The percentages of the realizations of RDA/AI were calculated according to American and Polish recommendations for middle-aged (40 years old) healthy woman [28,29] and are also presented in Tables 1 and 2. The RDA or AI values were: 1000 mg for Ca, 4700 mg for K, 320 mg for Mg, 1500 mg for Na, 0.9 mg for Cu, 18 mg for Fe, 1.8 mg for Mn, and 8 mg for Zn. The choice of another model person (man or child) would change %RDA or %AI values, but would not change the mutual relationships between the products being tested.

It was found that fulvic acid beverages differed within categories of products in the concentrations of minerals tested ($p < 0.05$), and eight out 14 of them were an excellent source of Fe. Although further studies on the bioavailability of Fe from these products are necessary, the content of this mineral needs to be underlined. The content of Fe in two out of three kinds of concentrates (product 1 and 2) was between 12 and 16 mg in 1 mL of the product, whereas for two kinds of ready-to-drink products was between 0.8 and 1.2 mg in 1 mL. One kind of concentrate and two ready-to-drink beverages contained trace amounts of this element. The maximum daily portion of products 1, 4, and 6 realized more than 100% of the RDA for Fe. Product 2 was also a good source of this element and realized approximately 45–50% of dietary requirement for iron. The presence of a significant amount of iron in commercially available fulvic acids was also confirmed by other scientists who studied the effect of fulvic acids on the growth of tomatoes, cucumbers, sunflowers, and lemon trees [30–33]. The important sources of other minerals were: product 3—Mg (approximately 40% of RDA); product 6—Mn and K (approximately 70% or 40% of RDA or AI, respectively); and product 7—Na (approximately 18% of AI).

Grant et al. [34] also underlined the potential benefit of fulvic acid dietary supplements as a source of some minerals. They investigated the elemental composition of four fulvic acid dietary supplements in a liquid (two fulvic acid mineral waters and fulvic mineral complex) and capsule form (fulvic acid dietary supplement). The origins of fulvic acids in the samples which they tested were not presented. Their results also confirmed the presence of Mg—the range of 0.89–7.20 mg/g, which was not as wide as in our study (from below 0.01 to 50 mg/mL). The content of Fe was also significantly higher for most of the products in our study (<0.01–16 mg/mL) than for samples from Grant et al.'s study (0.15–0.98 mg/g) [34]. On the other hand, our products mostly contained smaller amounts of Zn (Grant et al.: 0.16–2.2 mg/g; our study: <0.01–0.06 mg/mL), Mn (Grant et al.: 0–1.55 mg/g; our study: <0.01–0.21 mg/mL), and Cu (Grant et al.: 0.022–0.034 mg/g; our study: <0.01 mg/mL). The differences between products from different years or the same category or between our study and study of Grant et al. [34] may result from variety of fulvic acid materials, their origin from soils and plants growing in various conditions, and extraction methods used by producers to obtain them. Moreover, the compositions of the final products, including the amounts of fulvic acids, differ between producers.

Although in vitro assays for determination of the antioxidant activity of compounds do not reflect in vivo conditions, their application may give some view of the potential antioxidant activities in vivo. Therefore, Table 3 presents the antioxidant capacities of the products we tested, expressed as the TP, TF, FRAP, and TEAC values. It was found that fulvic acid beverages differed within categories of products in polyphenol and flavonoid contents, and in the TEAC and FRAP values ($p < 0.05$). TP content ranged from 12–67 µg/mL in ready-to-drink beverages to 12,814–19,844 µg/mL in concentrates. The concentration of TF in drinks ranged from 6.5 to 187 µg/mL, and in concentrates from 5886 to 7321 µg/mL. Only two kinds of concentrates and one kind of ready-to-drink had antioxidant activity expressed as the FRAP and/or TEAC values. Product 3 had no antioxidant activity. As it can be expected, concentrates had up to 1650-fold more antioxidants than ready-to-drink beverages. However, taking into account the maximum daily portion suggested by the producer, the differences were much lower (up to 93-fold for TP, 58-fold for TF, and 6.2-fold for FRAP value). The daily portion of product 7 was an even better source of TF than the daily portion of concentrates. Moreover, the concentrations of TP or TF in fulvic acid concentrates, and their TEAC and FRAP values, were much higher than reported for many polyphenol-rich beverages, such as red wine, fruit juices, antioxidant-enriched juices, and ice-teas [35–38].

Fulvic acids in a liquid form can be a good natural substitute for artificial isotonic beverages widely available on the global food market or an interesting option for people with iron deficiency. Nowadays, the market of beverages strongly benefits from the healthy lifestyles of contemporary consumers. Consumers tend to eat more food from the categories "natural," "organic," or "functional." Lal [39] emphasized that the sector of functional beverages could be the category where consumers look for innovations. Thus, fulvic acids drinks, due to their antioxidant properties and high contents of important microelements and macroelements (e.g., Fe and Mg), could be perceived as the functional beverages that do not contain artificial additives, such as sweeteners, colorants, preservatives, and flavour enhancers. They could be an interesting opportunity for both producers and consumers and may find a high acceptance among health-conscious people.

4. Conclusions

Nowadays, there is a growing interest among consumers for products made from natural ingredients, not containing preservatives, and having beneficial effects on humans. Besides economic factors, the taste and the health awareness of consumers on the importance of nutrients supplied with food to the human body have a great impact on the food market, including beverages.

The results of the present study on beverages containing fulvic acids, available in the form of concentrates and ready-to-drink beverages, showed that they may contain substantial amounts of Fe (up to about 130% of RDA), Mg (up to about 40% of RDA), and Mn (up to about 70% of RDA). They can also be a good source of polyphenolic compounds (up to about 19.8 mg/mL) with high antioxidant activity. Therefore, they may become interesting and valuable food products or food ingredients with potential effects on human health.

Author Contributions: Conceptualization, M.S., I.R., and A.G.-Ś.; methodology, I.R. and A.G.-Ś; investigation, M.S., I.R., and A.G.-Ś.; resources, M.S., I.R., and A.G.-Ś; data curation, M.S., I.R., and A.G.-Ś; writing—original draft preparation, M.S., I.R., and A.G.-Ś; writing—review and editing, M.S., I.R., and A.G.-Ś; supervision, I.R. and A.G.-Ś.

Funding: This research received no external funding.

Conflicts of Interest: The authors declare no conflict of interest.

References

1. Ji, F.; McGlone, J.J.; Kim, S.W. Effects of dietary humic substances on pig growth performance, carcass characteristics, and ammonia emission. *J. Anim. Sci.* **2006**, *84*, 2482–2490. [CrossRef] [PubMed]
2. Łomińska-Płatek, D.; Anielak, A.M. The content of fulvic acids in the primary effluent at the Płaszów WWTP in Kraków, E3S Web of Conferences 17. In Proceedings of the 9th Conference on Interdisciplinary Problems in Environmental Protection and Engineering EKO-DOK, Boguszow-Gorce, Poland, 23–25 April 2017. [CrossRef]

3. Malan, C. Review: Humic and fulvic acids. A Practical Approach. In *Sustainable Soil Management Symposium. Stellenbosch*; Agrilibrium Publisher: Cape Town, South Africa, 2015.
4. Pettit, R.E. Organic Matter, Humus, Humate, Humic Acid, Fulvic Acid and Humin: Their Importance in Soil Fertility and Plant Health. 2004. Available online: https://humates.com (accessed on 19 June 2018).
5. Sanmanee, N.; Areekijseree, M. The effects of fulvic acid on copper bioavailability to porcine oviductal epithelial cells. *Biol. Trace Elem. Res.* **2010**, *135*, 162–173. [CrossRef] [PubMed]
6. Reshi, Z.; Tyub, S. *Detritus and Decomposition in Ecosystems. Chapter 7: Humus Biosynthesis*; New India Publishing Agency: Pitam Pura, India, 2007; pp. 153–176.
7. Alvarez-Puebla, R.A.; Valenzuela-Calahorro, C.; Garrido, J.J. Theoretical study on fulvic acid structure, confirmation and aggregation, a molecular modelling approach. *Sci. Total Environ.* **2006**, *358*, 243–254. [CrossRef] [PubMed]
8. Kishor, P.; Bimala, S.; Nagendra, T. Shilajit: Humic matter panacea for cancer. *Int. J. Toxicol. Pharmacol. Res.* **2012**, *4*, 17–25.
9. Aydin, S.K.; Dalgic, S.; Karaman, M.; Kirlangic, O.F.; Yildirim, H. Effects of fulvic acid on different cancer cell lines. *Proceedings* **2017**, *1*, 1031. [CrossRef]
10. Christl, I.; Metzger, A.; Heidmann, I.; Kretzschma, R. Effect of humic and fulvic acid concentrations and ionic strength on copper and lead binding. *Environ. Sci. Technol.* **2005**, *39*, 5319–5326. [CrossRef]
11. Zhang, X.-F.; Yang, G.; Dong, Y.; Zhao, Y.-Q.; Sun, X.-R.; Chen, L.; Chen, H.-B. Studies on the binding of fulvic acid with transferrin by spectroscopic analysis. *Spectrochim. Acta A Mol. Biomol. Spectrosc.* **2015**, *137*, 1280–1285. [CrossRef]
12. Man, D.; Pisarek, I.; Braczkowski, M.; Pytel, B.; Olchawa, R. The impact of humic and fulvic acids on the dynamic properties of liposome membranes: The ESR method. *J. Liposome Res.* **2014**, *24*, 106–112. [CrossRef]
13. Cárdenas Rodríguez, N.; Coballase Urrutia, E.; Huerta Gertrudis, B.; Pedraza Chaverri, J.; Barragán Mejía, G. Antioxidant activity of fulvic acid: A living matter-derived bioactive compound. *J. Food, Agric. Environ.* **2011**, *9*, 123–127.
14. Carrasco-Gallardo, C.; Farías, G.A.; Fuentes, P.; Crespo, F.; Maccioni, R.B. Can nutraceuticals prevent Alzheimer's disease? Potential therapeutic role of a formulation containing shilajit and complex B vitamins. *Arch. Med. Res.* **2012**, *43*, 699–704. [CrossRef]
15. Feng, Y.; Wang, X. Antioxidant Therapies for Alzheimer's Disease. *Oxid. Med. Cell Longev.* **2012**, 17. [CrossRef] [PubMed]
16. Meena, H.; Pandey, H.K.; Arya, M.C.; Ahmed, Z. Shilajit: A panacea for high-altitude problems. *Int. J. Ayurveda Res.* **2010**, *1*, 37–40. [CrossRef] [PubMed]
17. Van Rensburg, C. The antiinflammatory properties of humic substances: A mini review. *Phytother. Res.* **2015**, *29*, 791–795. [CrossRef] [PubMed]
18. Winkler, J.; Ghosh, S. Therapeutic potential of fulvic acid in chronic inflammatory diseases and diabetes. *J. Diabetes Res.* **2018**, *2018*, 7. [CrossRef]
19. Baigorri, R.; Fuentes, M.; González-Gaitano, G.; García-Mina, J.M.; Almendros, G.; González-Vila, F.J. Complementary multianalytical approach to study the distinctive structural features of the main humic fractions in solution: Gray humic acid, brown humic acid, and fulvic acid. *J. Agric. Food Chem.* **2009**, *57*, 3266–3272. [CrossRef]
20. Shailesh, K.B.; Aswin, M.T.; Jitendra, K.M. Shilajit. In *Nutraceuticals Efficacy, Safety and Toxicity*; Academic Press: Cambridge, MA, USA, 2016; pp. 707–716.
21. Wilson, E.; Rajamanickam, G.V.; Dubey, G.P.; Klose, P.; Musial, F.; Saha, F.J.; Rampp, T.; Michalsen, A.; Dobosa, G.J. Review on shilajit used in traditional Indian medicine. *J. Ethnopharmacol.* **2011**, *136*, 1–9. [CrossRef]
22. Ozbek, N.; Akman, S. Method development for the determination of calcium, copper, magnesium, manganese, iron, potassium, phosphorus and zinc in different types of breads by microwave induced plasma-atomic emission spectrometry. *Food Chem.* **2016**, *200*, 245–248. [CrossRef]
23. Singleton, V.L.; Rossi, J.A. Colorimetry of total phenolics with phosphomolybdic-phosphotungstic acid reagents. *Am. J. Enol. Vitic.* **1965**, *16*, 144–158.
24. Karadeniz, F.; Burdurlu, H.S.; Koca, N.; Soyer, Y. Antioxidant activity of selected fruits and vegetables grown in Turkey. *Turk. J. Agric. For.* **2005**, *29*, 297–303.

25. Re, R.; Pellergini, N.; Proteggente, A.; Pannala, A.S.; Yang, M.; Rice-Evans, C. Antioxidant activity applying an improved ABTS radical cation decolorization assay. *Free Radic. Biol. Med.* **1999**, *26*, 1231–1237. [CrossRef]
26. Benzie, I.F.F.; Strain, J.J. The ferric reducing ability of plasma (FRAP) as a measure of "antioxidant power": The FRAP assay. *Anal. Biochem.* **1996**, *239*, 70–76. [CrossRef] [PubMed]
27. Enko, J.; Gliszczyńska-Świgło, A. Influence of the interactions between tea (Camellia sinensis) extracts and ascorbic acid on their antioxidant activity: Analysis with interaction indexes and isobolograms. *Food Addit. Contam. Part A* **2015**, *32*, 1234–1242. [CrossRef] [PubMed]
28. Jarosz, M. (Ed.) *Normy Żywienia dla Populacji Polskiej–Nowelizacja [Nutritional Requirements for the Polish Population–Upgrade]*; National Food and Nutrition Institute: Warsaw, Poland, 2017; p. 223.
29. U.S. Department of Health and Human Services; U.S. Department of Agriculture. *2015–2020 Dietary Guidelines for Americans*, 8th ed.; U.S. Department of Health and Human Services: Washington, DC, USA, 2015.
30. Adani, F.; Genevini, P.; Zaccheo, P.; Zocchi, G. The effect of commercial humic acid on tomato plant growth and mineral nutrition. *J. Plant Nutr.* **1998**, *21*, 561–575. [CrossRef]
31. Bocanegra, M.P.; Lobartini, J.C.; Orioli, G.A. Plant uptake of iron chelated by humic acids of different molecular weights. *Commun. Soil. Sci. Plant Anal.* **2006**, *37*, 1–2. [CrossRef]
32. Canellas, L.P.; Dantas, D.J.; Aguiar, N.O.; Peres, L.E.P.; Zsögön, A.; Olivares, F.L.; Dobbss, L.B.; Façanha, A.R.; Nebbioso, A.; Piccolo, A. Probing the hormonal activity of fractionated molecular humic components in tomato auxin mutants. *Ann. Appl. Biol.* **2011**, *159*, 202–211. [CrossRef]
33. Sánchez-Sánchez, A.; Sánchez-Andreu, J.; Juárez, M.; Jordá, J.; Bermúdez, D. Humic substances and amino acids improve effectiveness of chelate FeEDDHA in lemon trees. *J. Plant Nutr.* **2002**, *25*, 2433–2442. [CrossRef]
34. Grant, T.D.; Wuilloud, R.G.; Wuilloud, J.C.; Caruso, J.A. Investigation of the elemental composition and chemical association of several elements in fulvic acids dietary supplements by size-exclusion chromatography UV inductively coupled plasma mass spectrometric. *J. Chrom. A* **2004**, *1054*, 313–319. [CrossRef]
35. Abountiolas, M.; Nascimento Nunes, C.D. Polyphenols, ascorbic acid and antioxidant capacity of commercial nutritional drinks, fruit juices, smoothies and teas. *Int. J. Food Sci. Technol.* **2018**, *53*, 188–198. [CrossRef]
36. Aguiilar, T.; de Bruijn, J.; Loyola, C.; Bustamante, L.; Vergara, C.; von Baer, D.; Mardne, C.; Serra, I. Characterization of an Antioxidant-Enriched Beverage from Grape Musts and Extracts of Winery and Grapevine By-Products. *Beverages* **2018**, *4*, 4. [CrossRef]
37. Seeram, N.P.; Aviram, M.; Zhang, Y.; Henning, S.M.; Feng, L.; Dreher, M.; Heber, D. Comparison of antioxidant potency of commonly consumed polyphenol-rich beverages in the United States. *J. Agric. Food Chem.* **2008**, *56*, 1415–1422. [CrossRef]
38. Stella, S.P.; Ferrarezi, A.C.; dos Santos, K.O.; Monteiro, M. Antioxidant activity of commercial ready to drink orange juice and nectar. *J. Food Sci.* **2011**, *76*, 392–397. [CrossRef] [PubMed]
39. Lal, G.G. Processing of beverages for the health food market consumer. In *Nutraceutical and Functional Food Processing Technology*; Boye, J.I., Ed.; Wiley-Blackwell: Hoboken, NJ, USA, 2015; pp. 189–208.

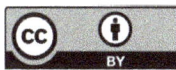

© 2019 by the authors. Licensee MDPI, Basel, Switzerland. This article is an open access article distributed under the terms and conditions of the Creative Commons Attribution (CC BY) license (http://creativecommons.org/licenses/by/4.0/).

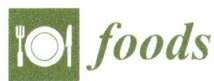

Communication

Grape Seeds: Chromatographic Profile of Fatty Acids and Phenolic Compounds and Qualitative Analysis by FTIR-ATR Spectroscopy

Massimo Lucarini [1,*], Alessandra Durazzo [1], Johannes Kiefer [2], Antonello Santini [3,*], Ginevra Lombardi-Boccia [1], Eliana B. Souto [4,5], Annalisa Romani [6], Anja Lampe [2], Stefano Ferrari Nicoli [1], Paolo Gabrielli [1], Noemi Bevilacqua [7], Margherita Campo [6], Massimo Morassut [7] and Francesca Cecchini [7]

1. CREA-Research Centre for Food and Nutrition, Via Ardeatina 546, 00178 Roma, Italy; alessandra.durazzo@crea.gov.it (A.D.); g.lombardiboccia@crea.gov.it (G.L.-B.); stefano.nicoli@crea.gov.it (S.F.N.); paolo.gabrielli@crea.gov.it (P.G.)
2. Technische Thermodynamik, University of Bremen, Badgasteiner Str. 1, 28359 Bremen, Germany; jkiefer@uni-bremen.de (J.K.); anjalampe@uni-bremen.de (A.L.)
3. Department of Pharmacy, University of Napoli Federico II, Via D. Montesano 49, 80131 Napoli, Italy
4. Department of Pharmaceutical Technology, Faculty of Pharmacy, University of Coimbra, 3000-548 Coimbra, Portugal; souto.eliana@gmail.com
5. CEB-Centre of Biological Engineering, University of Minho, Campus de Gualtar, 4710-057 Braga, Portugal
6. PHYTOLAB, University of Florence, 50019 Sesto Fiorentino (Firenze), Italy; annalisa.romani@unifi.it (A.R.); margherita.campo@unifi.it (M.C.)
7. CREA-Research Centre for Viticulture and Enology, 00049 Velletri (Roma), Italy; noemi.bevilacqua@crea.gov.it (N.B.); massimo.morassut@crea.gov.it (M.M.); francesca.cecchini@crea.gov.it (F.C.)
* Correspondence: massimo.lucarini@crea.gov.it (M.L.); asantini@unina.it (A.S.); Tel.: +39-06-5149-4430 (M.L.); +39-81-253-9517 (A.S.)

Received: 10 November 2019; Accepted: 18 December 2019; Published: 21 December 2019

Abstract: The primary product of the oenological sector is wine. Nonetheless, the grape processing produces large amounts of by-products and wastes, e.g., the grape seeds. In the context of a sustainable production, there is a strong push towards reutilizing these by-products and waste for making useful derivatives since they are rich of bioactive substances with high additional value. As it is true for the wine itself, bringing these by-products derivatives to the market calls for quality measures and analytical tools to assess quality itself. One of the main objectives is to collect analytical data regarding bioactive compounds using potentially green techniques. In the present work, the profile of fatty acids and the main phenolic compounds were investigated by conventional methods. The qualitative analysis of the main functional groups was carried out by Fourier Transform Infrared (FTIR) spectroscopy. Moreover, the successful use of FTIR technique in combination with chemometric data analysis is shown to be a suitable analytical tool for discriminating the grape seeds. Grape seeds of different origin have different content of bioactive substances, making this technique useful when planning to recover a certain substance with specific potential application in health area as food supplement or nutraceutical. For example, Cesanese d'Affile seeds were found to have a rather high fat content with a significant fraction of unsaturated fatty acids. On the other hand, the seeds of Nero d'Avola exhibit the highest amount of phenolic compounds.

Keywords: grape; grape seeds; FTIR spectroscopy; chemometrics; fatty acids; phenolic compounds; biorefinery; nutraceuticals

1. Introduction

The valorization of the agro-food waste represents an important goal for the preservation and support of a sustainable ecosystem and effective production. The new concept of circular economy applied to agricultural recycling perfectly fits to a modern "zero waste" lifestyle, and can be achieved by biorefineries, bioenergy plants, and environmentally friendly processes for the production of biomolecules on both small and large industrial scale [1–4]. Lucarini et al. [5] gave an overview of how by-products and wastes from the wine industry can be used as biorefinery feedstock.

The oenological sector's main product is the wine, and, to some extent, non-alcoholic juices. However, the process of winemaking produces wastewater, pomace (the solid residues of grapes), and lees, that require disposal or beneficial use, if possible. The winemaking process generates a considerable amount of organic solid waste [6], e.g., during the crashing-pressing processes and the wine clarification. Concerning the vinification process, the white vinification (without maceration step of the grape skins in the must) directly produces stalks and pomace. On the other hand, the red vinification process (with the grape skin maceration step in the must) leads to the immediate formation of steams and, only after a period of maceration, the pomace. Both vinification processes produce lees after the decanting [7]. After the pressing for juice/must, the pomace contains mainly: (i) skins; (ii) seeds; (iii) pulp residues of the grape. At the end of the fermentation, the lees that are separated from the wine during the clarification and decanting process, consist mainly of dead yeasts [8,9].

As aforesaid, the grape seeds are a relevant part of the waste. For this reason, in the last decade an ever-increasing interest in the seeds appeared, since they contain bioactive compounds such as fatty acids and polyphenols [5,10–14], which are attractive from a nutraceutical perspective [15–22]. Their potential benefits ranges from anti-platelet and anticoagulant activity, to antioxidant, hypoglycemic, and even activity against cancer [23–27].

The extracts obtained from processing the grape seeds can be useful ingredients for agronomic, food, nutraceutical, cosmetic, and pharmaceutical derivatives. For example, the oils that can be extracted from grape seeds are of high value, as they contain large fractions of polyunsaturated fatty acids [28]. Consequently, they can be brought to the market at relatively high prices. Hence, there is the need of analytical methods to confirm the authenticity and quality of by-products and wastes in the oenological sector.

While chromatographic techniques are still seen as the gold standard for analytical purposes in the winemaking industry, the spectroscopic methods are nowadays being reconsidered. They often do not require sample preparation steps and they are faster. Moreover, they can virtually provide information about all species present in the sample in one single step experiment without the need for any preliminary separation step as happens for other analytical techniques. Fourier-transform infrared (FTIR) spectroscopy is a very promising tool in this context. For example, applied to wine it is capable of determining a multitude of parameters including the alcohol content, the total acidity, the sugar content, the pH value, as well as the relative density [29,30].

Grape seeds were also studied by FTIR spectroscopy. Ismail et al. [31] used FTIR to study and quantify bioactive compounds in grape seeds. They identified carboxylate groups from gallic acid and proanthocyanidin gallate in the aqueous seed extract. Mohansrinivasan et al. [32] used FTIR analysis to identify the functional groups of the bioactive compounds present in grapeseed extracts obtained from ethyl acetate, water, and petroleum ether. Canbay and Bardakçı [33] applied a hexane extraction and further processing to grape seeds in order to yield fatty acid methyl esters (FAME), which were subsequently analyzed by FTIR spectroscopy. Nogales–Bueno et al. [34] utilized near-infrared (NIR) hyperspectral tools for the screening of extractable polyphenols in red grape skins. In further studies of their group [35,36], FTIR and Raman spectroscopy were applied to grape seed samples. They were able to find correlations between the spectral features and the phenolic extractability as well as other attributes in the grape skin and grape seed. From their studies [34–36], Nogales–Bueno et al. concluded that FTIR spectroscopy coupled with chemometrics represents a valuable tool for monitoring the composition of wine by-products. Such analysis can be utilized to identify the most suitable extraction process. Further applications of FTIR in the oenological sector included the investigation of the biodegradation of winery and distillery wastes during composting [37] and the analysis of grape seed oils [38,39].

The project behind the present study has a wider scope in the context of a circular economy in the oenological sector. One of its main objectives is to collect analytical data relating to the bioactive compounds present in the waste using potentially green techniques. In this connection, the present paper aims at extending the use of FTIR spectroscopy in the oenological sector by demonstrating that the method can also be used to discriminate grape seeds between different cultivars. For this purpose, grape seeds from Cesanese d'Affile (Lazio, Italy), Greco bianco (Campania, Italy), and Nero d'Avola (Sicilia, Italy) were characterized for their fatty acid content and the main phenolic compounds. Then, the attenuated total reflection (ATR) FTIR technique was applied for the qualitative analysis of the functional groups present in the extract and a multivariate analysis was carried out for the authentication and discrimination of the samples.

2. Materials and Methods

2.1. Plant Materials

The study was carried out using 3 *Vitis vinifera* (L.) cultivars (white and red grapes), grown in an experimental field in the Lazio region (Italy) (41°40′12″ N latitude, 12°46′48″ E longitude) at 332 m above sea level in 2017. The vineyard was 17 years old. The grapes were harvested at technological maturation. The cultivars had a Cordon Spur training system with a plant density of 2.60 × 1.5 m. The same cultural practices were applied in the vineyard. Cesanese d'Affile [40,41] cultivar autochthonous of the Lazio region (Central Italy) was characterized by a medium compact cluster and of cylindrical shape with small berries of spherical shape, and grape seeds of medium size and an average number of 1–2 per berry. Nero d'Avola [42] was a cultivar autochthonous of the Sicilia region (South Italy) with a medium cluster and of cylindrical shape with of medium size, rather oblong, regular, intense black color and seeds of medium size and an average number of 2–3 per berry. Greco Bianco was a cultivar grown in the region of the central-southern Italy, with a medium compact cluster and of cylindrical shape with 1–2 wings, with berries of medium-small size with ellipsoidal shape, green-yellow color, and large seeds with an average number of 2–3 per berry.

The procedure of seeds separation was carried out as follows: from 10 grape clusters for each cultivar, 400 berries were randomly detached. The seeds from these berries were manually separated from the pulp. Then, they underwent a homogenization procedure to improve the reproducibility before the resulting substance was frozen at −30 °C and then lyophilized for the subsequent analysis. The lyophilization process guarantees the samples homogencity and uniformity. In addition, this method allowed an optimal storage to protect the sample from oxidation and eventual possible contamination.

The lyophilized samples were ground in a refrigerated mill (Janke and Kunkec Ika Labortechnik, Germany) and the powder were sieved to obtain a granulometry of 0.5 mm.

2.2. Chemical Analysis

2.2.1. Fatty Acid Analysis

Fat was extracted through the method of Bligh and Dyer [43]. An aliquot of the extract was used for gas chromatographic (GC) analysis. The fatty acids were esterified using 5% anhydrous hydrogen chloride in methanol as esterification reagent [44]. The esterified fatty acids were quantified by gas chromatograph (Agilent 7890A), equipped with both FID (Flame Ionization Detector) and MS (Mass Spectrometry, Agilent 5975C) detectors [45]. The separation of the fatty acids was accomplished on a Mega-wax column (30 m × 0.32 mm i.d., 0.25 µm film thickness). The GC system allows to acquire and record in the same injection both the FID and MS signals, for qualitative and quantitative determinations respectively. Identification was also carried out by comparing the retention time of detected compounds in the sample with those from a standard FAME mix (Supelco TM 37 component FAME mix C4-C24; Sigma-Aldrich, St. Louis, MO, USA). Quantification was performed calculating the internal percentage distribution of FAME.

2.2.2. Phenolic Compound Analysis

For the extraction of phenolic compounds, the grape seeds were extracted with a solution EtOH:H_2O 70:30 (pH 3.2 by addition of HCOOH), in a p/V ratio of 15%, under stirring for 24 h, then the extract was separated from the solid matrix by low pressure filtration.

The High-Performance Liquid Chromatography with Diode-Array Detection coupled with a Mass Spectrometer (HPLC/DAD/MS) analyses were performed with a HP 1100 liquid chromatograph equipped with a Diode Array (DAD) detector and a Mass Selective Detector (MSD) and with an Atmospheric Pressure Ionization API-electrospray (Agilent Technologies, Palo Alto, CA, USA). Mass spectrometer operating conditions were the following: gas temperature 350 °C at a flow rate of 10.0 L/min, nebulizer pressure 30 psi, quadrupole temperature 30 °C and capillary voltage 3500 V. The mass spectrometer operated in positive and negative ionization mode at 80–120 eV. The analytical column was a LiChrosorb RP18 250 × 4.60 mm, 5 µm (LichroCART, Merck Darmstadt, Germany) maintained at 26 °C. The eluents were H_2O adjusted to pH 3.2 by HCOOH (A), and CH_3CN (B). A 7-step linear solvent gradient system, starting from 100% A up to 100% B was applied during a 117-min period at a flow rate of 0.8 mL/min [46].

The phenolic compounds were identified by using data from HPLC/DAD/MS analyses, by comparing and combining their retention times, UV/Vis and mass spectra with those of the available specific commercial standards and according to the available literature data. All the solvents (HPLC grade) and formic acid (ACS reagent) were purchased from Aldrich Chemical Company Inc. (Milwaukee, WI, USA). The standards gallic acid and (+) catechin were purchased from Extrasynthèse S.A. (Lyon, Nord-Genay, France). Each compound was quantified by HPLC/DAD, using a five-point regression curve built with the available standards. Calibration curves with $r^2 \geq 0.9998$ were considered. All polyphenolic derivatives showed good linearity over the range tested with correlation coefficients r^2 all above 0.9998.

The Limit of Detection (LOD) was obtained as the concentration corresponding to 3 times the noise recorded in the chromatograms; the Limit of Quantification (LOQ) was calculated as the concentration corresponding to 10 times the noise recorded in the chromatograms. The obtained values were: 0.21 µg/mL LOD and 0.68 µg/mL LOQ for catechin; 0.08 µg/mL LOD and 0.12 µg/mL LOQ for gallic acid. Gallic acid was calibrated at 280 nm using gallic acid as reference; catechin, epicatechin their oligomers were calibrated at 280 nm using (+) catechin as reference. In all cases, the actual concentrations of derivatives were calculated after making corrections for changes in molecular weight among compounds belonging to the same polyphenolic subclass.

2.2.3. Statistical Analysis

All analyses were performed in triplicate. Data are presented as mean ± standard deviation (s.d.). Statistica for Windows (Statistical package; release 4.5; StatSoft Inc., Vigonza, PD, Italy) was used to perform One-way Analysis of Variance (ANOVA).

2.3. *FTIR Analysis*

The FTIR spectra were recorded on a Nicolet iS10 FT-IR spectrometer (Thermo-Fisher Scientific, Waltam, MA, USA) equipped with a diamond crystal cell for attenuated total reflection (ATR) operation. The spectra were acquired (32 scans per sample or background) in the range of 4000–500 cm^{-1} at a nominal resolution of 4 cm^{-1}. The spectra were corrected using the background spectrum of air. The analysis was carried out at room temperature. For a measurement, a lyophilized sample was placed on the surface of the ATR crystal. Before acquiring a spectrum, the ATR crystal was carefully cleaned with wet cellulose tissue and dried using a flow of nitrogen gas. The cleaned crystal was checked spectrally to ensure that no residue was retained from the previous sample. For each sample, ten spectra were recorded. The spectrum of every sample was collected 10 times to check the reproducibility and do a statistical analysis. In addition to FTIR, the samples were analyzed conventionally to determine the fatty acid and phenolic compound profiles in order to aid the interpretation of the spectra, see next sub-sections for details.

The FTIR spectra were evaluated in two different ways: qualitative analysis of spectra and discrimination analysis.

2.3.1. Qualitative Analysis of the Spectra

As a first step, they were analyzed with respect to the spectral band positions in order to identify the signatures of the major functional groups. An assignment of the main bands was carried out by analyzing the acquired spectra and by comparing them with the literature.

2.3.2. Discrimination Analysis

In the second step, principal component analysis (PCA) was applied to the dataset. PCA is a statistical method that reduces the dimensionality of a data set by calculating the eigenvalue decomposition of the covariance matrix [47–50]. In other words, it identifies the spectral signatures that represent the variance of the data set. The results of a PCA are commonly discussed in terms of scores and loadings. The scores are the transformed variable values of a particular data point and the loadings represent the numbers by which each original variable should be multiplied to get the score. For a practical analysis, the scores and loadings plots are produced. The scores plot visualizes the scores with respect to the different principal components (PCs). A clustering of the data points in such a plot suggests that they exhibit spectral similarities and hence the corresponding samples can be assigned to a common category. The loadings of the individual PCs, on the other hand, can be plotted as a function wavenumber. The resulting spectra show characteristic signatures that allow a discrimination between the different categories. However, care must be taken when deciding how many PCs are to be considered. If a dataset's variance is mainly represented by two PCs, the higher components are predominantly noise and, as a consequence, the results may be over-interpreted. The signal-to-noise ratio of the loadings plot is a good indicator to decide whether or not a PC should be included in the analysis.

In the present work, the PCA algorithm implemented in Matlab R2012 was used without initial data centering in order to keep the method as simple as possible.

3. Results and Discussion

This section first presents the fatty acid and phenolic compound profiles of the grape seeds in order to provide a better description/characterization of matrices as reference for the subsequent discussion of the spectroscopic data and their qualitative and multivariate analysis. In order to validate the FTIR technique as a routine method for the characterization of grape seed extracts, the different samples were analyzed using HPLC/DAD/MS and GC/MS methods to identify and quantify both phenolic compounds and fatty acids that represent the main compounds present in the samples, and detectable by FTIR. This could be the basis for the interpretation of some bands present in the FTIR spectra.

3.1. Chemical Analysis

3.1.1. Fatty Acids

The fat content and the fatty acids profiles are summarized in Table 1 and an example chromatogram is shown in Figure A1. Cesanese d'Affile shows the highest value in fat content. It can be seen that the fatty acids profiles are reasonably similar within the margins of the measurement error. The main components are linoleic acid (C18:2 ω-6), oleic acid (C18:1), palmitic acid (C16:0), and stearic acid (C18:0). They add up to about 98% of the total fatty acids. Previous works have indicated grape seeds as a good source of the beneficial polyunsaturated fatty acids [51–53]. The current work of Pérez-Navarro et al. [51] reported a different profile of free fatty acids in the grape tissues, showing a higher proportion of unsaturated fatty acids in seeds (about 60%).

Table 1. Fat content (g/100 g) and fatty acid profiles (percent of total fatty acid content). The values in parentheses represent the standard deviation.

Compound	Nero d'Avola	Cesanese d' Affile	Greco Bianco
Fat content	8.66 (0.23) a	13.65 (0.71) b	8.06 (0.23) a
C12:0	0.24 (0.11) b	0.08 (0.03) ab	0.05 (0.02) a
C14:0	0.30 (0.09) a	0.19 (0.06) a	0.15 (0.05) a
C16:0	11.55 (1.18) a	12.19 (1.75) a	10.37 (0.72) a
C16:1	0.39 (0.17) a	0.25 (0.04) a	0.43 (0.07) a
C17:0	0.14 (0.03) a	0.12 (0.05) a	0.10 (0.03) a
C18:0	4.29 (0.21) a	5.01 (0.36) b	4.44 (0.09) ab
C18:1	23.09 (0.74) c	17.87 (0.11) a	21.07 (0.50) b
C18:2 ω-6	59.02 (0.97) a	63.71 (2.18) b	62.48 (1.68) ab
C18:3 ω-3	1.04 (0.19) a	0.69 (0.09) a	0.91 (0.23) a
C20:0	0.40 (0.15) c	n.d. *a	0.19 (0.13) b

Means within the same row with different superscripts letters (a, b and c) are significantly different ($p < 0.05$). * not detectable.

3.1.2. Phenolic Compounds

In Table 2 the main phenolic compounds present in grape seeds are summarized; a corresponding example chromatogram is shown in Figure A2. More distinct differences are observed for the phenolic compounds. The Nero D'Avola grape seed sample is rich both in flavan-3-ols (catechin and epicatechin) and their oligomeric or polymeric condensed derivatives (procyanidins). Instead, the Greco Bianco seeds exhibits the highest percentage of gallated compounds (35.78 mg/g on 46.70 total tannins, 76.6%) compared to Nero D'Avola (54.87 mg/g on 85.92 total tannins, 63.9%) and Cesanese d'Affile (39.32 mg/g on 57.80 total tannins, 68.0%). The highest weight oligomers, gallated trimers and tetramers, are more abundant in the Nero d'Avola sample (60.71 mg/g on 85.92 total tannins, 70.7%). Nero d'Avola seeds have also the highest content in total tannins and gallic acid (85.92 mg/g), followed by Cesanese d'Affile (57.80 mg/g) and Greco Bianco (46.70 mg/g). The results available in literature about grape seed extracts are not always consistent due to the different cultivars considered, areas of harvest, extraction techniques investigated and the use of solvents with different extraction capacities. Actually, grape seed extracts with variable titres from 15% up to 90% condensed tannins are available on the market for oenological, cosmetic or phytotherapic use, often lacking any information about characteristic of the raw material. In general, polyphenols and in particular condensed tannins and fatty acids are the most interesting and represented compounds in grape seeds [54–56]. The knowledge of the individual compounds and subclasses present in extracts with different polyphenolic contents has been used as a basis for the interpretation of some bands present in the FTIR spectra.

3.2. FTIR Data

3.2.1. Qualitative Analysis of FTIR Spectra

FTIR provides a characteristic signature of the chemical or biochemical substances present in a sample by featuring their molecular vibrations (stretching, bending, and torsions of the chemical bonds) [57]. Therefore, the FTIR spectrum represents a molecular fingerprint of the sample. The averaged spectra from the grape seed samples are shown in Figure 1. It is possible to discern numerous peaks, which correspond to functional groups and modes of vibration of the individual components. The broad band peaking at around 3270 cm^{-1} corresponds to the OH stretching modes. It can be attribute to the polysaccharides and/or lignins as reported by [36,58,59]. The peak at 3009 cm^{-1} is related to the C-H stretching vibration of the cis-double bond (=CH) groups. Asymmetric and symmetric stretching vibrations of CH$_2$ groups are found at 2923 and 2853 cm^{-1}, respectively. They are mainly associated with the hydrocarbon chains of the lipids or lignins [54]. The spectral band at 1744 cm^{-1} and the shoulder band at 1716 cm^{-1} is attributed to the absorption of the C=O bonds of the ester groups and it is related to the presence of the fatty acids and their glycerides, as well as pectins and lignins [60,61]. The bands around 1600 cm^{-1} are associated with the stretching of C=OO$^-$ and aromatic C=C groups, e.g., in pectins and phenolic compounds [61–63], but also with the bending vibrations of OH groups. The fingerprint region from 1500 to 800 cm^{-1} is very rich in peaks originating from various stretching, bending, rocking, scissoring, and torsional modes. This region is, on the one hand, very rich in information, but, on the other hand, difficult to analyze due to its complexity. This area provides important information about organic compounds, such as sugars, alcohols, and organic acids, present in the sample.

Table 2. HPLC/DAD/MS data expressed in mg/g of selected phenolic compounds present in the grape seeds. All results reported are the average of three replications and the relative standard deviation is less than 0.05.

Compound	Nero d'Avola	Cesanese d' Affile	Greco Bianco
gallic acid	0.04 (0.00) a	0.15 (0.01) c	0.11 (0.00) b
catechin dimer B3	1.32 (0.00) a	2.81 (0.01) c	1.91 (0.01) b
catechin	1.77 (0.01) a	4.89 (0.01) c	3.09 (0.08) b
procyanidin trimer	0.00 (0.00) a	0.88 (0.03) c	0.48 (0.01) b
catechin dimer B6	1.33 (0.01) b	1.62 (0.05) c	0.89 (0.02) a
catechin dimer B2	0.78 (0.01) a	1.86 (0.01) c	0.98 (0.01) b
epicatechin	0.60 (0.00) a	3.63 (0.03) c	2.01 (0.01) b
catechin trimer	0.41 (0.02) a	2.01 (0.01) c	1.15 (0.02) b
epicatechin gallate dimer	1.66 (0.01) a	5.46 (0.03) c	3.46 (0.07) b
catechin oligomers expressed as tetramers	24.80 (0.61) b	0.62 (0.02) a	0.29 (0.01) a
epicatechin gallate dimer	17.30 (0.41) b	1.16 (0.06) a	0.61 (0.01) a
catechin/epicatechin trimers digallate	30.90 (1.10) c	11.17 (0.08) b	9.17 (0.15) a
catechin/epicatechin trimers gallate	5.01 (0.02) a	21.53 (0.20) b	22.53 (0.24) c
total	85.92	57.80	46.68

Means within the same row with different superscripts letters (a, b and c) are significantly different ($p < 0.05$).

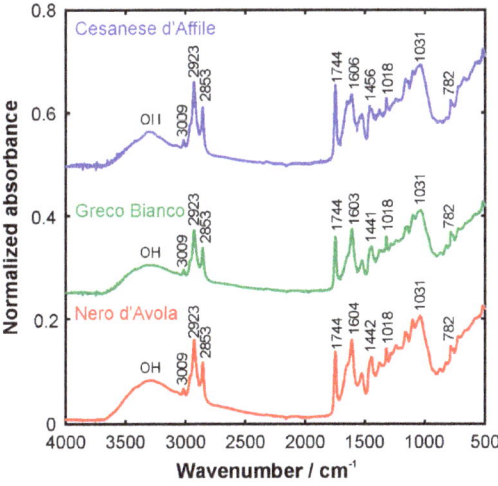

Figure 1. Averaged FTIR spectra of Cesanese d'Affile, Greco Bianco and Nero d'Avola grape seeds in the mid-infrared region (4000–500 cm^{-1}).

The aromatic C-C stretching at ~1520 and ~1443 cm^{-1} is related to phenolic compounds [58,59]. The CH$_3$ out of plane bending at 1377 cm^{-1}, the scissoring at 1318 cm^{-1}, and the C-O stretching at ~1035 cm^{-1} are related to polysaccharide structures [58,61]. The peak at 1143 cm^{-1} corresponds to aromatic C-H stretching and the band at 782 cm^{-1} is due to the rocking of CH$_2$, both in phenolic compounds [58].

3.2.2. Multivariate Analysis of FTIR Spectra

Overall, the spectra in Figure 1 appear very similar, which is reasonable due to the similarity in chemical composition. As we have seen in Section 3.1, the main differences appear in the phenolic compound profile, but the concentrations of these compounds are small. Nevertheless, small differences, e.g., in band shapes and relative intensities, can be observed in the spectra. In order to test, if an unsupervised classification of the individual spectra is possible, a PCA analysis of the full spectra was performed. This approach is commonly utilized for a classification of a data set. The first two principal components, PC1 and PC2, represent 99.4% of the variance of the data set. Out of this, PC1 accounts for 98.9%, which is in concert with the observation that the spectra appear very similar. In the score plot of PC1 and PC2, the seed from Cesanese d'Affile grape can already be distinguished from the Greco Bianco and Nero d'Avola seeds along the PC2 axis. Discriminating between the latter two requires further PCs. Therefore, Figure 2 presents the score plot of PC2 vs. PC4, in which all three grape seeds can be distinguished from each other. In this context, we note that PC3 and PC4 represent about 0.3 and 0.1% of the variance. This appears low at first glance, but their loadings vs. wavenumber plots exhibit relatively high signal-to-noise ratio with distinct spectral signatures. Therefore, utilizing them for the classification makes sense. For completeness, the normalized loadings plots are provided in the Appendix A, see Figure A3. We also note that applying the PCA to selected ranges of the spectra, e.g., the CH/OH stretching region, 2700–3700 cm^{-1}, allowed discrimination with less components. However, selecting an appropriate range requires *a priori* knowledge and therefore was not further considered in the framework of this study. The same is true for the application of hierarchical cluster analysis (HCA), which was also implemented in Matlab to test its capability. Feeding the full spectra into the algorithm did not allow a sufficiently clear clustering. Therefore, this is not further discussed here.

When we have a closer look at the PCA discrimination described above, the analysis of the loadings plots in Figure A3 provides further insights. As aforesaid, Cesanese d'Affile can be distinguished from the other two along the PC2 axis. The peak at 1646 cm^{-1} is a dominating signature of this component. Even in the raw spectra (cf. Figure 1) there is a shoulder band in the data of Greco Bianco and Nero d'Avola seeds, while it appears a rather clear peak in the Cesanese d'Affile spectrum. The chemical analysis would suggest that this signature originates from the fats and fatty acids as Cesanese d'Affile exhibits a higher content. However, previous FTIR studies of oils and pure fatty acids show no peaks in this region at all [64]. Given the fact that there is another characteristic feature in the OH stretching region of the PC2 loadings spectrum, it is likely that both signatures originate from hydroxyl groups. The narrow bandwidth indicates that these OH groups are distinctly bonded to their molecular surroundings via hydrogen bonds. Unravelling the molecular phenomena further requires advanced computational approaches such as molecular dynamics simulations and quantum chemistry. This is beyond the scope of the present work.

Nero d'Avola can be distinguished from the others along the PC4 axis. The PC4 loadings spectrum reveals characteristic signatures at 723 and 1014 cm^{-1} as well as a broad band in the OH stretching region. They can all be attributed to phenolic compounds, which makes sense given that Nero d´Avola exhibits the highest content of this category.

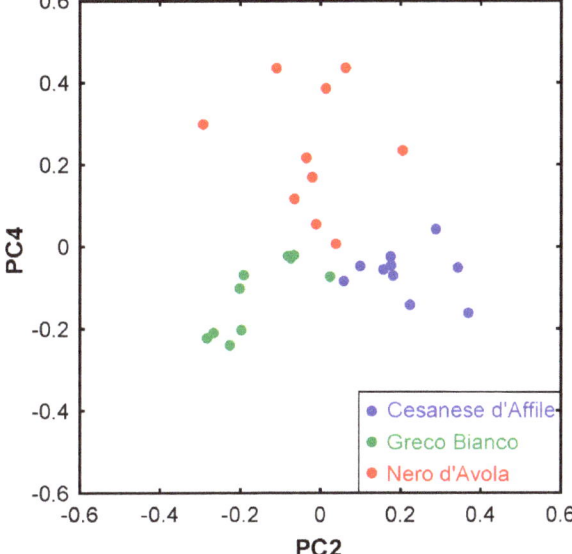

Figure 2. Score plot of the PCA of the FTIR spectra. Each dot represents the PC4 vs. PC2 scores of one spectrum recorded from an individual sample of grape seed.

4. Conclusions

This research showed that grape seeds are rich in beneficial polyunsaturated fatty acids and polyphenols and hence they can represent a promising source of nutraceuticals. The analysis of the chemical profiles of Cesanese d' Affile, Greco bianco, and Nero d'Avola seeds revealed that Cesanese d' Affile exhibits the highest fat content with a significant fraction of unsaturated fatty acids. On the other hand, the seeds of Nero D'Avola show the highest amount of phenolic compounds.

Moroever, we have shown that the grape seeds from different grape cultivars can be distinguished by FTIR-ATR spectroscopy using a chemometric data analysis. It was possible to link selected spectral signatures, which the principal component analysis picks up for the discrimination, with the chemical profiles. This is interesting as PCA is a purely mathematical tool, but to some extent it helps to understand the underlying physics. Overall, we conclude that FTIR spectroscopy is a suitable tool for applications in the oenological sector. This may facilitate the advanced detection of adulteration in the future. The term "advanced" in this context means that, e.g., the mixing of certain grape seeds with other "cheaper" ones from a minor quality cultivar can be revealed. In order to tap the full potential of FTIR spectroscopy it should be combined with multivariate data analysis. If the algorithms are trained with sufficiently large calibration data sets, such analyses can yield a multitude of parameters and make other (often more expensive and time consuming) analytical methods become redundant. Further FTIR/chemometrics studies on a huge number of samples will be addressed to the developed calibration models for the identification and quantification of the main bioactive compounds present in the waste.

The qualitative-quantitative knowledge of fatty acids and condensed tannins obtained with destructive analysis techniques can represent a first data-base useful to validate and make reliable the FTIR technique as quality and titre monitoring of active principles in grape seeds.

Author Contributions: M.L., A.S. and F.C. initiated the project and planned the experimental work; N.B., P.G., M.L., M.M., M.C., S.F.N., and A.D. performed the experiments; M.L., A.D., J.K. and A.L. processed and evaluated the data; A.D., M.L., A.L., and J.K. contributed to interpreting the data; M.L., A.D., J.K., A.S., G.L.-B., E.B.S., A.R., N.B., and F.C. wrote the first draft of the manuscript. All authors revised and improved the manuscript. All authors have read and agreed to the published version of the manuscript.

Funding: This research received funding from Italcol SpA, Consulente Enologica Srl and the support of the Project NATUR-BAKERY-INNOV" Innovative production of a bakery line, for well-being and sport, based on functional natural extracts"—POR FESR 2014–2020—CUP 7429.31052017.113000254. Authors thank the support of the project: Nutraceutica come supporto nutrizionale nel paziente oncologico; CUP: B83D18000140007.

Conflicts of Interest: The authors declare no conflict of interest.

Appendix A

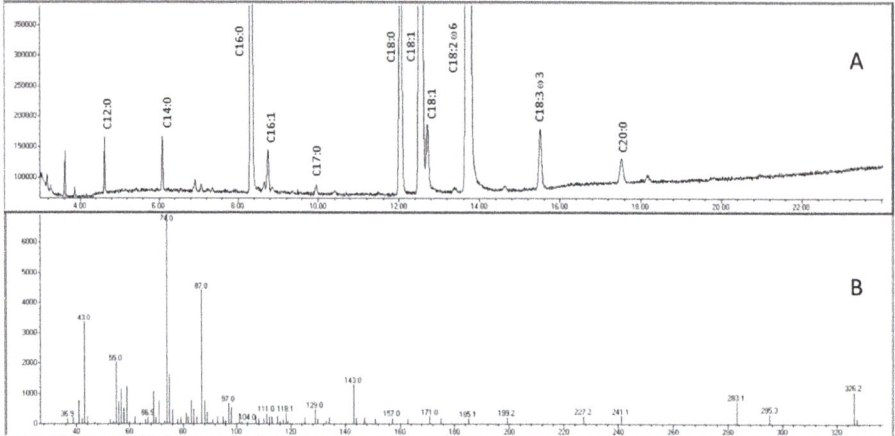

Figure A1. (**A**) Total Ion Chromatogram (TIC) of fatty acid profile of Nero d'Avola sample and (**B**) GC/MS spectrum used for peaks identification (example of arachidonic acid).

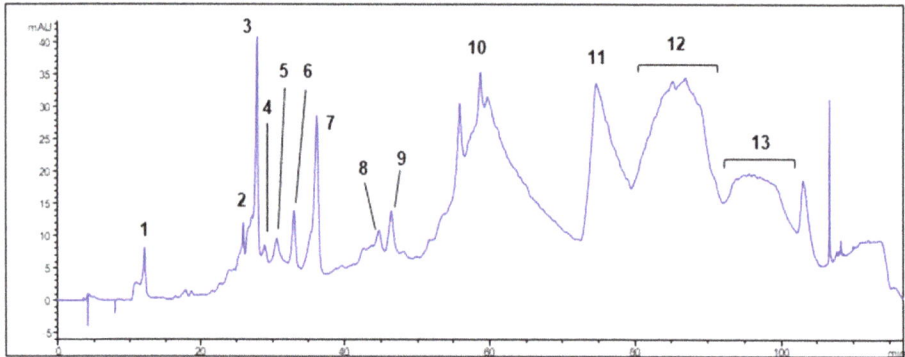

Figure A2. Chromatographic profile of Nero d'Avola seed extract, acquired at 280 nm. 1. Gallic acid; 2. Catechin dimer B3; 3. Catechin; 4. Procyanidin trimer; 5. Catechin dimer B6; 6. Catechin dimer B2; 7. Epicatechin; 8. Catechin trimer; 9. Epicatechin gallate dimer; 10. Catechin oligomers expressed as tetramers; 11. Epicatechin gallate dimer; 12. Catechin/epicatechin trimers digallate; 13. Catechin/epicatechin trimers gallate.

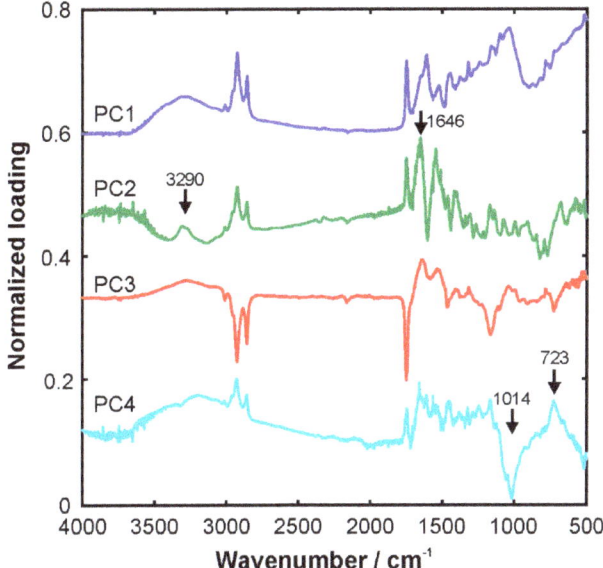

Figure A3. Loadings vs. wavenumber plot of the first 4 PCs of the FTIR spectra.

References

1. Tuck, C.O.; Perez, E.; Horvath, I.T.; Sheldon, R.A.; Poliakoff, M. Valorization of biomass: Deriving more value from waste. *Science* **2012**, *337*, 695–699. [CrossRef]
2. Lin, C.S.K.; Koutinas, A.A.; Stamatelatou, K.; Mubofu, E.B.; Matharu, A.S.; Kopsahelis, N.; Pfaltzgraff, L.A.; Clark, J.H.; Papanikolaou, S.; Kwan, T.H.; et al. Current and future trends in food waste valorization for the production of chemicals, materials and fuels: A global perspective. *Biofuels Bioprod. Biorefin.* **2014**, *8*, 686–715. [CrossRef]
3. Lin, C.S.K.; Luque, R. *Renewable Resources and Biorefineries*; Royal Society of Chemistry: Cambridge, UK, 2014.
4. Zuin, V.G.; Ramin, L.Z. Green and Sustainable Separation of Natural Products from Agro-Industrial Waste: Challenges, Potentialities and Perspectives on Emerging Approach. *Top. Curr. Chem.* **2018**, *376*, 1–54. [CrossRef]
5. Lucarini, M.; Durazzo, A.; Romani, A.; Campo, M.; Lombardi-Boccia, G.; Cecchini, F. Bio-Based Compounds from Grape Seeds: A Biorefinery Approach. *Molecules* **2018**, *23*, 1888. [CrossRef]
6. Ruggieri, L.; Cadena, E.; Martínez-Blanco, J.; Gasol, C.M.; Rieradevall, J.; Gabarrell, X.; Gea, T.; Sort, X.; Sánchez, A. Recovery of organic wastes in the Spanish wine industry. Technical, economic and environmental analyses of the composting process. *J. Clean. Prod.* **2009**, *17*, 830–838. [CrossRef]
7. Ribéreau-Gayon, P.; Glories, Y.; Maujean, A.; Dubourdieu, D. *Trattato di Enologia*, 3rd ed.; Edagricole: Bologna, Italy, 2007.
8. Devesa-Rey, R.; Vecino, X.; Varela-Alende, J.L.; Barral, M.T.; Cruz, J.M.; Moldes, A.B. Valorization of winery waste vs. the costs of not recycling. *Waste Manag.* **2011**, *11*, 2327–2335. [CrossRef]
9. Xu, C.; Zhang, Y.; Zhang, Y.; Jun, W.; Lu, J. Extraction, distribution and characterisation of phenolic compounds and oil in grapeseeds. *Food Chem.* **2010**, *122*, 688–694. [CrossRef]
10. Romani, A.; Campo, C.; Pinelli, P. HPLC/DAD/ESI-MS analyses and antiradical activity of hydrolyzable tannins from different vegetal species. *Food Chem.* **2012**, *130*, 214–221. [CrossRef]
11. Garavaglia, J.; Markoski, M.M.; Oliveira, A.; Marcadenti, A. Grape Seed Oil Compounds: Biological and Chemical Actions for Health. *Nutr. Metab. Insights* **2016**, *9*, 59–64. [CrossRef]
12. Durante, M.; Montefusco, A.; Marrese, P.P.; Soccio, M.; Pastore, D.; Piro, G.; Mita, G.; Lenucci, M.S. Seeds of pomegranate, tomato and grapes: An underestimated source of natural bioactive molecules and antioxidants from agri-food by-products. *J. Agric. Food Chem.* **2017**, *63*, 65–72. [CrossRef]

13. Shinagawa, F.B.; de Santana, F.C.; Araujo, E.; Purgatto, E.; Mancini-Filho, J. Chemical composition of cold pressed Brazilian grape seed oil. *Food Sci. Technol.* **2017**, *38*, 164–171. [CrossRef]
14. Durazzo, A.; Lucarini, M. Editorial: The state of science and innovation of bioactive research and applications, health, and diseases. *Front. Nutr.* **2019**, *6*, 178. [CrossRef]
15. Santini, A.; Tenore, G.C.; Novellino, E. Nutraceuticals: A paradigm of proactive medicine. *Eur. J. Pharm. Sci.* **2017**, *96*, 53–61. [CrossRef]
16. Santini, A.; Novellino, E. Nutraceuticals: Shedding light on the grey area between pharmaceuticals and food. *Expert Rev. Clin. Pharmacol.* **2018**, *11*, 545–547. [CrossRef]
17. Abenavoli, L.; Izzo, A.A.; Milić, N.; Cicala, C.; Santini, A.; Capasso, R. Milk thistle (*Silybum marianum*): A concise overview on its chemistry, pharmacological, and nutraceutical uses in liver diseases. *Phytother. Res.* **2018**, *32*, 2202–2213. [CrossRef]
18. Daliu, P.; Santini, A.; Novellino, E. A decade of nutraceutical patents: Where are we now in 2018? *Expert Opin. Ther. Pat.* **2018**, *28*, 875–882. [CrossRef]
19. Durazzo, A.; Lucarini, M.A. Current shot and re-thinking of antioxidant research strategy. *Braz. J. Anal. Chem.* **2018**, *5*, 9–11. [CrossRef]
20. Daliu, P.; Santini, A.; Novellino, E. From pharmaceuticals to nutraceuticals: Bridging disease prevention and management. *Expert Rev. Clin. Pharm.* **2019**, *12*, 1–7. [CrossRef]
21. Durazzo, A.; Lucarini, M.; Souto, E.B.; Cicala, C.; Caiazzo, E.; Izzo, A.A.; Novellino, E.; Santini, A. Polyphenols: A concise overview on the chemistry, occurrence and human health. *Phytother. Res.* **2019**, *33*, 2221–2243. [CrossRef]
22. Ferhi, S.; Santaniello, S.; Zerizer, S.; Cruciani, S.; Fadda, A.; Sanna, D.; Dore, A.; Maioli, M.; D'hallewin, G. Total phenols from grape leaves counteract cell proliferation and modulate apoptosis-related gene expression in MCF-7 and HepG2 human cancer cell lines. *Molecules* **2019**, *24*, 612. [CrossRef]
23. Di Meo, F.; Aversano, R.; Diretto, G.; Demurtas, O.C.; Villano, C.; Cozzolino, S.; Filosa, S.; Carputo, D.; Crispi, S. Anti-cancer activity of grape seed semi-polar extracts in human mesothelioma cell lines. *J. Funct. Foods* **2019**, *61*, 103515. [CrossRef]
24. Bijak, M.; Sut, A.; Kosiorek, A.; Saluk-Bijak, J.; Golanski, J. Dual Anticoagulant/Antiplatelet Activity of Polyphenolic Grape Seeds Extract. *Nutrients* **2019**, *11*, 93. [CrossRef]
25. Burcova, Z.; Kreps, F.; Schmidt, S.; Strizincova, P.; Jablonsky, M.; Kyselka, J.; Haz, A.; Surina, I. Antioxidant Activity and the Tocopherol and Phenol Contents of Grape Residues. *Bioresources* **2019**, *14*, 4146–4156.
26. Kong, F.; Qin, Y.; Su, Z.; Ning, Z.; Yu, S. Optimization of Extraction of Hypoglycemic Ingredients from Grape Seeds and Evaluation of α-Glucosidase and α-Amylase Inhibitory Effects In Vitro. *J. Food Sci.* **2018**, *83*, 1422–1429. [CrossRef]
27. Sabir, A.; Unver, A.; Kara, Z. The fatty acid and tocopherol constituents of the seed oil extracted from 21 grape varieties (*Vitis* spp.). *J. Sci. Food Agric.* **2012**, *92*, 1982–1987. [CrossRef]
28. Friedel, M.; Patz, C.D.; Dietrich, H. Comparison of different measurement techniques and variable selection methods for FT-MIR in wine analysis. *Food Chem.* **2013**, *141*, 4200–4207. [CrossRef]
29. He, Z.H.; Duan, X.R.; Ma, Z.H. Measuring Routine Parameters of Wine by ATR-MIR Spectroscopy. *Appl. Mech. Mater.* **2013**, *397*, 1749–1752. [CrossRef]
30. Ismail, E.H.; Khalil, M.M.H.; Al Seif, F.A.; El-Magdoub, F. Biosynthesis of gold nanoparticles using extract of grape (*Vitis vinifera*) leaves and seeds. *Prog. Nanotechnol. Nanomater.* **2014**, *3*, 1–12.
31. Mohansrinivasan, V.; Devi, C.; Deori, M.; Biswas, A.; Naine, J.S. Exploring the anticancer activity of grape seed extract on skin cancer cell lines A431. *Braz. Arch. Biol. Technol.* **2015**, *58*, 540–546. [CrossRef]
32. Canbay, H.S.; Bardakçı, B. Determination of fatty acid, C, H, N and trace element composition in grape seed by GC/MS, FTIR, elemental analyzer and ICP/OES. *SDU J. Sci.* **2011**, *6*, 140–148.
33. Nogales-Bueno, J.; Baca-Bocanegra, B.; Rodríguez-Pulido, F.J.; Heredia, F.J.; Hernández-Hierro, J.M. Use of near infrared hyperspectral tools for the screening of extractable polyphenols in red grape skins. *Food Chem.* **2015**, *172*, 559–564. [CrossRef]
34. Nogales-Bueno, J.; Baca-Bocanegra, B.; Rooney, A.; Hernández-Hierro, J.M.; Heredia, F.J.; Byrne, H.J. Linking ATR-FTIR and Raman features to phenolic extractability and other attributes in grape skin. *Talanta* **2017**, *167*, 44–50. [CrossRef]

35. Nogales-Bueno, J.; Baca-Bocanegra, B.; Rooney, A.; Hernández-Hierro, J.M.; Byrne, H.J.; Heredia, F.J. Study of phenolic extractability in grape seeds by means of ATR-FTIR and Raman spectroscopy. *Food Chem.* **2017**, *232*, 602–609. [CrossRef]
36. Torres-Climent, A.; Gomis, P.; Martín-Mata, J.; Bustamante, M.A.; Marhuenda-Egea, F.C.; Pérez-Murcia, M.D.; Pérez-Espinosa, A.; Paredes, C.; Moral, R. Chemical, thermal and spectroscopic methods to assess biodegradation of winery-distillery wastes during composting. *PLoS ONE* **2015**, *10*, e0138925. [CrossRef]
37. Hanganu, A.; Todasca, M.C.; Chira, N.A.; Maganu, M.; Rosca, S. The compositional characterisation of Romanian grape seed oils using spectroscopic methods. *Food Chem.* **2012**, *134*, 2453–2458. [CrossRef]
38. Nurrulhidayah, A.F.; Che Man, Y.B.; Al-Kahtani, H.A.; Rohman, A. Application of FTIR spectroscopy coupled with chemometrics for authentication of Nigella sativa seed oil. *Spectroscopy* **2011**, *25*, 243–250. [CrossRef]
39. Moretti, S.; Giannini, B.; Cecchini, F.; Garofolo, M. Cambiamenti dell'attività antiossidante, durante il periodo di maturazione della bacca, in due diverse varietà di uva e loro relazione con il contenuto polifenolico. In Proceedings of the Atti del XXXIII Congresso Mondiale Della Vigna e del Vino (OIV), Tbilisi, GA, USA, 20–27 June 2010.
40. Cecchini, F.; Bevilacqua, N.; Morassut, M. Bioactive compounds of winery by-products: The sustainable development of oenological field. In Proceedings of the 6th International Virtual Conference on Advanced Scientific Results, Ziina, Slovakia, 25–29 June 2018; pp. 236–240.
41. Giannini, B.; Cecchini, F.; Moretti, S. Nutraceutic property of Italian red and white grape cultivar and wine. In *Proceedings of the 2nd International Symposium of Wine Active Compounds, Dijon, France, March 2011*; Chassagne, D., Ed.; Oenoplurimédia, Chaintré: Bourgogne, France, 2011; pp. 321–322.
42. Bligh, E.G.; Dyer, W.J. A rapid method of total lipid extraction and purification. *Can. J. Biochem. Physiol.* **1959**, *37*, 911–917. [CrossRef]
43. Christie, W.W. Preparation of ester derivatives of fatty acids for chromatographic analysis. *Adv. Lipid Methodol.* **1993**, *2*, 69–111.
44. Lucarini, M.; Durazzo, A.; Sánchez del Pulgar, V.; Gabrielli, P.; Lombardi-Boccia, G. Determination of fatty acid content in meat and meat products: The FTIR-ATR approach. *Food Chem.* **2018**, *267*, 223–230. [CrossRef]
45. Romani, A.; Ieri, F.; Turchetti, B.; Mulinacci, N.; Vincieri, F.F.; Buzzini, P. Analysis of condensed and hydrolyzable tannins from commercial plant extracts. *J. Pharm. Biomed. Anal.* **2006**, *41*, 415–420. [CrossRef]
46. Hotelling, H. Analysis of a complex of statistical variables into principal components. *J. Educ. Psychol.* **1933**, *24*, 417. [CrossRef]
47. Jolliffe, I. *Principal Component Analysis*; John Wiley & Sons: Hoboken, NJ, USA, 2002.
48. Pearson, K. Principal components analysis. *Lond. Edinb. Dublin Philos. Mag. J. Sci.* **1901**, *6*, 559. [CrossRef]
49. Wold, S.; Esbensen, K.; Geladi, P. Principal Component Analysis. *Chemom. Intell. Lab. Syst.* **1987**, *2*, 37–52. [CrossRef]
50. Pérez-Navarro, J.; Da Ros, A.; Masuero, D.; Izquierdo-Cañas, P.M.; Hermosín-Gutiérrez, I.; Gómez-Alonso, S.; Mattivi, F.; Vrhovsek, U. LC-MS/MS analysis of free fatty acid composition and other lipids in skins and seeds of Vitis vinifera grape cultivars. *Food Res. Int.* **2019**, *125*, 108556. [CrossRef]
51. Messina, C.M.; Manuguerra, S.; Catalano, G.; Arena, R.; Cocchi, M.; Morghese, M.; Montenegro, L.; Santulli, A. Green biotechnology for valorisation of residual biomasses in nutraceutic sector: Characterization and extraction of bioactive compounds from grape pomace and evaluation of the protective effects in vitro. *Nat. Prod. Res.* **2019**, *6*, 1–6. [CrossRef]
52. Zdunić, G.; Godevac, D.; Šavikin, K.; Krivokuća, D.; Mihailović, M.; Pržić, Z.; Marković, N. Grape Seed Polyphenols and Fatty Acids of Autochthonous Prokupac Vine Variety from Serbia. *Chem. Biodivers.* **2019**, *16*, e1900053, Epub 2019 May 29. [CrossRef]
53. Giannini, B.; Mulinacci, N.; Pasqua, G.; Innocenti, M.; Valletta, A.; Cecchini, F. Phenolics and antioxidant activity in different cultivars/clones of *Vitis vinifera* L. seeds over two years. *Plant Biosyst.* **2016**, *150*, 1408–1416. [CrossRef]
54. Kennedy, J.A.; Troup, G.J.; Pilbrow, J.R.; Hutton, D.R.; Hewitt, D.; Hunter, C.R.; Jones, G.P. Development of seed polyphenols in berries from *Vitis vinifera* L. cv. Shiraz. *Aust. J. Grape Wine Res.* **2000**, *6*, 244–254. [CrossRef]
55. Sorolla, S.; Flores, A.; Canals, T.; Cantero, R.; Font, J.; Ollé, L.; Bacardit, A. Study of the Qualitative and Semi-quantitative Analysis of Grape Seed Extract by HPLC. *J. Am. Leather Chem. Assoc.* **2018**, *113*, 3.

56. Smith, B.C. *Infrared Spectra Interpretation. A Systematic Approach*, 1st ed.; CRC Press LLC: Boca Raton, FL, USA, 1999.
57. Lupoi, J.S.; Singh, S.; Parthasarathi, R.; Simmons, B.A.; Henry, R.J. Recent innovations in analytical methods for the qualitative and quantitative assessment of lignin. *Renew. Sustain. Energy Rev.* **2015**, *49*, 871–906. [CrossRef]
58. Heredia-Guerrero, J.A.; Benítez, J.J.; Domínguez, E.; Bayer, I.; Cingolani, R.; Athanassiou, A.; Heredia, A. Infrared and Raman spectroscopic features of plant cuticles: A review. *Front. Plant Sci.* **2014**, *5*, 305. [CrossRef] [PubMed]
59. Fasoli, M.; Dell'Anna, R.; Dal Santo, S.; Balestrini, R.; Sanson, A.; Pezzotti, M.; Zenoni, S. Pectins, hemicelluloses and celluloses show specific dynamics in the internal and external surfaces of grape berry skin during ripening. *Plant Cell Physiol.* **2016**, *57*, 1332–1349. [CrossRef] [PubMed]
60. Wilson, R.H.; Smith, A.C.; Kačuráková, M.; Saunders, P.K.; Wellner, N.; Waldron, K.W. The mechanical properties and molecular dynamics of plant cell wall polysaccharides studied by Fourier-transform infrared spectroscopy. *Plant Physiol.* **2000**, *124*, 397–406. [CrossRef] [PubMed]
61. Gao, Y.; Fangel, J.U.; Willats, W.G.T.; Vivier, M.A.; Moore, J.P. Dissecting the polysaccharide-rich grape cell wall changes during winemaking using combined high-throughput and fractionation methods. *Carbohydr. Polym.* **2015**, *133*, 567–577. [CrossRef]
62. Ricci, A.; Olejar, K.J.; Parpinello, G.P.; Kilmartin, P.A.; Versari, A. Application of Fourier transform infrared (FTIR) spectroscopy in the characterization of tannins. *Appl. Spectrosc. Rev.* **2015**, *50*, 407–442. [CrossRef]
63. Mahesar, S.A.; Lucarini, M.; Durazzo, A.; Santini, A.; Lampe, A.I.; Kiefer, J. Application of Infrared Spectroscopy for Functional Compounds Evaluation in Olive Oil: A Current Snapshot. *J. Spectrosc.* **2019**, *2019*, 5319024. [CrossRef]
64. Kiefer, J.; Noack, K.; Bartelmess, J.; Walter, C.; Dörnenburg, H.; Leipertz, A. Vibrational structure of the polyunsaturated fatty acids eicosapentaenoic acid and arachidonic acid studied by infrared spectroscopy. *J. Mol. Struct.* **2010**, *965*, 121–124. [CrossRef]

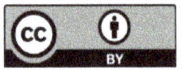

© 2019 by the authors. Licensee MDPI, Basel, Switzerland. This article is an open access article distributed under the terms and conditions of the Creative Commons Attribution (CC BY) license (http://creativecommons.org/licenses/by/4.0/).

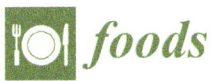

Communication

Anti-adipogenic Effect of β-Carboline Alkaloids from Garlic (*Allium sativum*)

Su Cheol Baek [†], Ki Hong Nam [†], Sang Ah Yi [†], Mun Seok Jo, Kwang Ho Lee, Yong Hoon Lee, Jaecheol Lee * and Ki Hyun Kim *

School of Pharmacy, Sungkyunkwan University, Suwon 16419, Korea; schii513@daum.net (S.C.B.); nam6422@hanmail.net (K.H.N.); angelna1023@hanmail.net (S.A.Y.); anstjr920827@gmail.com (M.S.J.); sholaly@naver.com (K.H.L.); yhl2090@naver.com (Y.H.L.)
* Correspondence: jaecheol@skku.edu (J.L.); khkim83@skku.edu (K.H.K.); Tel.: +82-31-290-7726 (J.L.); +82-31-290-7700 (K.H.K.)
† These authors contributed equally to this work.

Received: 16 November 2019; Accepted: 10 December 2019; Published: 12 December 2019

Abstract: Garlic (*Allium sativum* L.) is utilized worldwide for culinary and medicinal use and has diverse health benefits. As part of our ongoing research to identify bioactive components from natural resources, phytochemical analysis of the methanolic extract of garlic led to the isolation and characterization of six compounds: Three eugenol diglycosides (**1–3**) and three β-carboline alkaloids (**4–6**). In particular, the absolute configurations of β-carboline alkaloids (**5** and **6**) were established by gauge-including atomic orbital nuclear magnetic resonance chemical shift calculations, followed by DP4+ analysis. Here, we evaluated the effects of compounds **1–6** on 3T3-L1 preadipocyte adipogenesis and lipid metabolism. 3T3-L1 adipocyte differentiation was evaluated using Oil Red O staining; the expression of adipogenic genes was detected using RT-qPCR. Among compounds **1–6**, (1*R*,3*S*)-1-methyl-1,2,3,4-tetrahydro-β-carboline-3-carboxylic acid (**6**) inhibited 3T3-L1 preadipocyte adipogenesis and reduced the expression of adipogenic genes (*Fabp4*, *PPARγ*, *C/EBPβ*, *Adipsin*, and *Adipoq*). Moreover, it markedly decreased the actylation of α-tubulin, which is crucial for cytoskeletal remodeling during adipogenesis. Anti-adipogenic effects were observed upon treatment with compound **6**, not only during the entire process, but also on the first two days of adipogenesis. Additionally, treatment with compound **6** regulated the expression of genes involved in adipocyte lipid metabolism, decreasing the lipogenic gene (*SREBP1*) and increasing lipolytic genes (*ATGL* and *HSL*). We provide experimental evidence of the health benefits of using (1*R*,3*S*) 1-methyl-1,2,3,4-tetrahydro-β-carboline-3-carboxylic acid obtained from garlic to prevent excessive adipogenesis in obesity.

Keywords: *Allium sativum*; β-carboline alkaloids; anti-adipogenic effects; 3T3-L1 preadipocytes; Ac-α-tubulin

---

1. Introduction

Garlic (*Allium sativum* L.) is one of the bulbous plants in the family Liliaceae, more recently attributed to the family Amaryllidaceae [1]. Since ancient times and to date, garlic has been a part of people's lives as a condiment or culinary spice, therapeutic agent against common diseases, cleansing aid, and energy booster for athletes. Interestingly, in ancient Greece and Rome, the consumption of garlic was believed to give courage to soldiers and sailors, respectively. [2]. The most commonly utilized part of garlic is its bulb, which has a characteristic spicy and pungent flavor and is a fundamental component in several cuisines from Southern, Eastern, and Southeastern Asia, Northern Africa, Middle East, and Southern Europe. Since ancient times, garlic has been used in traditional medicine to treat fevers, headaches, intestinal worms, and dysentery [3]. In Asia, garlic is used as a food preservative, a remedy for fever or indigestion, and an antimicrobial agent [4]. Garlic is well-known for its effects against cancer and for increasing immunity; therefore, it is sold as a functional food worldwide [5]. Further, garlic extracts exhibit antifungal, antibacterial, antiviral, antioxidant, immuno-stimulating, and cholesterol-lowering properties [6,7]; the therapeutic functions of garlic in chronic diseases include the prevention of diabetes and platelet aggregation [8–11]. Several literatures demonstrated the correlation between the consumption of garlic and the decreased risk of cancer development in various organs [12–14]. The anticancer potential of garlic has been known to be due to the interaction of bioactive components in garlic with specific molecular targets, which range from cell cycle control to the expression of antioxidants and detoxification enzymes [15,16]. Owing to the health benefits of garlic, its phytochemical constituents have been actively investigated. Garlic is predominantly composed of organosulfur compounds, which give it its pungent smell and spicy taste. A major sulfur-containing compound in garlic is S-allyl-L-cysteine sulfoxide (alliin) [17], which forms complexes with the enzyme alliinase, following crushing, cutting, or grinding of garlic bulbs [3]. Alliinase causes the breakdown of alliin to form various volatile sulfur compounds like diallyl sulfide and diallyl disulfide [18,19]. Other reported compounds in the alliums are saponins and polyphenols, which contribute to the bioactivity of allium plant extracts [18–20]. In addition, previous phytochemical studies of garlic revealed the presence of eugenol diglycosides and β-carboline alkaloids with biological activities [20,21].

As part of our ongoing research to identify bioactive components from Korean natural resources [22–24], we explored the potential bioactive constituents of garlic. The phytochemical analysis of the methanolic (MeOH) extract of garlic led to the isolation of six compounds: Three eugenol diglycosides (**1–3**) and three β-carboline alkaloids (**4–6**). They were identified via a comparison of their nuclear magnetic resonance (NMR) spectroscopic data with reported values, as well as by LC/MS analysis. Absolute configurations of the β-carboline alkaloids (**5** and **6**) were established using gauge-including atomic orbital (GIAO) NMR chemical shift calculations, followed by DP4+ analysis. Several studies have identified garlic-derived organosulfur compounds that display anti-obesity effects [25–28]. However, there is limited information about the metabolic effects of other active compounds isolated from garlic compared to that of the organosulfur compounds. In this study, we evaluated the effects of compounds **1–6** on the adipogenesis of 3T3-L1 preadipocytes and lipid metabolism, suggesting the potential therapeutic activity of these compounds against obesity and metabolic diseases. Here, we provide details on the extract, isolation, and structural clarity of the compounds, as well as their biological effects on the lipid metabolism of adipocytes.

2. Materials and Methods

2.1. Extraction of Garlic Sample and Isolation of Compounds

General experimental procedures and information regarding the garlic sample used in this study are included in Supplementary Materials. Minced *A. sativum* (1 kg) was extracted three times with 100% MeOH (18 L) in a day at room temperature and filtered. The resultant filtrate was evaporated using a rotavapor, which gave the MeOH extract (101.7 g). The MeOH extract was successively subjected to solvent-partitioning with *n*-hexane, CH_2Cl_2 (MC), ethyl acetate (EA), and *n*-butanol (BuOH), yielding residues weighing 1.4, 0.287, 0.153, and 4.5 g, respectively. A detailed description of the phytochemical analysis and isolation of the six compounds (**1-6**) from *n*-BuOH-soluble fraction are included in Supplementary Materials.

2.2. Cell Culture and Differentiation

3T3-L1 preadipocytes were maintained in DMEM containing 10% bovine calf serum (BCS) and 1% P/S. For the differentiation of 3T3-L1 cells into mature adipocytes, the cells were incubated in DMEM with 10% FBS, 1% P/S, 0.5 mM of 3-isobuyl-1-methylxanthine (IBMX), 1 μM of dexamethasone, and 1 μg/mL of insulin. Then, the medium was replaced every 2 days with DMEM with 10% FBS, 1% P/S, and 1 μg/mL of insulin. To assess the effects of compounds **1–6** on adipogenesis, we treated 3T3-L1 cells with compounds **1–6** during the entire process of adipogenesis. Eight days after starting differentiation (day 8), the cells were harvested and subjected to further experiments, including immunoblotting and RT-qPCR.

2.3. Cell Counting

3T3-L1 cells were treated with compounds **1–6** for 24 h, then detached from the plate with EDTA. The detached cells were diluted with PBS, and the cell number was counted using LUNA-II™ Automated Cell Counter (Logos Biosystems, Anyang, Korea).

2.4. Immunoblotting

Proteins in the adipocytes were extracted using Pro-Prep (Intron Biotechnology, Seongnam, Korea), and 20 µg of each protein was separated by SDS-polyacrylamide gel (12%) electrophoresis. Separated proteins were transferred to polyvinylidene difluoride (PVDF, Millipore, Burlington, MA, USA) membranes via a semi-dry transfer (Bio-Rad, Hercules, CA, USA). The membranes were blocked with non-fat dry milk for 1 h and incubated with the indicated primary antibodies (dilution 1:2000) overnight, followed by incubation with horseradish peroxidase (HRP)-conjugated secondary antibodies for 1 h (Abcam, Cambridge, UK). HRP signals reacting with chemiluminescence reagents (Abclon, Guro, Korea) were detected on AGFA x-ray film CP-Bu NEW and quantified using ImageJ. Anti-acetylated α tubulin (Santa Cruz Biotechnology, SC-23950, Dallas, TX, USA) and anti-tubulin (Santa Cruz Biotechnology, SC-32293, Dallas, TX, USA) were used for the immunoblotting assay.

2.5. Reverse Transcription and Quantitative Real-Time PCR (RT-qPCR)

Total RNA from the adipocytes was extracted with Easy-Blue reagent (Intron Biotechnology). Then, cDNA was generated from 1 µg of extracted RNA using the Maxim RT-PreMix Kit (Intron Biotechnology). For quantitative real-time PCR (qPCR), cDNA was mixed with KAPA SYBR® FAST qPCR Master Mix (Kapa Biosystems) and each primer is mentioned below. The qPCR reaction was detected using a CFX96 Touch™ real-time PCR detector (Bio-Rad). Relative mRNA levels for each reaction were normalized to that of *β-Actin*. Relative expression differences were calculated using the ΔΔCT method [29]. The qPCR primer sequences used in this study are listed in Table 1.

Table 1. Sequences of primers for mRNA used in RT-qPCR.

Gene	Forward	Reverse
β-Actin	5′-ACGGCCAGGTCATCACTATTG-3′	5′-TGGATGCCACAGGATTCCA-3′
Adipsin	5′-CATGCTCGGCCCTACATG-3′	5′-CACAGAGTCGTCATCCGTCAC-3′
Adipoq	5′-TGTTCCTCTTAATCCTGCCCA-3′	5′-CCAACCTGCACAAGTTCCCTT 3′
ATGL	5′-TTCACCATCCGCTTGTTGGAG-3′	5′-AGATGGTCACCCAATTTCCTC-3′
C/EBPα	5′-CTCCCAGAGGACCAATGAAA-3′	5′-AAGTCTTAGCCGGAGGAAGC-3′
C/EBPβ	5′-GGACAAGCTGAGCGACGAGTA-3′	5′-CAGCTGCTCCACCTTCTTCTG-3′
Fabp4	5′-AAGGTGAAGAGCATCATAACCCT-3′	5′-TCACGCCTTTCATAACACATTCC-3′
HSL	5′-CACAAAGGCTGCTTCTACGG-3′	5′-GGAGAGAGTCTGCAGGAACG-3′
PPARγ	5′-GCATGGTGCCTTCGCTGA-3′	5′-TGGCATCTCTGTGTCAACCATG-3′
SREBP1	5′-AACGTCACTTCCAGCTAGAC-3′	5′-CCACTAAGGTGCCTACAGAGC-3′

2.6. Oil Red O Staining

Oil Red O staining was performed to visualize lipid droplets in the adipocytes. Mature adipocytes were fixed with 10% formaldehyde for 1 h and washed with 60% isopropanol. Then, the cells were incubated with the Oil Red O working solution for 1 h, followed by washing twice with distilled water. To prepare the Oil Red O stock solution, 300 mg of Oil Red O powder was dissolved in 100 mL of 99% isopropanol. The Oil Red O working solution, prepared just before use, contained three parts of Oil Red O stock solution and two parts of distilled water.

2.7. Statistical Analysis

Statistical significance was evaluated using Student's two-tailed t-test with Excel and assessed based on the *p*-value. Data represent the means ± SEM for n = 3. * $p < 0.05$, ** $p < 0.01$, and *** $p < 0.001$.

3. Results and Discussion

3.1. Identification of Compounds

The phytochemical analysis of the *n*-BuOH-soluble fraction from the methanol extract of garlic was performed using column chromatography and HPLC purification along with LC/MS-based analysis. The analysis led to the isolation of six compounds (**1–6**), including three eugenol diglycosides (**1–3**) and three β-carboline alkaloids (**4–6**) (Figure 1). The compounds were identified as eugenyl-*O*-β-D-glucopyranosyl-(1→6)-β-D-glucopyranoside (**1**) [30], 4-*O*-β-D-glucopyranosyl(1→6)-β-D-glucopyranosyl 5-methoxy eugenol (**2**) [30], eugenyl *O*-α-D-rhamnopyranosyl-(1→6)-β-D-glucopyranoside (**3**) [31], (3*S*)-1,2,3,4-tetrahydro-β-carboline-3-carboxylic acid (**4**) [32], (1*S*,3*S*)-1-methyl-1,2,3,4-tetrahydro-β-carboline-3-carboxylic acid (**5**) [32], and (1*R*,3*S*)-1-methyl-1,2,3,4-tetrahydro-β-carboline-3-carboxylic acid (**6**) [32], by comparing their NMR spectroscopic data with reported values as well as by LC/MS analysis. In particular, the absolute configurations of β-carboline alkaloids (**5** and **6**) were established by GIAO NMR chemical shift calculations, followed by DP4+ analysis [33]. Given that the β-carboline alkaloids (**5** and **6**) were likely biosynthetically produced from L-tryptophan, a naturally occurring product, the computationally calculated ^{1}H NMR chemical shifts of two possible diastereomers (1*S*,3*S*)-**5/6** and (1*R*,3*S*)-**5/6** were compared with the experimental values of **5** and **6** using the results of the DP4+ analysis. The comparison indicated a structural equality of **5** to (1*S*,3*S*)-**5** with 98.54% probability and **6** to (1*R*,3*S*)-**6** with 99.46% probability (Figures S1 and S2). Further, according to the formula $\Delta\delta = \delta_{calcd} - \delta_{exptl}$, differences (Δδ) were calculated (Tables S1 and S2). The correlation coefficient (R^2) from linear regression analysis, largest absolute deviation (LAD), and the mean absolute deviation (MAD) for the ^{1}H NMR data of (1*S*,3*S*)-**5** were 0.9884 (Figure 2A), 1.18, and 0.22 (Figure 2B), respectively, whereas R^2, LAD, and MAD values for the data of (1*R*,3*S*)-**5** were 0.9860, 1.26, and 0.25, respectively. These obtained data supported the result from DP4+ probability analysis to be (1*S*,3*S*) in **5**. In the case of **6**, R^2, LAD, and MAD for ^{1}H NMR data of (1*S*,3*S*)-**6** were 0.9855 (Figure 2C), 1.38, and 0.25 (Figure 2D), respectively, whereas R^2, LAD, and MAD values for the data of (1*R*,3*S*)-**6** were 0.9858, 1.25, and 0.28, respectively. Accordingly, the absolute configuration of **6** was assigned to be (1*R*,3*S*), which was in agreement with the DP4+ probability analysis of **6**.

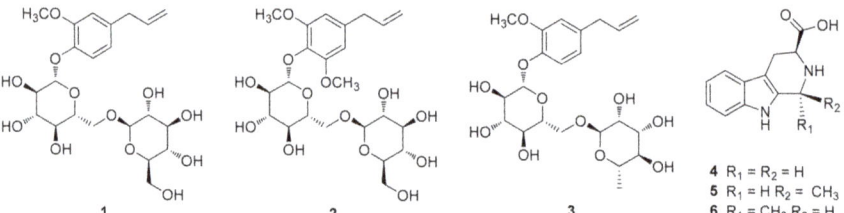

Figure 1. Chemical structures of compounds **1–6**.

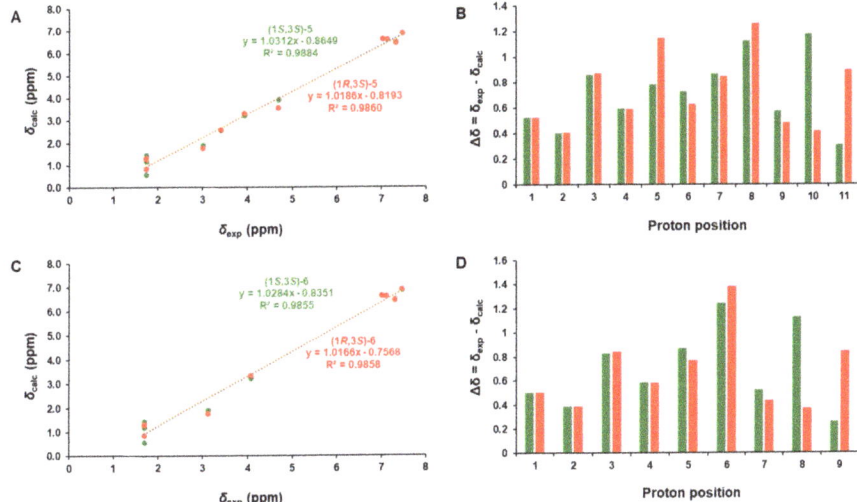

Figure 2. (**A**) Regression analysis of experimentally versus computationally calculated ^{1}H NMR chemical shifts of (1S,3S)-**5** and (1R,3S)-**5** with linear fitting shown as a line. (**B**) Relative chemical shift errors between calculated and experimental ^{1}H NMR data for (1S,3S)-**5** and (1R,3S)-**5**. (**C**) The regression analysis of experimentally versus computationally calculated ^{1}H NMR chemical shifts of (1S,3S)-**6** and (1R,3S)-**6** with linear fitting is shown as a line. (**D**) Relative chemical shift errors between computationally calculated and experimental ^{1}H NMR data for (1S,3S)-**6** and (1R,3S)-**6**.

3.2. Effects of Compounds 1–6 on Adipogenesis

To evaluate the influence of compounds **1–6** on adipogenesis, we first assessed the cytotoxicity of compounds **1–6** in 3T3-L1 preadipocytes. All compounds exhibited no cytotoxic effects up to 20 μM, but 40 μM of compounds **4** and **5** reduced the viability of 3T3-L1 cells (Figure 3). Thus, we treated 3T3-L1 cells with 20 μM of compounds **1–6** during adipogenesis (Figure 4A). The staining of lipid droplets with Oil Red O solution showed that compounds **1–6** inhibited lipid droplet accumulation in the adipocytes (Figure 4B). The transcription levels of the adipocyte marker genes (*Fabp4*, *PPARγ*, *C/EBPβ*, *Adipsin*, and *Adipoq*) were reduced upon treatment with compounds **1–6** (Figure 4C). During the maturation of adipocytes, the accumulation and fusion of lipid droplets accompany microtubule-dependent cytoskeletal reorganization facilitated by the acetylation of α-tubulin [34]. Thus, we examined whether compounds **1–6** influenced the level of the acetylated α-tubulin. As expected, the acetylation of α-tubulin was ablated upon exposure to compounds **1–6** during adipogenesis (Figure 4D), implying the failure of cytoskeletal remodeling required for adipogenesis. Among compounds **1–6**, compound **6** exhibited the highest anti-adipogenic effect (Figure 4); this enabled us to focus on the activity of compound **6**.

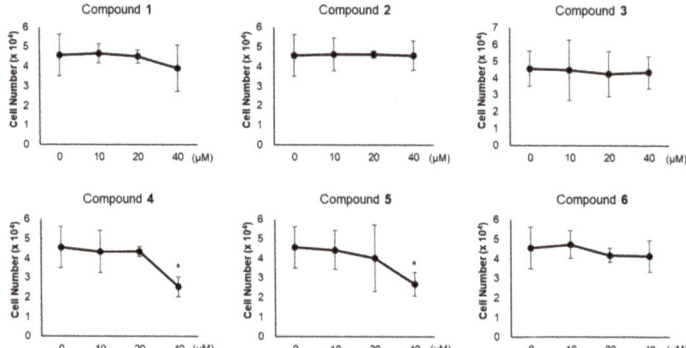

Figure 3. Cytotoxicity of compounds **1–6**. Cell viability in 3T3-L1 treated with compounds **1–6** (10, 20, 40 µM) for 24 h were determined. Data represent the means ± SD for n = 3. * $p < 0.05$.

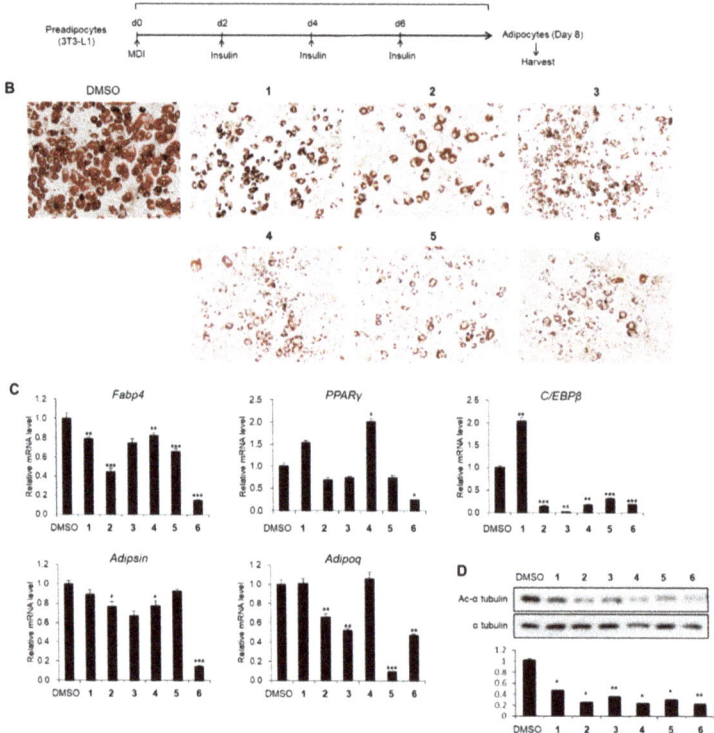

Figure 4. The inhibitory effects of compounds **1–6** on adipogenesis. (**A**) Schematic representation of 3T3-L1 differentiation into adipocytes. Cells were treated with compounds **1–6** during the entire process of differentiation. (**B**) The Oil Red O staining of 3T3-L1 adipocytes incubated with compounds **1–6** (20 µM) during adipogenesis. (**C**) The mRNA levels of *Fabp4*, *PPARγ*, *C/EBPβ*, *Adipsin*, and *Adipoq* genes in 3T3-L1 adipocytes incubated with compounds **1–6** (20 µM) during adipogenesis. Data represent the means ± SEM for n = 3. * $p < 0.05$, ** $p < 0.01$, and *** $p < 0.001$. (**D**) Immunoblot analysis of 3T3-L1 adipocytes incubated with compounds **1–6** (20 µM) during adipogenesis.

3.3. Effects of Compound 6 on the Early Stages of Adipogenesis

As cytoskeletal changes are early events during adipogenic differentiation [35], we hypothesized that the anti-adipogenic activity of (1R,3S)-1-methyl-1,2,3,4-tetrahydro-β-carboline-3-carboxylic acid (**6**) would be critical in the early stages of adipogenesis (Figure 5A). Treatment with compound **6** during the first 2 days interfered with the generation of adipocytes containing large lipid drops to a level comparable to that of the entire process of treatment with compound **6** (Figure 5B). Magnified images showed that lipid accumulation and fusion were considerably impaired with a big nucleus in the center of the cells upon exposure to compound **6**, whereas most of the cytosolic parts of the control cells were occupied by lipids with a peripheral nucleus (Figure 5B). Inhibitory effects on adipogenic gene expression were consistently observed upon treatment with compound **6** during the early stages as well as the entire process of adipogenesis (Figure 5C). These data indicate that the early stages of adipogenesis were impaired by compound **6**.

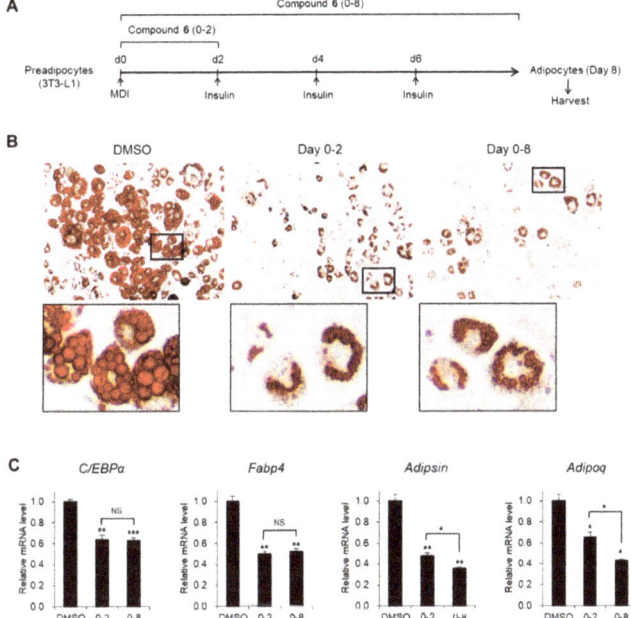

Figure 5. Inhibitory effects of compound **6** on the early stages of adipogenesis. (**A**) Schematic representation of 3T3-L1 differentiation into adipocytes. Cells were treated with compound **6** during the early days (day 0–2) or the entire process of differentiation. (**B**) Oil Red O staining of 3T3-L1 adipocytes incubated with compound **6** (20 µM) during adipogenesis. (**C**) The mRNA levels of *C/EBPα*, *Fabp4*, *Adipsin*, and *Adipoq* genes in 3T3-L1 adipocytes incubated with compound **6** (20 µM) during adipogenesis. Data represent the means ± SEM for n = 3. * $p < 0.05$, ** $p < 0.01$, and *** $p < 0.001$. NS: not significant.

3.4. Effects of Compound 6 on Lipid Metabolism

Next, we assessed the effects of compound **6** under diverse concentrations (5, 10, 20, and 40 µM) on adipogenesis (Figure 6A). As detected by the Oil Red O staining, adipogenesis and lipid accumulation were markedly inhibited by treatment with compound **6**, even at a low concentration (5 µM; Figure 6B). Moreover, the expression levels of adipogenic genes were significantly reduced upon incubation with a low concentration of compound **6** (Figure 6C), suggesting that compound **6** is a potent modulator of adipogenesis. As the magnified images of stained adipocytes showed lipid dispersion of compound **6** compared to the control (Figures 5B and 6B), we evaluated the capacity of compound **6** to regulate lipid metabolism. The mRNA expression of lipogenic gene *SREBP1* was significantly reduced upon exposure to compound **6** during the maturation of adipocytes, whereas the transcription of lipolytic genes, *ATGL* and *HSL*, was elevated (Figure 6D). These data demonstrate that the interruption of lipid drop enlargement by compound **6** was mediated by the regulation of the gene involved in the lipid metabolism.

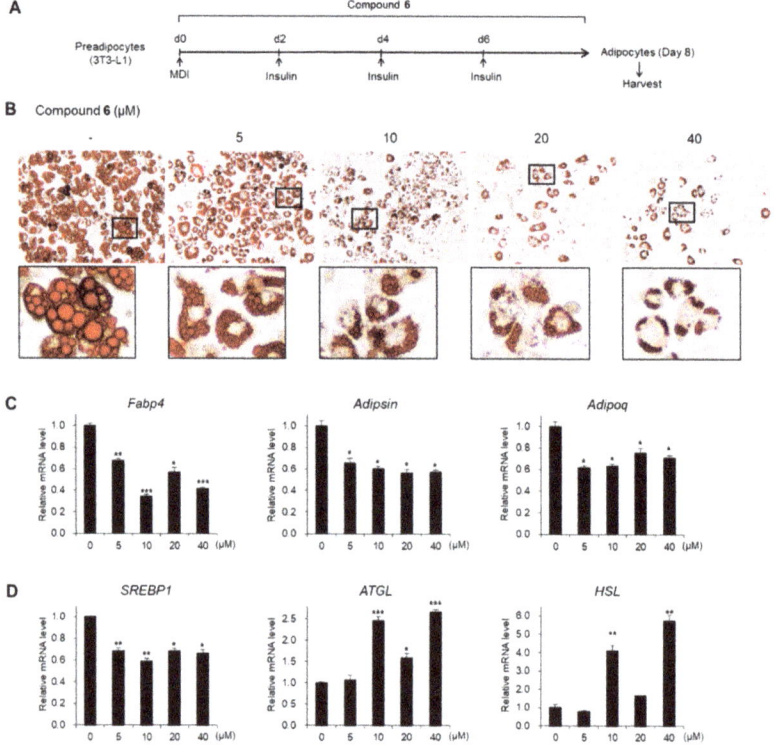

Figure 6. Effects of compound **6** on adipogenesis and lipid metabolism. (**A**) Schematic representation of 3T3-L1 differentiation into adipocytes. Cells were treated with compound **6** during the entire process of differentiation. (**B**) The Oil Red O staining of 3T3-L1 adipocytes incubated with compound **6** during adipogenesis. (**C**) The mRNA levels of *Fabp4*, *Adipsin*, and *Adipoq* genes in 3T3-L1 adipocytes incubated with compound **6** during adipogenesis. (**D**) The mRNA levels of *SREBP1*, *ATGL*, and *HSL* genes in 3T3-L1 adipocytes incubated with compound **6** during adipogenesis. Data represent the means ± SEM for n = 3. * $p < 0.05$, ** $p < 0.01$, and *** $p < 0.001$.

Obesity, a major cause of diverse metabolic disorders including type-2 diabetes, is characterized by the excessive expansion of white adipose tissue [36]. This process is accompanied by the differentiation of precursor cells into adipocytes (adipogenesis) and lipid drop accumulation in adipocytes (lipogenesis) [37]. Therefore, a pharmacological approach to block adipogenesis and lipogenesis has been considered effective to ameliorate metabolic disorders. In this study, we screened the effects of compounds **1–6** obtained from garlic on adipocyte differentiation and identified that (1*R*,3*S*)-1-methyl-1,2,3,4-tetrahydro-β-carboline-3-carboxylic acid (compound **6**) can disrupt lipid accumulation in adipocytes by promoting lipolysis and disturbing lipogenesis (Figure 7). While there is abundant evidence demonstrating the neuroprotective and anticancer effects of bioactive β-carbolines from diverse natural products [38–41], the metabolic effects of β-carbolines are not well defined. To the best of our knowledge, we report, for the first time, the effects of garlic-derived β-carboline alkaloids on adipogenesis and lipid metabolism.

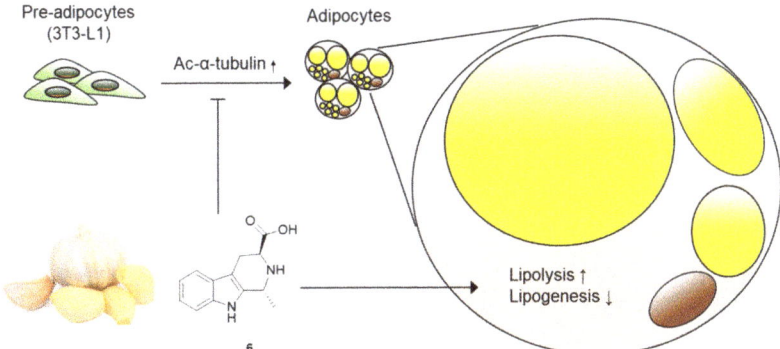

Figure 7. Molecular model underlying the mechanism of action of compound **6**. Compound **6** inhibits adipogenesis from 3T3-L1 preadipocytes, suppresses acetylation of α-tubulin, and regulates lipid metabolism, enhancing lipolysis and reducing lipogenesis.

In the early stages of adipogenic differentiation from preadipocytes, the acetylation of α-tubulin mediates cytoskeletal remodeling and elongation of primary cilia [34,42]. A defect in the acetylation of α-tubulin results in the disappearance of primary cilia, which impairs the generation of mature adipocytes [42,43]. Treatment with compound **6** effectively disturbed the acetylation of α-tubulin during adipogenesis, which is apparently responsible for the anti-adipogenic activity of compound **6**. These data offer better understanding of the manner in which compound **6** prevents adipogenesis from 3T3-L1 cells.

4. Conclusions

We provide experimental evidence of the potential role of (1*R*,3*S*)-1-methyl-1,2,3,4-tetrahydro-β-carboline-3-carboxylic acid (**6**) in adipogenesis from preadipocytes. The active compound was isolated from garlic (*A. sativum*), one of the most popular seasoning agents or condiments used worldwide; it is a β-carboline alkaloid, which is not a common constituent of garlic. Compound **6** repressed adipocyte differentiation from 3T3-L1 preadipocytes by preventing cytoskeletal remodeling, which is essential for adipogenesis. Moreover, compound **6** inhibited lipid accumulation by regulating lipolytic and lipogenic gene expression. Our findings provide a potential therapeutic strategy that uses a novel active compound from garlic to prevent excessive adipogenesis in obesity.

Supplementary Materials: The following are available online at http://www.mdpi.com/2304-8158/8/12/673/s1, Figure S1: DP4+ analysis of compound **5** with isomers (1*S*,3*S*)-**5** (Isomer 1) and (1*R*,3*S*)-**5** (Isomer 2), Figure S2: DP4+ analysis of compound **6** with isomers (1*S*,3*S*)-**6** (Isomer 1) and (1*R*,3*S*)-**6** (Isomer 2), Table S1: The computed ^{1}H NMR data for (1*S*,3*S*)-**5** and (1*R*,3*S*)-**5**, Table S2: The computed ^{1}H NMR data for (1*S*,3*S*)-**6** and (1*R*,3*S*)-**6**. General experimental procedures, plant material, extraction and isolation, computational NMR chemical shift calculation procedures for DP4+ analysis, DP4+ analysis results of compounds **5** and **6**, and the computed ^{1}H NMR data for (1*S*,3*S*)-**5/6** and (1*R*,3*S*)-**5/6** are available free of charge on the internet.

Author Contributions: Conceptualization, J.L. and K.H.K.; Formal analysis, S.C.B., K.H.N., S.A.Y., M.S.J., K.H.L., Y.H.L., and K.H.K.; Investigation, S.C.B., K.H.N., and S.A.Y.; Writing-Original draft preparation, S.C.B., K.H.N., S.A.Y., and K.H.K.; Writing-review & edit, S.C.B., K.H.N., S.A.Y., J.L., and K.H.K.; Project administration, J.L. and K.H.K.; Funding acquisition, J.L. and K.H.K.

Funding: This work was supported by a National Research Foundation of Korea (NRF) grant, funded by the Korean government (MSIT) (2018R1A2B2006879, 2019R1A5A2027340, 2017R1A6A3A04001986, and 2019R1I1A1A01058903).

Acknowledgments: We would like to thank Editage (www.editage.co.kr) for English language editing. We would like to thank Dr. Young Hye Kim (KBSI) for the ESIMS analysis.

Conflicts of Interest: The authors have no conflicts of interest to declare.

References

1. Angiosperm Phylogeny Group. An update of the Angiosperm phylogeny group classification for the orders and families of flowering plants: APG III. *Bot. J. Linn. Soc.* **2009**, *161*, 105–121. [CrossRef]
2. Rivlin, R.S. Historical perspective on the use of garlic. *J. Nutr.* **2001**, *132*, 951S–954S. [CrossRef] [PubMed]
3. Iciek, M.; Kwiecieri, I.; Wlodek, L. Biological properties of garlic and garlic-derived organosulfur compounds. *Environ. Mol. Mutagen.* **2009**, *50*, 247–265. [CrossRef] [PubMed]
4. Shamseer, L.; Charrois, T.L.; Vohra, S. Complementary, holistic and integrative medicine: Garlic. *Pediatr. Rev.* **2006**, *27*, 77–80. [CrossRef] [PubMed]
5. Jacob, B.; Narendhirakannan, R.T. Role of medicinal plants in the management of diabetes mellitus: A review. *3 Biotech.* **2019**, *9*, 4. [CrossRef] [PubMed]
6. Pittler, M.H.; Ernst, E. Clinical effectiveness of garlic (*Allium sativum*). *Mol. Nutr. Food Res.* **2007**, *51*, 1382–1385. [CrossRef]
7. Štajner, D.; Milić, N.; Čanadanović-Brunet, J.; Kapor, A.; Štajner, M.; Popović, B.M. Exploring *Allium* species as a source of potential medicinal agents. *Phytother. Res.* **2006**, *20*, 581–584. [CrossRef]
8. Lanzotti, V. The analysis of onion and garlic. *J. Chromatogr. A* **2006**, *1112*, 3–22. [CrossRef]
9. Amagase, H.; Petesch, B.L.; Matsuura, H.; Kasuga, S.; Itakura, Y. Intake of garlic and its bioactive components. *J. Nutr.* **2001**, *131*, 955S–962S. [CrossRef]
10. Lawson, L.D.; Ransom, D.K.; Hughes, B.G. Inhibition of whole blood platelet-aggregation by compounds in garlic clove extracts and commercial garlic products. *Thromb. Res.* **1992**, *65*, 141–156. [CrossRef]
11. Hussain, S.P.; Jannu, L.N.; Rao, A.R. Chemopreventive action of garlic on methylcholanthrene-induced carcinogenesis in the uterine cervix of mice. *Cancer Lett.* **1990**, *49*, 175–180. [CrossRef]
12. Pinto, J.T.; Lapsia, S.; Shah, A.; Santiago, H.; Kim, G. Antiproliferative effects of garlic-derived and other allium related compounds. *Adv. Exp. Med. Biol.* **2001**, *492*, 83–106. [PubMed]
13. Key, T.J.; Silcocks, P.B.; Davey, G.K.; Appleby, P.N.; Bishop, D.T. A case-control study of diet and prostate cancer. *Br. J. Cancer* **1997**, *76*, 678–687. [CrossRef] [PubMed]
14. Milner, J.A. Garlic: Its anticarcinogenic and antitumorigenic properties. *Nutr. Rev.* **1996**, *54*, S82–S86. [CrossRef] [PubMed]
15. Agarwal, K.C. Therapeutic actions of garlic constituents. *Med. Res. Rev.* **1996**, *16*, 111–124. [CrossRef]
16. Yeh, Y.Y. Garlic phytochemicals in disease prevention and health promotion: An overview. *New Drug Clin.* **1996**, *45*, 441–450.
17. Hirsch, K.; Danilenko, M.; Giat, J.; Miron, T.; Rabinkov, A.; Wilchek, M.; Mirelman, D.; Levy, H.; Sharoni, Y. Effect of purified allicin, the major ingredient of freshly crushed garlic, on cancer cell proliferation. *Nutr. Cancer* **2000**, *38*, 245–254. [CrossRef]
18. Shang, A.; Cao, S.; Xu, X.; Gan, R.; Tang, G.; Corke, H.; Mavumengwana, V.; Li, H. Bioactive compounds and biological functions of garlic (*Allium sativum* L.). *Foods* **2019**, *8*, 246. [CrossRef]
19. Corzo-Martınez, M.; Corzo, N.; Villamiel, M. Biological properties of onions and garlic. *Trends Food Sci. Technol.* **2007**, *18*, 609–625. [CrossRef]
20. Lanzotti, V.; Barile, E.; Antignani, V.; Bonanomi, G.; Scala, F. Antifungal saponins from bulbs of garlic, *Allium sativum* L. var. Voghiera. *Phytochemistry* **2012**, *78*, 126–134. [CrossRef]
21. Ichikawa, M.; Yoshida, J.; Ide, N.; Sasaoka, T.; Yamaguchi, H.; Ono, K. Tetrahydro-beta-carboline derivatives in aged garlic extract show antioxidant properties. *J. Nutr.* **2006**, *136*, 726S–731S. [CrossRef] [PubMed]
22. So, H.M.; Eom, H.J.; Lee, D.; Kim, S.; Kang, K.S.; Lee, I.K.; Baek, K.-H.; Park, J.Y.; Kim, K.H. Bioactivity evaluations of betulin identified from the bark of *Betula platyphylla* var. *japonica* for cancer therapy. *Arch. Pharm. Res.* **2018**, *41*, 815–822. [PubMed]
23. Baek, S.C.; Choi, E.; Eom, H.J.; Jo, M.S.; Kim, S.; So, H.M.; Kim, S.H.; Kang, K.S.; Kim, K.H. LC/MS-based analysis of bioactive compounds from the bark of *Betula platyphylla* var *japonica* and their effects on regulation of adipocyte and osteoblast differentiation. *Nat. Prod. Sci.* **2018**, *24*, 235–240.
24. Yu, J.S.; Roh, H.-S.; Baek, K.-H.; Lee, S.; Kim, S.; So, H.M.; Moon, E.; Pang, C.; Jang, T.S.; Kim, K.H. Bioactivity-guided isolation of ginsenosides from Korean Red Ginseng with cytotoxic activity against human lung adenocarcinoma cells. *J. Ginseng Res.* **2018**, *42*, 562–570. [CrossRef] [PubMed]

25. Ambati, S.; Yang, J.Y.; Rayalam, S.; Park, H.J.; Della-Fera, M.A.; Baile, C.A. Ajoene exerts potent effects in 3T3-L1 adipocytes by inhibiting adipogenesis and inducing apoptosis. *Phytother. Res.* **2009**, *23*, 513–518. [CrossRef]
26. Lii, C.K.; Huang, C.Y.; Chen, H.W.; Chow, M.Y.; Lin, Y.R.; Huang, C.S.; Tsai, C.W. Diallyl trisulfide suppresses the adipogenesis of 3T3-L1 preadipocytes through ERK activation. *Food Chem. Toxicol.* **2012**, *50*, 478–484. [CrossRef]
27. Ban, J.O.; Lee, D.H.; Kim, E.J.; Kang, J.W.; Kim, M.S.; Cho, M.C.; Jeong, H.S.; Kim, J.W.; Yang, Y.; Hong, J.T.; et al. Antiobesity effects of a sulfur compound thiacremonone mediated via down-regulation of serum triglyceride and glucose levels and lipid accumulation in the liver of db/db mice. *Phytother. Res.* **2012**, *26*, 1265–1271. [CrossRef]
28. Kim, E.J.; Lee, D.H.; Kim, H.J.; Lee, S.J.; Ban, J.O.; Cho, M.C.; Jeong, H.S.; Yang, Y.; Hong, J.T.; Yoon, D.Y. Thiacremonone, a sulfur compound isolated from garlic, attenuates lipid accumulation partially mediated via AMPK activation in 3T3-L1 adipocytes. *J. Nutr. Biochem.* **2012**, *23*, 1552–1558. [CrossRef]
29. Livak, K.J.; Schmittgen, T.D. Analysis of relative gene expression data using real-time quantitative PCR and the 2(-Delta Delta C(T)) Method. *Methods* **2001**, *25*, 402–408. [CrossRef]
30. Yahara, S.; Kato, K.; Nohara, T. Studies on the constituents of the water soluble portion in Asiasari radix. *Shoyakugaku Zasshi* **1990**, *44*, 331–334.
31. Orihara, Y.; Furuya, T.; Hashimoto, N.; Deguchi, Y.; Tokoro, K.; Kanisawa, T. Biotransformation of isoeugenol and eugenol by cultured cells of *Eucalyptus perriniana*. *Phytochemistry* **1992**, *31*, 827–831. [CrossRef]
32. Wang, X.; Liu, R.; Yang, Y.; Zhang, M. Isolation, purification and identification of antioxidants in an aqueous aged garlic extract. *Food Chem.* **2015**, *187*, 37–43. [CrossRef]
33. Grimblat, N.; Zanardi, M.M.; Sarotti, A.M. Beyond DP4: An improved probability for the stereochemical assignment of isomeric compounds using quantum chemical calculations of NMR shifts. *J. Org. Chem.* **2015**, *80*, 12526–12534. [CrossRef]
34. Yang, W.; Guo, X.; Thein, S.; Xu, F.; Sugii, S.; Baas, P.W.; Radda, G.K.; Han, W. Regulation of adipogenesis by cytoskeleton remodelling is facilitated by acetyltransferase MEC-17-dependent acetylation of α-tubulin. *Biochem. J.* **2013**, *449*, 605–612. [CrossRef]
35. Spiegelman, B.M.; Farmer, S.R. Decreases in tubulin and actin gene expression prior to morphological differentiation of 3T3 adipocytes. *Cell* **1982**, *29*, 53–60. [CrossRef]
36. Spiegelman, B.M.; Flier, J.S. Obesity and the Regulation of Energy Balance. *Cell* **2001**, *104*, 531–543. [CrossRef]
37. Smith, U.; Kahn, B.B. Adipose tissue regulates insulin sensitivity: Role of adipogenesis, de novo lipogenesis and novel lipids. *J. Intern. Med.* **2016**, *280*, 465–475. [CrossRef]
38. Piechowska, P.; Zawirska-Wojtasiak, R.; Mildner-Szkudlarz, S. Bioactive β-Carbolines in Food: A Review. *Nutrients* **2019**, *11*, 814. [CrossRef]
39. Ferraz, C.A.A.; de Oliveira Júnior, R.G.; Picot, L.; da Silva Almeida, J.R.G.; Nunes, X.P. Pre-clinical investigations of β-carboline alkaloids as antidepressant agents: A systematic review. *Fitoterapia* **2019**, *137*, 104196. [CrossRef]
40. Zhao, W.Y.; Zhou, W.Y.; Chen, J.J.; Yao, G.D.; Lin, B.; Wang, X.B.; Huang, X.X.; Song, S.J. Enantiomeric β-carboline dimers from Picrasma quassioides and their anti-hepatoma potential. *Phytochemistry* **2019**, *159*, 39–45. [CrossRef]
41. Zhang, M.; Sun, D. Recent Advances of Natural and Synthetic β-Carbolines as Anticancer Agents. *Anticancer Agents Med. Chem.* **2015**, *15*, 537–547. [CrossRef] [PubMed]
42. Forcioli-Conti, N.; Estève, D.; Bouloumié, A.; Dani, C.; Peraldi, P. The size of the primary cilium and acetylated tubulin are modulated during adipocyte differentiation: Analysis of HDAC6 functions in these processes. *Biochimie* **2016**, *124*, 112–123. [CrossRef] [PubMed]
43. Zhu, D.; Shi, S.; Wang, H.; Liao, K. Growth arrest induces primary-cilium formation and sensitizes IGF-1-receptor signaling during differentiation induction of 3T3-L1 preadipocytes. *J. Cell Sci.* **2009**, *122*, 2760–2768. [CrossRef] [PubMed]

© 2019 by the authors. Licensee MDPI, Basel, Switzerland. This article is an open access article distributed under the terms and conditions of the Creative Commons Attribution (CC BY) license (http://creativecommons.org/licenses/by/4.0/).

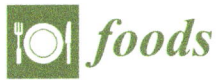

Article

The Stability and Activity Changes of Apigenin and Luteolin in Human Cervical Cancer Hela Cells in Response to Heat Treatment and Fe^{2+}/Cu^{2+} Addition

Wan-Ning Liu [1], Jia Shi [1], Yu Fu [2] and Xin-Huai Zhao [1,*]

[1] Key Laboratory of Dairy Science, Ministry of Education, Northeast Agricultural University, Harbin 150030, Heilongjiang, China
[2] College of Food Science, Southwest University, Chongqing 400715, China
* Correspondence: zhaoxh@neau.edu.cn; Tel.: +86-451-5519-1813

Received: 14 July 2019; Accepted: 12 August 2019; Published: 14 August 2019

Abstract: Flavonoids are natural polyphenolic compounds with desired bio-functions but with chemical instability and sensitivity to temperature, oxygen, and other factors. Apigenin and luteolin, two flavones of the flavonoid family in plant foods, were; thus, assessed and compared for their stability, especially the changes in anti-cancer activity in response to the conducted heat treatments and the addition of ferrous or cupric ions. The two flavones in aqueous solutions showed first-order degradation at 20 and 37 °C. The addition of ferrous or cupric ions (except for Cu^{2+} at 37 °C) enhanced luteolin stability via forming the luteolin–metal complexes; however, Fe/Cu addition (especially at 37 °C) consistently impaired apigenin stability. Using the human cervical cancer Hela cells and two cell treatment times (24 and 48 h), it was evident that heat treatments (37 and 100 °C) or Fe/Cu addition could endow apigenin and luteolin with decreased activities in growth inhibition, DNA damage, intracellular reactive oxygen species (ROS) generation, and apoptosis induction. In general, higher temperature led to greater decrease in these activities, while Fe^{2+} was more effective than Cu^{2+} to decrease these activities. The correlation analysis also suggested that the decreased ROS generation of the two flavones in the Hela cells was positively correlated with their decreased apoptosis induction. It is; thus, concluded that the two treatments can influence the two flavones' stability and especially exert an adverse impact on their anti-cancer activities.

Keywords: apigenin; luteolin; degradation; ferrous ions; cupric ions; cervical cancer cells; growth inhibition; apoptosis

1. Introduction

Flavonoids are a class of secondary plant phenolic compounds existing in a wide range of human diets. Flavonoids are interesting target compounds to many researchers because they have anti-oxidative, anti-microbial, anti-inflammatory, and anti-cancer effects [1]. Flavonoids, as natural anti-oxidants, even can exert stronger anti-oxidant activity than that of anti-oxidative vitamins and synthetic phenols [2]. Flavonoid compounds, such as hesperetin, naringenin, ponciretin, and diosmetin, are effective to inhibit harmful microorganisms; for example, they can inhibit the growth of *Helicobacter pylori* [3]. Furthermore, flavonoids have profound immune-regulatory and anti-inflammatory effects [4]. Cocoa flavonoids had immuno-regulation in the EL4.BU.OU6 cells by increasing the release of interleukin-4 [5]. Rutin, hesperidin, hesperetin, and quercetin were effective for both chronic and neurogenic inflammation [6]. Moreover, many researchers have paid special attention to the anti-cancer functions of flavonoids and flavonoid extracts. Quercetin, luteolin, chrysin, kaempferol, apigenin, and myricetin have cytotoxic effects on the human esophageal adenocarcinoma OE33 cells, resulting in growth inhibition, cell-cycle arrest, and apoptosis [7]. Baicalin could inhibit the growth of several human prostate cancer cells, including DU145, PC-3, LNCaP, and CA-HPV-10 cells [8]. Naringenin from citrus fruits could inhibit the proliferation of human colon cancer HT29 cells [9]. All results suggest that dietary flavonoids are promising natural compounds with desired ability to reduce cancer risk. Subsequently, an inverse correlation between flavonoid intake and the incidence of laryngeal and esophageal cancers has been reported [10].

Fe and Cu are two essential trace elements in the body, and are widely found in human diets. Fe/Cu ions have active redox property and thus can easily react with dietary flavonoids, which might alter chemical structures, especially the bio-functions of flavonoids. When flavonoids interact with Fe/Cu ions, they are oxidized by the two ions with decreased absorbance at their maximum absorption peaks [11]. Flavonoids can chelate with the two ions and thus form complexes with changed properties. Flavonoid–Fe^{2+} complexes showed enhanced stability, while flavonoid–Cu^{2+} complexes had auto-oxidation [12,13]. Furthermore, flavonoid oxidation by Cu^{2+} was irreversible [13]. However, superoxide scavenging capacities of rutin, taxifolin, epicatechin, and luteolin were weaker than their respective Fe/Cu complexes [14]. Overall, it is reasonable to believe that the anti-cancer potentials of flavonoids could be affected by these transition metal ions.

During food processing, Fe/Cu ions may easily enter food matrices, as food matrices have the opportunity to contact the surfaces of pipes and equipment made from the two metals. Furthermore, some treatments used in food processing might exert potential impacts on dietary flavonoids; for example, heat treatment is necessary or unavoidable. In general, flavonoids are sensitive to high temperature [15], because high temperature can promote their degradation. The higher temperature of elderberry anthocyanins gave rise to higher degradation rate constants [16], while flavonoids in cloudy apple juice at 80 to 145 °C also experienced increased degradation rates [17]. Dietary flavonoids at higher temperatures; therefore, might be endowed with changed bio-functions, mainly due to flavonoid degradation. Brazilian bean after boiling and draining had decreased flavonoid content and lower anti-oxidant capacity [18]. Thermal treatment of galangin, kaempferol, morin, and myricetin led to weakened growth inhibition on the human colon carcinoma HCT-116 cells [19,20]. Thus, the effects of heat treatment and metal entrance on anti-cancer functions of flavonoids in other cancer cells, like the human cervical cancer Hela cells, deserve further study.

The flavones are commonly found flavonoid compounds in natural foods, among those flavone members are apigenin and luteolin. Apigenin is rich in Chinese cabbage, bell pepper, garlic, bilimbi fruit, guava, wolfberry leaves, and local celery, while luteolin is rich in bird chili, onion leaves, and bilimbi fruit and its leaves [21]. Normally, flavones had been reported to have stronger anti-cancer activities due to their high lipophilicity [22]. Apigenin is a promising anti-cancer compound, because it could inhibit the growth of several cancer cells [23]. Luteolin also is served as a potential and emerging anti-cancer compound, due to its clear toxic effect on eukaryotic DNA topoisomerase I [24]. From a chemical point of view, apigenin and luteolin have several –OH groups in their molecules (Figure 1) and thus have different stability once they are heated or mixed with Fe/Cu ions. Whether apigenin and luteolin after these treatments still have good anti-cancer functions is important but unsolved at present. Such a study; thus, deserves consideration.

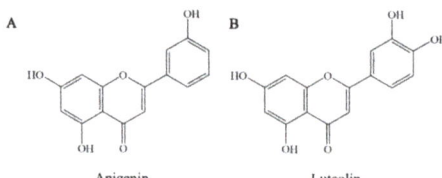

Figure 1. The chemical structures of flavone compounds apigenin and luteolin.

In this study, both apigenin and luteolin were measured for their stability under two temperatures (20 and 37 °C) or Fe^{2+}/Cu^{2+} addition. The two temperatures are regarded as room temperature of diet storage and average temperature of the body, respectively. Moreover, the latter is also the culture temperature of most cells. Afterwards, the two flavones were subjected to heat treatments at 37 and 100 °C or Fe/Cu addition, and then evaluated for their changes in anti-cancer activity using the human cervical cancer Hela cells as a cell model. Four indices including growth inhibition, cell morphology (or DNA damage), reactive oxygen species (ROS) generation, and apoptosis induction were used to clarify or compare activity changes. The study aimed to reveal whether the two treatments (heat treatment and Fe/Cu addition) could affect the stability of apigenin and luteolin as well as their anti-cancer effects in Hela cells.

2. Materials and Methods

2.1. Chemicals and Reagents

The apigenin and luteolin (purity >98%) were bought from Dalian Meilun Biological Technology Co. Ltd. (Dalian, Liaoning, China). The cell counting kit-8 (CCK-8) was purchased from Dojindo Molecular Technologies Inc. (Kyushu, Japan). The reactive oxygen species (ROS) assay kit, Annexin V-FITC apoptosis detection kit, and Hoechst 33258 kit were obtained from Beyotime Institute of Biotechnology (Shanghai, China). 5-Fluorouracil (5-Fu) was bought from Tianjin Jinyao Pharmaceutical Co. Ltd. (Tianjin, China). All other chemicals used were of analytical grade. The water used in this study was ultrapure water generated with Milli-Q PLUS (Millipore Corporation, New York, NY, USA).

2.2. Cell Line and Culture Conditions

The Hela cells (STR: Amelogenin: X; CSF1PO: 9,10; D13S317: 12,13.3; D16S539: 9,10; D18S51: 16; D19S433: 13, 14; D21S11: 27,28; D2S1338: 17; D3S1358: 15, 18; D5S818: 11, 12; D7S820: 8,12; D8S1179: 12, 13; FGA: 18,21; TH01: 7; TPOX: 8,12; vWA: 16,18) used in this study were purchased from the Cell Bank of Shanghai Institute of Biochemistry and Cell Biology (Shanghai, China). As recommended by the cell supplier, the cells were cultured in the Dulbecco's modified eagle's medium (DMEM) (Sigma-Aldrich, Co. St. Louis, MO, USA) supplemented with 10% fetal bovine serum (FBS) (Hyclone, Logan, UT, USA) and 1% penicillin/streptomycin solution at 37 °C in a 5% CO_2 atmosphere.

2.3. Assays of Degradation Rates of the Two Flavones

Both apigenin and luteolin were dissolved in dimethyl sulfoxide (DMSO) to prepare stock solutions of 0.1 mol/L. The stock solutions were diluted with ethanol and then with 0.1 mol/L phosphate buffer solution (PBS, pH 7.3) to two final concentrations of 20 and 30 µmol/L, using respective dilution factors of 5000 and 3333. Otherwise, the stock solutions were diluted with ethanol and PBS similarly but with addition of $CuCl_2$ or $FeCl_2$, which resulted in a fixed molar ratio of flavones to Fe/Cu (3:1). All prepared solutions were incubated at two temperatures (20 and 37 °C) for 6 h, and measured for their absorbance values at various time points using two wavelengths (apigenin 354 nm; luteolin 360 nm) and a UV-visible spectrophotometer (UV-2401 PC, Shimadzu Co., Kyoto, Japan). PBS was used as blank in this assay. Residual levels of apigenin and luteolin were estimated using the respective standard curves generated from a serial of standard solutions.

Based on the established first-order reaction model of flavonoid degradation [25], the degradation rate constants (k, h^{-1}) of apigenin and luteolin were calculated using a derived linear regression equation.

2.4. Treatments of the Two Flavones for Cell Experiments

Apigenin and luteolin were dissolved in DMSO to obtain 0.3 moL/L stock solutions, and diluted by the DMEM supplemented with 5% FBS to yield flavone concentrations of 20 to 80 µmoL/L using the dilution factors ranging from 15,000 to 3750. The stock solutions were also diluted by DMEM without FBS to a fixed flavone concentration of 42.1 µmoL/L (using dilution factor of 7126), and heated in the dark with a thermostatic water bath operated at 37 °C (or 100 °C) for 6 h (or 0.5 h). After heat treatment, the two solutions were immediately cooled in the ice water and added with the FBS to yield a final flavone concentration of 40 µmoL/L. The FBS was not involved in these thermal treatments. Or else, the stock solutions were diluted with DMEM supplemented with 5% FBS, and added with 100 mmoL/L $CuCl_2$ or $FeCl_2$ solution to yield a final flavone concentration (40 µmoL/L) together with a fixed molar ratio (3:1) of flavones to Fe/Cu.

2.5. Assay of Growth Inhibition

The cells (1×10^4 cells per 100 µL per well) were seeded onto the 96-well plates and incubated for 12 h. After removal of cell medium, the cells were treated with 0.1% DMSO (negative control), 100 µmol/L 5-Fu (positive control), and the prepared flavone samples for 24 and 48 h, respectively, and then washed twice with the PBS. The CCK-8 solution of 100 µL (10 µL CCK-8 plus 90 µL DMEM containing 5% FBS) was added to each well, and the cells were further incubated at 37 °C for 1.5 h. A microplate reader (Bio-Rad Laboratories, Hercules, CA, USA) was then used to measure the optical density values at 450 nm, which were used to calculate the percentages of growth inhibition as previously described [26].

2.6. Hoechst 33258 Staining

The cells in 6-well plates were grown to 70% confluence and incubated with the untreated or treated flavone samples (40 µmol/L) for 24 h. After discarding cell media, 4% methanol of 1 mL was added into each well to fix the cells at 4 °C for 10 min. After washing twice with the PBS buffer, the Hoechst 33258 (200 mg/mL) of 1 mL was added into each well to stain the cells for 10 min. The cells were then observed under a fluorescence microscope (Zeiss Axio Observer A1m, Carl Zeiss, Oberkochen, Germany), while cell images were taken at 350 nm using an objective of 40-fold.

2.7. Assay of Apoptosis Induction

The proportions of the apoptotic cells in different cell groups were detected using flow cytometry technique and Annexin V-fluorescein isothiocyanate (FITC)/propidium iodide (PI) double staining as previously described [27]. The cells were grown to 70% confluence in 6-well plates, incubated with the untreated and treated flavones at 40 µmol/L for 24 and 48 h, harvested, washed with the cold PBS, and centrifuged at $110 \times g$ for 5 min to discard the supernatants. The pellets were re-suspended gently in the Annexin V-FITC binding buffer of 200 µL, and incubated with the Annexin V-FITC of 10 µL for 15 min in the dark at 20 °C. The binding buffer (300 µL) and PI (5 µL) were added into each well and mixed gently. The stained cells were assayed with a flow cytometer (FACS Calibur, Becton Dickson, San Jose, CA, USA), to detect the percentages of necrotic, late apoptotic, intact, and early apoptotic cells (Q1–Q4).

2.8. Assay of Intracellular Reactive Oxygen Species

In this assay, the cells were treated similarly as those in the assay of apoptosis induction. After cell harvesting and PBS washing, the cells were re-incubated with 20,70-dichlorofluorescein (DCF-DA, 5 mmoL/L) at 37 °C for 30 min in the dark, washed three times with the PBS, and re-suspended in the PBS of 1 mL. The cell suspension was seeded onto the 96-well plates and measured for their fluorescence intensities using a fluorescence microplate reader (Infinite 200, Tecan, Männedorf, Switzerland) and respective emission and excitation wavelengths of 488 and 525 nm. The relative ROS levels were expressed as the percentages of the control cells as previously described [28].

2.9. Statistical Analysis

All reported data collected from three independent experiments or assays were expressed as means or means ± standard deviations, and compared using the SPSS 20.0 software (SPSS Inc., Chicago, IL, USA). All obtained data meet the assumptions of normality and constant variance. Significant differences ($p < 0.05$) between the means of multiple groups were evaluated by the one-way analysis of variance with Duncan's multiple range tests and two-way analysis of variance (ANOVA). The Pearson's correlation coefficient was also calculated using this software.

3. Results

3.1. Instability of Apigenin and Luteolin at Two Temperatures or in the Presence of Fe^{2+}/Cu^{2+}

Apigenin and luteolin showed typical UV-spectra with maximum absorption peaks around 354 and 360 nm, respectively. This study; thus, used two wavelengths to detect residual apigenin and luteolin, which were exposed to two temperatures or Fe^{2+}/Cu^{2+} for different time periods. The results indicated that both apigenin and luteolin were chemically instable in these cases, because their residual levels showed a decreasing trend (Figure 2). The calculated degradation rate constants (k) revealed how the higher temperature (37 °C) and the two ions affected the stability of apigenin and luteolin (Table 1). When their solutions were kept at 20 or 37 °C, apigenin and luteolin showed k values of 0.0207 and 0.0214 or 0.0226 and 0.0245 h^{-1}, respectively. Higher temperature clearly led to higher k value (i.e., decreased stability). In the presence of Fe^{2+}/Cu^{2+}, apigenin gave greater degradation, because the measured k values were increased to 0.0395–0.0728 h^{-1}. More importantly, higher temperature (37 °C) combined with Cu^{2+} brought about more drastic apigenin degradation. As for luteolin, Fe^{2+} resulted in lower k values (i.e., decreased degradation), while Cu^{2+} at 37 °C led to enhanced degradation (i.e., larger k value). These results suggested that: (1) Both higher temperature and Fe^{2+}/Cu^{2+} caused structural instability for apigenin; and (2) only higher temperature and Cu^{2+} could increase the instability of luteolin. Both heat treatments and Cu/Fe addition; therefore, might alter the anti-cancer activities of these two flavones.

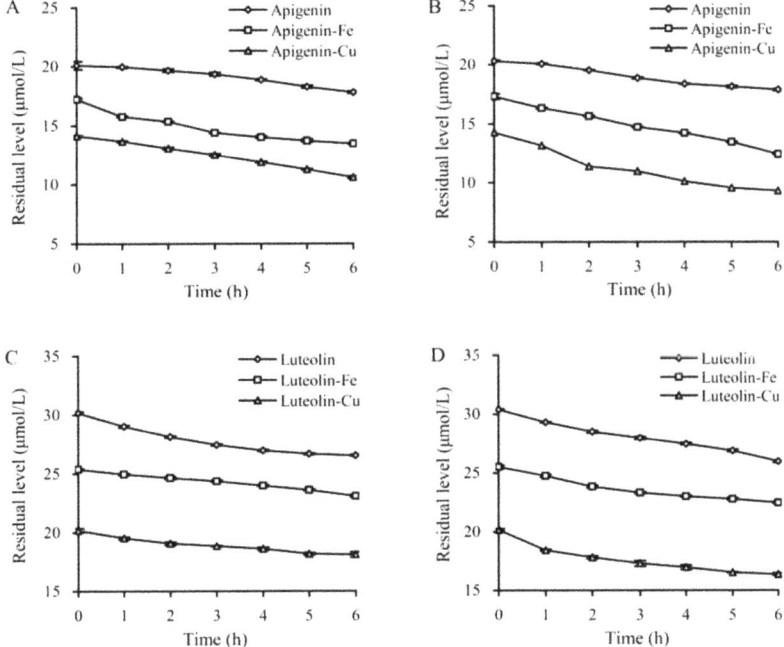

Figure 2. Residual levels of apigenin and luteolin in the solutions incubated at 20 °C (**A**,**C**) and 37 °C (**B**,**D**) for different time periods.

Table 1. Degradation rate constants (k, h^{-1}) of apigenin and luteolin in solutions treated with two temperatures or added with Fe^{2+}/Cu^{2+} s.

	Indices	Added Metals (Flavones:Metals 3:1)	Apigenin	Luteolin
Temperature	37 °C	None	0.0207 ± 0.0012 [F]	0.0214 ± 0.0004 [c]
		Fe^{2+}	0.0395 ± 0.0011 [D]	0.0149 ± 0.0009 [f]
		Cu^{2+}	0.0480 ± 0.0015 [C]	0.0176 ± 0.0021 [e]
	100 °C	None	0.0226 ± 0.0001 [E]	0.0245 ± 0.0006 [b]
		Fe^{2+}	0.0520 ± 0.0002 [B]	0.0203 ± 0.0005 [d]
		Cu^{2+}	0.0728 ± 0.0010 [A]	0.0317 ± 0.0004 [a]
Significance		Temperature	**	**
		Metals	**	**
		Temperature × Metals	**	**

Different lowercase or capital letter superscripts after the values in the same column indicate that the means differ significantly according to one-way ANOVA ($p < 0.05$). The two asterisks indicate that the means differ significantly according to two-way ANOVA ($p < 0.05$).

3.2. Growth Inhibition of the Flavone Samples on Hela Cells

The CCK-8 assaying results indicated that both apigenin and luteolin at 20–80 µmoL/L dose- and time-dependently had cytotoxic effects on the Hela cells (Figure 3), resulting in inhibition percentages of 30.6%–62.7% and 33.8%–70.6% (24 h) or 59.5%–76.4% and 62.3%–88.6% (48 h), respectively. Both apigenin and luteolin at 40 µmoL/L caused corresponding inhibition percentages of 52.0% and 57.9% (24 h) or 65.7% and 73.2% (48 h) in the cells. Thus, flavone concentration of 40 µmol/L was used in later study, because this concentration led to growth inhibition up to 50%–70%.

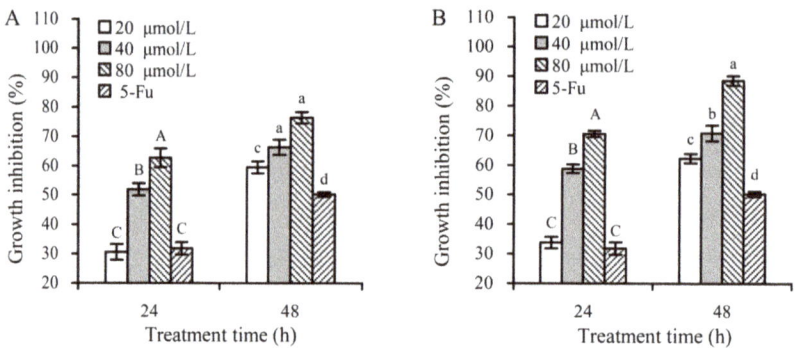

Figure 3. Growth inhibition of apigenin (**A**) and luteolin (**B**) of various concentrations on the Hela cells at treatment times of 24 and 48 h. 5-Fu, 5-fluorouracil as a positive control. Different capital or lowercase letters above the columns indicate that the means within the same group differ significantly according to one-way ANOVA ($p < 0.05$).

This flavone concentration was then used to compare different growth inhibition of these flavone samples with or without heat treatment or Fe/Cu addition in the Hela cells (Figure 4). Heat treatment at 37 °C decreased the inhibition percentages of apigenin and luteolin to 50.5% and 55.0% (24 h) or 63.2% and 67.5% (48 h), respectively. Heat treatment at 100 °C brought about much decreased growth inhibition, because the measured inhibition percentages of apigenin and luteolin were reduced to 48.4% and 51.1% (24 h) or 59.0% and 64.0% (48 h), respectively. Overall, heat treatment at 100 °C and Fe addition showed greater potential to decrease growth inhibition of the two flavones.

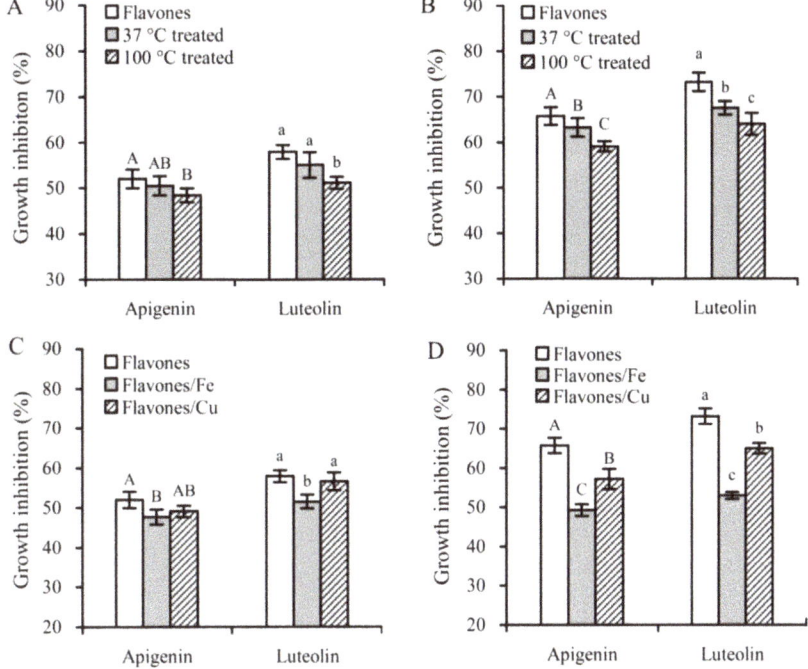

Figure 4. Growth inhibition of 40 μmoL/L flavonols (with or without thermal treatments and Fe/Cu addition) on the Hela cells with treatment times of 24 (**A,C**) and 48 h (**B,D**). Different capital or lowercase letters above the columns indicate that the means within the same group differ significantly according to one-way ANOVA ($p < 0.05$).

3.3. Morphological Alteration of Hela Cells Treated by the Flavone Samples

Morphological alteration of the treated cells can reflect potential apoptosis induction of the target substances. Morphological features of the treated Hela cells were; thus, observed using the Hoechst 33258 staining and fluorescence microscopy. In these results, the cell nuclei were dyed and observed in the fluorescent images. The apoptotic cells were observed as light blue while the viable cells were observed as dark blue. Moreover, the apoptotic cells often showed apoptotic morphology as the condensation and fragmentation of nuclei shrinkage as well as the formation of apoptotic bodies. In general, the untreated flavones were more effective than the treated ones to alter the morphological features of Hela cells, while 100 °C treatment and Fe addition brought about relatively higher cell density (Figure 5). Compared with the control cells without any treatment, the treated cells showed the typical apoptotic morphology and decreased cell density in the observation field. These results suggested that these assessed samples could damage DNA and thus had potential (but different) apoptosis induction towards the Hela cells.

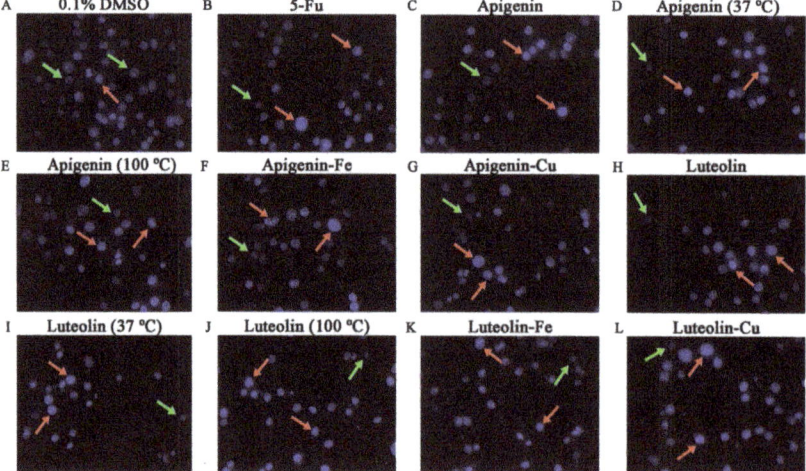

Figure 5. Morphological features of the Hela cells treated with 0.1% DMSO, 100 μmol/L 5-fluorouracil (5-Fu), and 40 μmol/L flavone samples (with or without thermal treatment and Fe/Cu addition) for 24 h. A fluorescence microscope was used to photograph images (40×). The red and green arrows indicate the corresponding apoptotic and intact cells.

3.4. Pro-Oxidation of the Flavone Samples

The Hela cells treated with or without these flavone samples were; thus, detected for their ROS levels (Table 2). The results indicated that all assessed samples had pro-oxidation in the cells, as the treated cells showed increased relative ROS levels (larger than 200%) than in the control cells ($p < 0.05$). The untreated apigenin and luteolin brought about relative ROS levels of 229% and 284% (24 h) or 263% and 281% (48 h), respectively. The apigenin and luteolin treated at 37 °C for 6 h resulted in lower ROS levels of 212% and 272% (24 h) or 260% and 263% (48 h), respectively. Apigenin and luteolin treated at 100 °C for 0.5 h showed much weaker ability to increase ROS generation than those heated at 37 °C for 6 h. For apigenin and luteolin, Fe addition led to the highest ROS reduction in the cells; however, Cu addition only decreased ROS levels to a slight extent, compared with Fe addition. Overall, both heat treatment and Fe/Cu addition consistently led to decreased ROS generation in the Hela cells.

Table 2. The measured reactive oxygen species (ROS) levels in the Hela cells treated with different samples for 24 and 48 h.

Flavones	Heat Treatment (°C)	Added Ions (Flavones:Metals 3:1)	ROS Levels (% of Control)	
			24 h	48 h
Apigenin	None	None	228.6 ± 2.4 [A]	262.8 ± 1.5 [A]
	37	None	211.7 ± 3.8 [B]	260.0 ± 6.4 [B]
	100	None	206.9 ± 3.4 [C]	245.3 ± 1.6 [C]
	None	Fe^{2+}	205.6 ± 3.8 [C]	223.6 ± 1.0 [E]
	None	Cu^{2+}	212.1 ± 1.6 [B]	237.4 ± 1.9 [D]
Luteolin	None	None	284.1 ± 8.2 [a]	280.9 ± 3.8 [a]
	37	None	271.8 ± 5.0 [b]	262.9 ± 3.5 [b]
	100	None	234.2 ± 7.7 [c]	256.8 ± 2.5 [c]
	None	Fe^{2+}	232.1 ± 1.0 [c]	225.1 ± 5.7 [e]
	None	Cu^{2+}	268.4 ± 2.7 [b]	246.4 ± 0.7 [d]

Different lowercase or capital letter superscripts after the values in the same column indicate that the means are significantly different according to one-way ANOVA ($p < 0.05$).

However, ROS generation of luteolin at 48 h was lower than that at 24 h (except 100 °C heat treatment) (Table 2). In these cases, the respective samples had stronger pro-oxidation, could enhance

ROS to much higher levels and, thereby, caused greater cell apoptosis, which led to a lower number of viable cells. After a longer period, only a few viable cells continued to generate ROS. Finally, ROS generation with incubation time of 48 h was less than that with incubation time of 24 h.

3.5. Apoptosis Induction of the Flavone Samples

Apoptosis induction of the untreated and treated flavones were then assessed with the flow cytometry technique using the Annexin V-FITC/PI double staining and treatment times of 24 and 48 h (Figures 6 and 7).

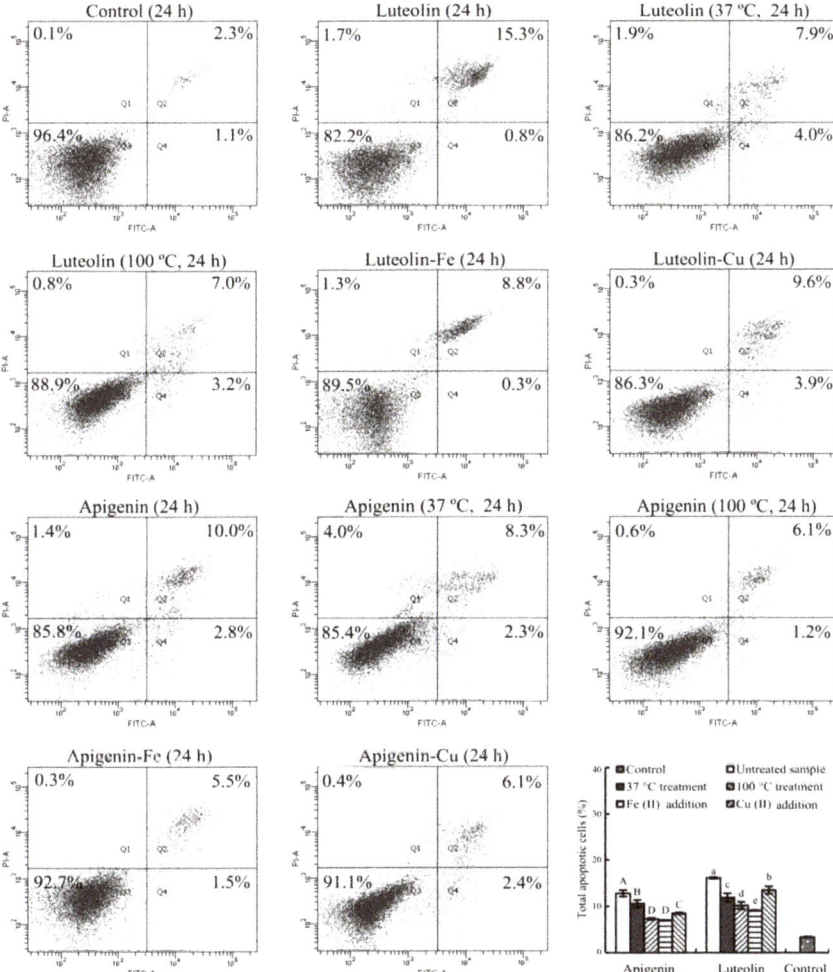

Figure 6. Cell percentages of the Hela cells treated with 0.1% DMSO (control) and 40 µmoL/L flavone samples with or without thermal treatments and Fe/Cu addition for 24 h.

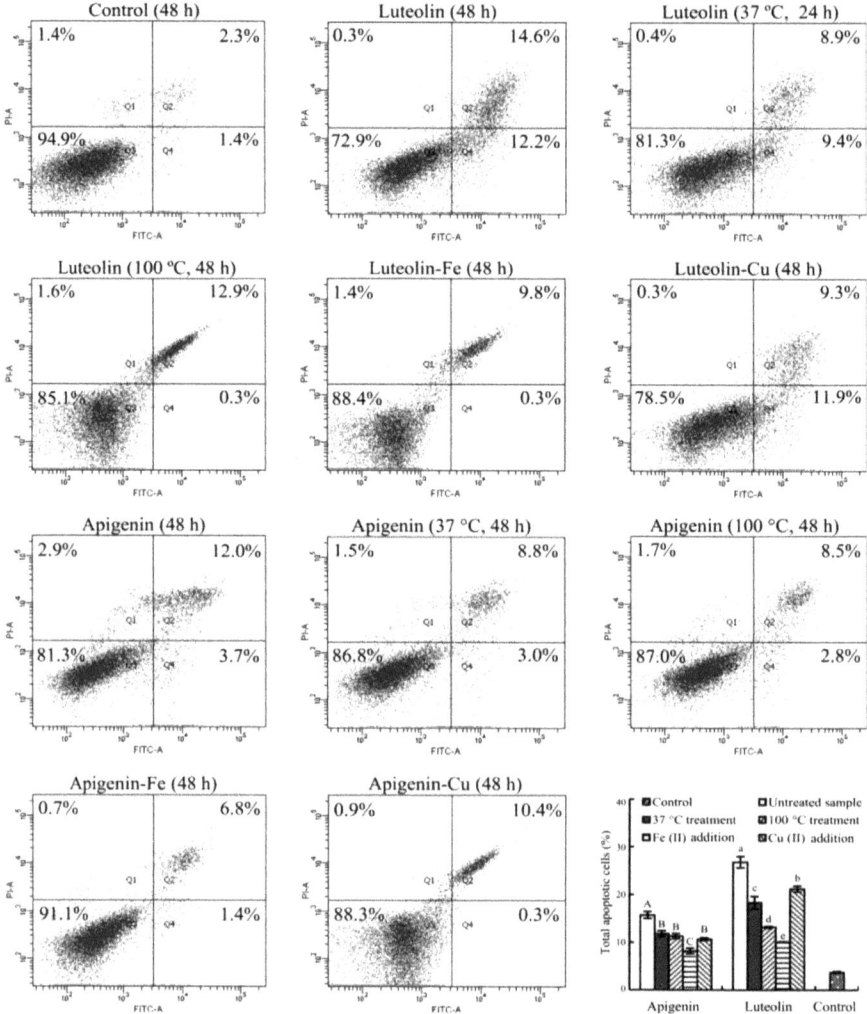

Figure 7. Cell percentages of the Hela cells treated with 0.1% DMSO (control) and 40 μmol/L flavone samples with or without thermal treatments and Fe/Cu addition for 48 h.

The control cells at 24 or 48 h only had total apoptotic cells (Q2 + Q4) of 3.4% or 3.7%. The cells treated with the untreated apigenin and luteolin for 24 (or 48) h led to increased total apoptotic cells about 12.8% and 16.1% (or 15.7% and 26.8%). If the cells were treated with the heated flavones, the total apoptotic cells were measured with the reduced percentages, especially using heat treatment at 100 °C. Subsequently, the total apoptotic cells were 7.3% and 10.2% (24 h) or 11.3% and 13.2% (48 h) with corresponding apigenin and luteolin treatments. When the two flavones were added with Fe^{2+}, the respective apigenin and luteolin treatments resulted in the total apoptotic cells of 7.0% and 9.1% (24 h) or 8.2% and 10.1% (48 h). When the two flavones were added with Cu^{2+}, the measured total apoptotic cells were 8.5% and 13.5% (24 h) or 10.7% and 21.2% (48 h) with respective apigenin and luteolin treatments. Data comparison further revealed how these treatments had positive or negative impacts on the apoptosis induction of the two flavones. Overall, the conducted heat treatment (especially at 100 °C) caused decreased total apoptotic cell proportions, while Fe addition also resulted in much decreased total apoptotic cell proportions than Cu addition did.

Further data analysis revealed that the measured ROS levels (Table 2) in the cells with a treatment time of 24 h were positively and significantly correlated with the detected total apoptotic cell percentages (Figures 6 and 7), because the calculated Pearson's correlation coefficient (i.e., r-value) of the two indices was 0.854 ($p < 0.05$). This correlation meant that the decreased abilities in ROS generation of apigenin and luteolin possibly resulted in decreased apoptosis induction. In other words, the used treatments brought about flavone degradation and lower abilities to generate ROS in Hela cells, and thereby led to decreased apoptosis induction. However, this phenomenon was no longer observed when the cells were treated with a longer time of 48 h. The treatment time of 48 h led to too much cell death or the lower number of viable cells (Figure 4). Consequently, only fewer viable cells in the media were able to generate ROS. This fact meant that much higher extent of apoptosis induction of apigenin and luteolin led to lower ROS generation. Therefore, the calculated Pearson's correlation coefficient (r-value) of the two indices (i.e., ROS levels versus apoptotic cell percentages) decreased to 0.589 ($p > 0.05$). In this case, the measured apoptosis induction and ROS generation were positively but insignificantly correlated.

4. Discussion

Flavones, in general, have several –OH groups in their molecules, and; therefore, they as phenolic compounds are susceptible to oxidation. Heat treatment; thus, promotes flavone degradation, and is adverse to the stability and bio-activities of flavonoids. Polyphenols in the solid grape marc were degraded at 100–150 °C, leading to decreased anti-oxidation [29]. At the temperature of 250 °C, catechins might lose their DPPH radical scavenging ability completely due to the thermal degradation of catechins [30]. The anti-cancer activities of flavonoids (e.g., growth inhibition) are governed by their chemical structures [31,32]. Subsequently, structure changes of flavonoids will result in increased or decreased activity. It was found that heat treatment of cymaroside (i.e., luteolin-7-O-β-glucoside) led to the increased immuno-modulation by enhancing NK cells activity [33]. Additionally, the heated flavonoids showed decreased activities in the human colon carcinoma HCT-116 cells [19,20]. Thus, heat treatments (especially using 100 °C) in the present study caused greater degradation and decreased growth inhibition for both apigenin and luteolin.

It is well-known that Fe/Cu are capable of oxidizing flavonoids in solutions, resulting in flavonoid degradation [34]. However, flavonoids also can complex with multi-valent metal ions [35], resulting in changed stability. Thus, Fe/Cu added to apigenin and luteolin solutions might bring two major reactions: forming flavone–metal complexes and catalyzing flavone degradation [12,13]. From a chemical point of view, the redox cycling exists between transition metals and ligands [36]. Quercetin, rutin, and 3-hydroxyflavone in the presence of Fe^{2+}/Cu^{2+} exhibited a significant decomposition, yielding semiquinone compounds [36]. Both apigenin and luteolin; thus, could be oxidized by the added Fe/Cu, resulting in changed chemical stability. However, apigenin and luteolin are different in their chemical structures that; thus, govern their stability changes in the presence of Fe^{2+}/Cu^{2+}. Normally, one luteolin molecule can chelate 1.5 Fe^{2+}/Cu^{2+}, but apigenin without two adjacent –OH groups is almost unable to chelate the two ions [11]. Apigenin in the present study; thus, was instable in the presence of Fe^{2+}/Cu^{2+} (Table 1). On the contrary, luteolin has two adjacent –OH groups in its C-ring and thus can chelate the two ions; subsequently, it mainly showed enhanced stability in the presence of Fe^{2+}/Cu^{2+} (Table 1). Moreover, the Cu-added luteolin also showed decreased stability at 37 °C (but not at 20 °C), which was attributed to the stronger oxidation of Cu^{2+} at this temperature. Consistent with the present finding, it was also found that quercetin bound with Fe^{2+} had inhibited oxidation, while that bound with Cu^{2+} received promoted oxidation [12]. In methanol medium, Cu^{2+} also promoted quercetin oxidation [13]. It was reasonable in the present study that the two flavones showed worse stability in the presence of Cu^{2+}, especially at the higher temperature.

Hela cells have the potential to proliferate indefinitely and have been widely used for cancer research. It was reported that many flavonoids and their derivatives had the ability to inhibit Hela cells. Natural flavone eupatorine inhibited Hela cells through inducing cell-cycle arrest and apoptosis [37]. Wang and coauthors reported that quercetin could induce the apoptosis and autophagy of Hela cells [38]. Other researchers proved that quercetin had anti-cancer effects on HeLa cells via the adenosine 5′-monophosphate -activated protein kinase (AMPK)-induced HSP70 and down-regulation of epidermal growth factor receptor (EGFR) [39]. In this study, Fe^{2+}/Cu^{2+} showed different behaviors to affect the growth inhibition of apigenin and luteolin in the cells. Fe is one of the required nutritive elements for tumor growth [40], and is also reported to influence cell-cycle regulation at multiple sites [41]. Fe^{2+} chelation of flavonoids is one of the important mechanisms in response to their growth inhibition in cancer cells. Fe addition thereby decreased luteolin's Fe-chelating activities, promoted apigenin oxidation, thus reasonably reduced its growth inhibition. Cu^{2+} is capable of inducing cellular oxidative stress, bringing DNA damage, and then initiating cell apoptosis [42]. Cu addition for the two flavones; thus, gave rise to two chemical reactions: enhancing flavone degradation and increasing cellular Cu content. The enhanced flavone degradation led to decreased growth inhibition, whilst the increased Cu content brought about extra oxidative stress or higher cytotoxic effect on the Hela cells. Subsequently, Cu addition of the two flavones in this study was observed with less decreased growth inhibition than Fe addition. The bio-activity changes of flavonoids in the presence of transition metal ions had been observed in other studies; for example, the complexes of rutin and dihydroquercetin with Fe, Cu, and Zn had higher anti-oxidation than the free counterparts as the inhibitors of asbestos-induced cell injury [43]. Similarly, the free radical scavenging ability of quercetin–Cu complex was higher than free quercetin [44]. Metal ions such as Cu, Fe, and Zn also had been evidenced to impact anti-microbial, anti-viral, and anti-inflammatory activities of flavonoids [45]. The present results also provided another evidence to show different effects of Fe^{2+}/Cu^{2+} on anti-cancer activities of the two flavones.

Flavonoids have both anti- and pro-oxidation in cells, depending on flavonoid concentrations and free radical sources [46]. The pro-oxidation of flavonoids plays an important role in their anti-cancer activities, via promoting the generation of intracellular ROS in cancer cells [47]. In general, a relative higher flavonoid level in cancer cells leads to pro-oxidation, promotes ROS generation, and, thereby, induces DNA damage [48]. Pro-oxidation of a tea polyphenolic compound, epigallocatechin-3-gallate, has been proved to govern its growth inhibition on colorectal HT29 cells, oral squamous carcinoma SCC-25 and SCC-9 cells, and premalignant leukoplakia MSK-Leuk1cells [49], while cytotoxic effects of quercetin, morin, and kaempferol on promyelocytic leukemia HL-60 cells were found to be caused by their pro-oxidation [22]. Both heat treatment and Fe/Cu addition of apigenin and luteolin led to oxidation and, thereby, altered the redox potential of the two flavones; the assessed samples; thus, had different abilities to generate intracellular ROS, and then showed different growth inhibition on Hela cells. Moreover, the enhanced ROS generation in cells suggests cell apoptosis, because this phenomenon is regarded as a classic way to trigger cell apoptosis [50]. Thus, flavonoids such as quercetin, luteolin, chrysin, kaempferol, apigenin, myricetin, and baicalin showed clear apoptosis induction to the human esophageal adenocarcinoma OE33 cells and three human prostate cancer cells, resulting in increased total apoptotic cells [7,8]. The conducted treatments in this study; thus, decreased ROS generation and apoptosis induction of the two flavones in the cells. It is reasonable that decreased ROS generation of the two flavones with treatment time of 24 h was positively and significantly consistent with their decreased apoptosis induction, as the correlation analysis results showed.

5. Conclusions

Two flavones, apigenin and luteolin, in aqueous solutions, had degradation to different extents, while Fe^{2+}/Cu^{2+} addition mainly resulted in stability (i.e., decreased degradation) for luteolin due to the formation of luteolin–metal complexes, but also led to instability (i.e., increased degradation) for apigenin. The flavone degradation was clearly enhanced at 37 °C (the classic temperature of cell culture) rather than 20 °C. The used heat treatments (37 and 100 °C) and Fe^{2+}/Cu^{2+} addition were adverse to the anti-cancer activities of the two flavones against human cervical cancer Hela cells; subsequently, growth inhibition, DNA damage, and especially apoptosis induction (positively correlated with the intracellular ROS generation) of the two flavones were decreased. It is; thus, proposed that more attention should be paid to both heat treatment and some metal ions like Fe^{2+}/Cu^{2+} due to their negative effects when assessing the bio-activities of flavonoid compounds. However, this study only aimed to verify how the used heating treatments and two metal ions impacted flavone stability and anti-cancer activities in vitro. The related molecular mechanisms and an in vivo investigation will be carried out in a further study.

Author Contributions: W.-N.L. and J.S. performed the experiments; X.-H.Z. obtained the funding, designed the experiments, and analyzed the data; and Y.F. and X.-H.Z. wrote and revised the paper.

Funding: This research was funded by the Key Research Project in Science and Technology of the Education Department of Heilongjiang Province, grant number Project No. 11551z018.

Acknowledgments: The authors thank the anonymous reviewers for their valuable advice.

Conflicts of Interest: The authors declare no conflicts of interest.

References

1. Robak, J.; Gryglewski, R.J. Bioactivity of flavonoids. *Pol. J. Pharmacol.* **1996**, *48*, 555–564. [PubMed]
2. Bogdanski, P.; Suliburska, J.; Szulinska, M.; Stepien, M.; Pupek-Musialik, D.; Jablecka, A. Green tea extract reduces blood pressure, inflammatory biomarkers, and oxidative stress and improves parameters associated with insulin resistance in obese, hypertensive patients. *Nutr. Res.* **2012**, *32*, 421–427. [CrossRef] [PubMed]
3. Bae, E.A.; Han, M.J.; Kim, D.H. In vitro anti-helicobacter pylori activity of some flavonoids and their metabolites. *Planta. Med.* **1999**, *65*, 442–443. [CrossRef] [PubMed]
4. Middleton, E. Effects of flavonoids on immune and inflammatory cell functions. *Biochem. Pharmacol.* **1992**, *43*, 1167–1179. [CrossRef]
5. Ramiro, E.; Franch, A.; Castellote, C.; Andrés-Lacueva, C.; Izquierdo-Pulido, M.; Castell, M. Effect of theobroma cacao flavonoids on immune activation of a lymphoid cell line. *Br. J. Nutr.* **2005**, *93*, 859–866. [CrossRef] [PubMed]
6. Rotelli, A.E.; Guardia, T.; Juárez, A.O.; de La Rocha, N.E.; Pelzer, L.E. Comparative study of flavonoids in experimental models of inflammation. *Pharmacol. Res.* **2003**, *48*, 601–606. [CrossRef]
7. Zhang, Q.; Zhao, X.H.; Wang, Z.J. Flavones and flavonols exert cytotoxic effects on a human oesophageal adenocarcinoma cell line (OE33) by causing G2/M arrest and inducing apoptosis. *Food Chem. Toxicol.* **2008**, *46*, 2042–2053. [CrossRef] [PubMed]
8. Chan, F.L.; Choi, H.L.; Chen, Z.Y.; Chan, P.S.F.; Huang, Y. Induction of apoptosis in prostate cancer cell lines by a flavonoid, baicalin. *Cancer Lett.* **2000**, *160*, 219–228. [CrossRef]
9. Frydoonfar, H.R.; Mcgrath, D.R.; Spigelman, A.D. The variable effect on proliferation of a colon cancer cell line by the citrus fruit flavonoid naringenin. *Colorectal Dis.* **2010**, *5*, 149–152. [CrossRef]
10. Batra, P.; Sharma, A.K. Anti-cancer potential of flavonoids: Recent trends and future perspectives. *3 Biotech* **2013**, *3*, 439–459. [CrossRef]
11. Mira, L.; Fernandez, M.T.; Santos, M.; Rocha, R.; Florêncio, M.H.; Jennings, K.R. Interactions of flavonoids with iron and copper ions: A mechanism for their antioxidant activity. *Free Radic. Res.* **2002**, *36*, 1199–1208. [CrossRef] [PubMed]
12. Hajji, H.E.; Nkhili, E.; Tomao, V.; Dangles, O. Interactions of quercetin with iron and copper ions: Complexation and autoxidation. *Free Radic. Res.* **2006**, *40*, 303–320. [CrossRef] [PubMed]
13. Pękal, A.; Biesaga, M.; Pyrzynska, K. Interaction of quercetin with copper ions: Complexation, oxidation and reactivity towards radicals. *Bio. Met.* **2010**, *24*, 41–49. [CrossRef] [PubMed]
14. Kostyuk, V.A.; Potapovich, A.I.; Strigunova, E.N.; Kostyuk, T.V.; Afanas'ev, I.B. Experimental evidence that flavonoid metal complexes may act as mimics of superoxide dismutase. *Arch. Biochem. Biophys.* **2004**, *428*, 204–208. [CrossRef] [PubMed]
15. Barnes, J.S.; Foss, F.W.; Schug, K.A. Thermally accelerated oxidative degradation of quercetin using continuous flow kinetic electrospray-ion trap-time of flight mass spectrometry. *J. Am. Soc. Mass Spectrom.* **2013**, *24*, 1513–1522. [CrossRef] [PubMed]

16. Oancea, A.M.; Onofrei, C.; Turturică, M.; Bahrim, G.; Râpeanu, G.; Stănciuc, N. The kinetics of thermal degradation of polyphenolic compounds from elderberry (*Sambucus nigra* L.) extract. *Food Sci. Technol. Int.* **2018**, *24*, 361–369. [CrossRef]
17. De Paepe, D.; Valkenborg, D.; Coudijzer, K.; Noten, B.; Servaes, K.; De Loose, M.; Voorspoels, S.; Diels, L.; Van Droogenbroeck, B. Thermal degradation of cloudy apple juice phenolic constituents. *Food Chem.* **2014**, *162*, 176–185. [CrossRef] [PubMed]
18. Ranilla, L.G.; Genovese, M.I.; Lajolo, F.M. Effect of different cooking conditions on phenolic compounds and antioxidant capacity of some selected brazilian bean (*Phaseolus vulgaris* L.) cultivars. *J. Agric. Food Chem.* **2009**, *57*, 5734–5742. [CrossRef]
19. Wang, B.; Wang, J.; Zhao, X.H. In vitro activities of the four structurally similar flavonols weakened by the prior thermal and oxidative treatments to a human colorectal cancer line. *J. Food Biochem.* **2016**, *41*, e12310. [CrossRef]
20. Wang, B.; Zhao, X.H. Four in vitro activities of apigenin to human colorectal carcinoma cells susceptible to air-oxidative and heating treatments. *Emir. J. Food Agri.* **2017**, *29*, 69–77. [CrossRef]
21. Miean, K.H.; Mohamed, S. Flavonoid (myricetin, quercetin, kaempferol, luteolin, and apigenin) content of edible tropical plants. *J. Agric. Food Chem.* **2001**, *49*, 3106–3112. [CrossRef]
22. Sergediene, E.; Jönsson, K.; Szymusiak, H.; Tyrakowska, B.; Rietjens, I.M.; Cenas, N. Prooxidant toxicity of polyphenolic antioxidants to HL-60 cells: Description of quantitative structure-activity relationships. *FEBS Lett.* **1999**, *462*, 392–396. [CrossRef]
23. Shukla, S.; Gupta, S. Apigenin: A promising molecule for cancer prevention. *Pharm. Res.* **2010**, *27*, 962–978. [CrossRef] [PubMed]
24. Chowdhury, A.R.; Sharma, S.; Mandal, S.; Goswami, A.; Mukhopadhyay, S.; Majumder, H.K. Luteolin, an emerging anti-cancer flavonoid, poisons eukaryotic DNA topoisomerase I. *Biochem. J.* **2002**, *366*, 653–661. [CrossRef] [PubMed]
25. Wang, W.D.; Xu, S.Y. Degradation kinetics of anthocyanins in blackberry juice and concentrate. *J. Food Eng.* **2007**, *82*, 271–275. [CrossRef]
26. Lou, J.L.; Chu, G.H.; Zhou, G.J.; Jiang, J.; Huang, F.F.; Xu, J.J.; Zheng, S.; Jiang, W.; Lu, Y.Z.; Li, X.X.; et al. Comparison between two kinds of cigarette smoke condensates (CSCs) of the cytogenotoxicity and protein expression in a human B-cell lymphoblastoid cell line using CCK-8 assay, comet assay and protein microarray. *Mutat. Res. Genet. Toxicol. Environ. Mutagenesis* **2010**, *697*, 55–59. [CrossRef] [PubMed]
27. Vermes, I.; Haanen, C.; Steffensnakken, H.; Reutelingsperger, C. A novel assay for apoptosis flow cytometric detection of phosphatidylserine expression on early apoptotic cells using fluorescein labelled Annexin V. *J. Immunol. Methods* **1995**, *184*, 39–51. [CrossRef]
28. Li, J.; Tang, Q.; Li, Y.; Hu, B.; Ming, Z.; Fu, Q.; Qian, J.Q.; Xiang, J.Z. Role of oxidative stress in the apoptosis of hepatocellular carcinoma induced by combination of arsenic trioxide and ascorbic acid. *Acta Pharmacol. Sin.* **2010**, *27*, 1078–1084. [CrossRef]
29. Sólyom, K.; Solá, R.; Cocero, M.J.; Mato, R.B. Thermal degradation of grape marc polyphenols. *Food Chem.* **2014**, *159*, 361–366. [CrossRef]
30. Khuwijitjaru, P.; Plernjit, J.; Suaylam, B.; Samuhaseneetoo, S.; Pongsawatmanit, R.; Adachi, S. Degradation kinetics of some phenolic compounds in subcritical water and radical scavenging activity of their degradation products. *Can. J. Chem. Eng.* **2013**, *92*, 810–815. [CrossRef]
31. Ramanouskaya, T.V.; Smolnykova, V.V.; Grinev, V.V. Relationship between structure and antiproliferative, proapoptotic, and differentiation effects of flavonoids on chronic myeloid leukemia cells. *Anticancer Drugs* **2009**, *20*, 573–583. [CrossRef] [PubMed]
32. López-Lázaro, M. Flavonoids as anticancer agents: Structure-activity relationship study. *Curr. Med. Chem. Anticancer Agents* **2002**, *2*, 691–714. [CrossRef] [PubMed]
33. Maatouk, M.; Mustapha, N.; Mokdad-Bzeouich, I.; Chaaban, H.; Abed, B.; Iaonnou, I.; Ghedira, K.; Ghoul, M.; Ghedira, L.C. Thermal treatment of luteolin-7-O-β-glucoside improves its immunomodulatory and antioxidant potencies. *Cell Stress Chaperones* **2017**, *22*, 775–785. [CrossRef] [PubMed]
34. Makris, D.P.; Rossiter, J.T. Heat-induced, metal-catalyzed oxidative degradation of quercetin and rutin (quercetin 3-o-rhamnosylglucoside) in aqueous model systems. *J. Agric. Food Chem.* **2000**, *48*, 3830–3838. [CrossRef] [PubMed]

35. Selvaraj, S.; Krishnaswamy, S.; Devashya, V.; Sethuraman, S.; Krishnan, U.M. Flavonoid-metal ion complexes: A novel class of therapeutic agents. *Med. Res. Rev.* **2014**, *34*, 677–702. [CrossRef] [PubMed]
36. De Souza, R.F.V.; Sussuchi, E.M.; De Giovani, W.F. Synthesis, Electrochemical, Spectral, and Antioxidant Properties of Complexes of Flavonoids with Metal Ions. *Redox Rep.* **2003**, *33*, 1125–1144. [CrossRef]
37. Lee, K.; Hyun Lee, D.; Jung, Y.J.; Shin, S.Y.; Lee, Y.H. The natural flavone eupatorin induces cell cycle arrest at the G2/M phase and apoptosis in Hela cells. *Appl. Biol. Chem.* **2016**, *59*, 193–199. [CrossRef]
38. Wang, Y.; Zhang, W.; Lv, Q.; Zhang, J.; Zhu, D. The critical role of quercetin in autophagy and apoptosis in Hela cells. *Tumor Biol.* **2015**, *37*, 925–929. [CrossRef]
39. Jung, J.H.; Lee, J.O.; Kim, J.H.; Lee, S.K.; You, G.Y.; Park, S.H.; Park, J.M.; Kim, E.K.; Suh, P.G.; An, J.K.; et al. Quercetin suppresses Hela cell viability via AMPK-induced HSP70 and EGFR down-regulation. *J. Cell Physiol.* **2010**, *223*, 408–414. [CrossRef]
40. Hann, H.W.; Stahlhut, M.W.; Blumberg, B.S. Iron nutrition and tumor growth: Decreased tumor growth in iron-deficient mice. *Cancer Res.* **1988**, *48*, 4168–4170.
41. Yu, Y.; Kovacevic, Z.; Richardson, D.R. Tuning cell cycle regulation with an iron key. *Cell Cycle* **2007**, *6*, 1982–1994. [CrossRef] [PubMed]
42. Kim, R.H.; Lee, S.M.; Park, J.W. Enhancement by copper, zinc superoxide dismutase of DNA damage and mutagenicity with hydrogen peroxide. *IUBMB Life* **2010**, *45*, 635–642. [CrossRef]
43. Kostyuk, V.A.; Potapovich, A.I.; Vladykovskaya, E.N.; Korkina, L.G.; Afanas'ev, I.B. Influence of metal ions on flavonoid protection against asbestos-induced cell injury. *Arch. Biochem. Biophys.* **2001**, *385*, 129–137. [CrossRef] [PubMed]
44. Bukhari, S.B.; Memon, S.; Mahroof-Tahir, M.; Bhanger, M.I. Synthesis, characterization and antioxidant activity copper-quercetin complex. *Spectrochim. Acta A Mol. Biomol. Spectrosc.* **2009**, *71*, 1901–1906. [CrossRef] [PubMed]
45. Kasprzak, M.M.; Erxleben, A.; Ochocki, J. Properties and applications of flavonoid metal complexes. *RSC Adv.* **2015**, *57*, 45853–45877. [CrossRef]
46. Cao, G.; Sofic, E.; Prior, R.L. Antioxidant and prooxidant behavior of flavonoids: Structure-activity relationships. *Free Radic. Biol. Med.* **1997**, *22*, 749–760. [CrossRef]
47. Galati, G.; Sabzevari, O.; Wilson, J.X.; O'Brien, P.J. Prooxidant activity and cellular effects of the phenoxyl radicals of dietary flavonoids and other polyphenolics. *Toxicology* **2002**, *177*, 91–104. [CrossRef]
48. Stepanic, V.; Gasparovic, A.C.; Troselj, K.G.; Amic, D.; Zarkovic, N. Selected attributes of polyphenols in targeting oxidative stress in cancer. *Curr. Top Med. Chem.* **2015**, *15*, 496–509. [CrossRef]
49. Tao, L.; Park, J.Y.; Lambert, J.D. Differential prooxidative effects of the green tea polyphenol, (-)-epigallocatechin-3-gallate, in normal and oral cancer cells are related to differences in sirtuin 3 signaling. *Mol. Nutr. Food Res.* **2014**, *59*, 203–211. [CrossRef]
50. Sabharwal, S.S.; Schumacker, P.T. Mitochondrial ROS in cancer: Initiators, amplifiers or an Achilles' heel? *Nat. Rev. Cancer* **2014**, *14*, 709–721. [CrossRef]

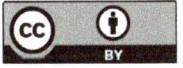

© 2019 by the authors. Licensee MDPI, Basel, Switzerland. This article is an open access article distributed under the terms and conditions of the Creative Commons Attribution (CC BY) license (http://creativecommons.org/licenses/by/4.0/).

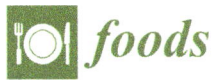

Article

Ginger Water Reduces Body Weight Gain and Improves Energy Expenditure in Rats

Samy Sayed [1,2], Mohamed Ahmed [3], Ahmed El-Shehawi [1,4], Mohamed Alkafafy [1,3], Saqer Al-Otaibi [1], Hanan El-Sawy [5], Samy Farouk [1] and Samir El-Shazly [1,6,*]

1. Department of Biotechnology, Faculty of Science, Taif University, Taif 21974, Saudi Arabia; samy_mahmoud@hotmail.com (S.S.); elshehawi@hotmail.com (A.E.-S.); dr_alkafafy@yahoo.com (M.A.); saqer-20@hotmail.com (S.A.-O.); dmrasamy@yahoo.com (S.F.)
2. Faculty of Agriculture, Cairo University, Giza 12613, Egypt
3. Faculty of Veterinary Medicine, University of Sadat City, Sadat City 32958, Egypt; m_m_ahmed2000@yahoo.com
4. Department of Genetics, Faculty of Agriculture, University of Alexandria, Alexandria 21526, Egypt
5. Department of Nutrition and Clinical Nutrition, Faculty of Veterinary Medicine, Kafrelsheikh University, Kafrelsheikh 33516, Egypt; hananelsawy2011@yahoo.com
6. Department of Biochemistry, Faculty of Veterinary Medicine, Kafrelsheikh University, Kafr Elsheikh 33511, Egypt
* Correspondence: elshazlysamir@yahoo.com

Received: 19 November 2019; Accepted: 30 December 2019; Published: 2 January 2020

Abstract: Obesity is a serious global problem that causes predisposition to numerous serious diseases. The current study aims to investigate the effect of ginger water on body weight and energy expenditure through modulation of mRNA expression of carbohydrate and lipid metabolism. A white colored liquid obtained during freeze-drying of fresh rhizomes of *Zingiber officinal* was collected and named ginger water. It was used to treat rats, then blood and tissue samples were collected from the liver and white adipose at the end of the experiment. The serum was prepared and used for biochemical assays, while tissue samples were used for RNA isolation and gene expression analysis via Reverse transcription polymerase chain reaction (RT-PCR). Results of High Performance Liquid Chromatography (HPLC) analysis of ginger water revealed the presence of chrysin and galangin at concentrations of 0.24 µg/mL and 0.53 µg/mL, respectively. Average body weight gain decreased significantly in groups that received ginger water. In addition, both total cholesterol and serum triacylglycerol were reduced in the groups that received ginger water. Furthermore, mRNA expression of Sterol regulatory element-binding protein 1 (SREBP-1c) in the liver and leptin in adipose tissues were downregulated, while those of adiponectin, hepatic carnitine palmitoyltransferase1 (CPT-1), acyl coA oxidase (ACO), Glucose transporter 2 (GLUT-2), and pyruvate kinase (PK) were upregulated in ginger water-treated groups. These results clearly revealed the lowering body weight gain effect of ginger water, which most likely occurs at the transcriptional level of energy metabolizing proteins.

Keywords: ginger water; obesity; energy homeostasis; gene expression; rat

1. Introduction

Obesity is a complex metabolic disorder that is currently a serious global problem. Obesity has been considered a fatal lifestyle disease during the past few decades because of increasingly high-fat and caloric-rich diets as well as genetic background [1,2]. The main reason for obesity is the energy imbalance in which the energy intake is higher than the energy expenditure. The main features of obesity include excessive fat mass and raised blood lipid concentration [3]. Obesity can lead to a wide range of diseases, such as type-2 diabetes, hypertension and hyperlipidemia, and cardiovascular diseases [4]. Therefore, prevention and treatment of obesity are a great health concern worldwide.

Although physical exercise and dieting are the preferred treatments for weight loss, in practice, this method is not effectively maintained, due to busy schedules. On the other hand, surgery is not preferable due to the risk factors and high cost. Therefore, there is a shift towards an increased use of medications to reduce weight with consideration of the side effects of these medications. Currently available antiobesity drugs attack body fat in various manners. They may promote metabolism and diminish appetite or they can affect fat digestion. Consequently, both health systems and researchers targeted the advancement of effective and safe therapies for obesity [5].

Natural products have been defined with different terms in various studies; functional food [6], food supplement [7], and the recently preferred definition "nutraceuticals" [8]. Although extensive research and patenting of nutraceuticals have been going for more than a decade, they do not have precise definition [9]. Nutraceuticals, when supported by clinical trials and known mode of action, have a major role in preventing as well as supporting the drug therapy of chronic diseases. In addition, the market of nutraceuticals is growing very fast with an expected market value of $578.23 billion in 2025, although it faces challenges due to the absence of clear regulations and marking difference from food supplements. It is expected that nutraceuticals, in the future, will be approved and marketed side by side with the pharmaceuticals [10]. This indicates the need for an international consensus of regulatory framework for research, approval, safety, labelling, marketing, and use of nutraceuticals [9].

Natural plant compounds and their derivatives have been reported to treat obesity without mortality or obvious adverse impacts [11]. Plants that contain components with antiobesity activity have been used all over the world as alternative and complementary herbal therapies [12]. Herbal medicines are plant-derived raw or refined products that are used for the treatment of diseases. The antiobesity effects of many combinations of plant extracts were investigated. Most of these investigations indicated antiobesity effects, for example, decreasing body weight gain in both animals and humans. *Arachis hypogaea* decreased body weight gain, liver size, and liver triglyceride content, with an increase of fecal lipid excretion [13]. A reduction in food intake as a result of reducing appetite and an impacted hormonal status was shown with pomegranate [14].

Ginger (*Zingiber officinale* Roscoe, Zingiberaceae) is a well-known spice and flavoring material that has also been used in traditional medicine in many areas. Ethanolic extract of ginger had a reducing impact on the levels of blood glucose in rats fed on a high fat diet [15]. In addition, ginger ameliorates hyperlipidemia in diabetic rats by decreasing serum cholesterol and serum triglycerides [16,17]. Studies showed that ginger supplement improves fructose utilization-incited fatty liver [18] and adipose tissue insulin resistance in rats [19]. Ginger extract weakened the kidney injury induced by chronic fructose consumption. This was mediated by suppressing renal over-expression of proinflammatory cytokines [20]. The important active component of ginger root is the unpredictable oil and impactful phenol compounds, for example, gingerol, which is a very powerful anti-inflammatory compound [21]. Gingerol has appeared to stabilize adipocyte hormones, plasma, lipases, and lipid profiles in high fat diet induced obese rats [22].

Modern scientific research has revealed that ginger possesses various therapeutic properties, such as antioxidant effects and anti-inflammatory impacts [23]. Ginger water is obtained during the freeze-drying of ginger rhizomes as a byproduct. Its strong smell and milky color raised our attention to its potential similar biological effects to ginger extract. Most previous studies have focused on the effects of the main constituents of ginger extracts; however, there are no investigations that have specifically addressed the efficacy of the byproduct, ginger water. Therefore, this investigation aimed to study the lowering body weight gain effect of ginger water and to explore the molecular mechanisms underlying this impact through investigating the ability of ginger water to adjust mRNA expression of different genes related to carbohydrate and lipid metabolism.

2. Materials and Methods

2.1. Experimental Design

A total of fifteen ten weeks-old adult male Wistar rats were used in this study. Animals were obtained from the Experimental Animal Research Center, University of King Abdulaziz, Saudi Arabia. The animals were kept in polyethylene cages and held under laboratory conditions of 22 °C and 55% H in the animal house of Taif University, Saudi Arabia with a 12 h/12 h light/dark cycle. All animal groups were fed standard laboratory chow with free access to water. The Committee of Taif University for animal care and use has approved all procedures under the authorization number of 1-440-6145.

2.2. Preparation of the Ginger Water

Ginger water is not a ginger extract, but it is a byproduct obtained during lyophilization (freeze-drying) of ginger rhizomes. Fresh rhizomes of the ginger plant were washed, sliced, and freeze-dried at −60 °C. During the freeze-drying process, the condensed white colored liquid in the freeze-dryer was collected, named as ginger water, analyzed using High Performance Liquid Chromatography (HPLC), and used for the experiment.

2.3. HPLC Analysis of Ginger Water

The obtained ginger water was subjected to analysis using HPLC. Briefly, ginger water was filtered through syringe filters and used for HPLC analysis against nine flavonoid standards (Cyanidine chloride, Myrecitine, Quercetine, Chrysine, Malvidine chloride, Delphinidine chloride, Naringenine, Caffeic acid, and Galangin). The HPLC conditions were similar to those mentioned previously by the authors in [24]. Samples were assayed on an HPLC Hewlett-Packard Phenomenex Luna C18 column (4.6 × 250 mm, 10 μm particle size, Hewlett-Packard, Palo Alto, CA, USA). Separation was done at 12 min linear gradient from 100% of 100 mM ammonium acetate (pH 5.5) to 100% methanol. The flow rate was 1.5 mL/min and oven temperature of 35 °C with injection volume of 20 μL. Sample components were monitored at 260 nm. For calibration, standard compounds were dissolved in ethyl alcohol. Then, each peak area was converted to micrograms per mL.

2.4. Animal Treatment

The animals were randomly distributed into three groups of five animals each. The first group received tap water and feed ad libitum throughout the experimental period and considered as a control group. The second and third groups received ginger water at a rate of 25% and 50% (v/v) in their drinking water, respectively. Treatment proceeded for approximately a month. Body weight and the average of daily food consumption were measured weekly until the experimental period ended.

2.5. Sampling

By the end of treatment and before animal sacrifice, animals were fasted for 10 h. Blood samples were directly collected from retro-orbital puncture after diethyl ether anesthesia. Serum samples were arranged and stored at −80 °C until use in subsequent analysis. Then, rats were killed by decapitation. Specimens for RNA isolation were collected from liver and white adipose tissue. Samples were kept in QiaZol (Qiagen Inc., Valencia, CA, USA) and stored at −80 °C for using in gene expression analysis.

2.6. Biochemical Assays

Total cholesterol (TC) and serum triacylglycerol (TAG) were measured cholorametrically using commercial kits (HUMAN Gesellschaft für Biochemica und Diagnostica mbH, Wiesbaden, Germany) according to the manufacturer's instructions.

2.7. Gene Expression Analysis

2.7.1. RNA Extraction and cDNA Synthesis

Tissue, 100 mg, was used for isolation of total RNA using QIAzol reagent (QIAGEN Inc., Valencia, CA, USA) as explained previously [14]. RNA quality was tested by agarose gel electrophoresis. Concentration and purity of RNA were evaluated at 260 nm and by determination of $OD_{260/280}$ ratio, respectively. For cDNA synthesis, 4 µg of RNA were used with oligo-dT primer and M-MuLV reverse transcriptase (GoScript™ Reverse Transcriptase Promega, Fitchburg, WI, USA) as described previously [25] in the PeX 0.5 Thermal Cycler (Thermo Electronic Corporation, Milford, MA, USA). The obtained cDNA was directly used for Reverse transcription polymerase chain reaction (RT-PCR) or kept at −20 °C for future use.

2.7.2. Semi-Quantitative-PCR

Expression of different genes related to energy metabolism was estimated by semi-quantitative PCR using their corresponding primers (Table 1). The tested genes included pyruvate kinase (PK), sterol regulatory element-binding protein-1c (SREBP-1c), glucose transporter-2 (GLUT-2), carnitine palmitoyl transferase-1 (CPT-1), acyl-CoA oxidase (ACO), and hormone sensitive lipase (HSL). The expression of leptin as well as adiponectin was also tested. Primers were designed using the Oligo-4 computer program and nucleotide sequence published in GeneBank (Table 1). PCR was conducted in 25 µL volume using PCR GoTaq®Master Mix (Promega Co., Fitchburg, WI, USA) as detailed previously [14]. The number of cycles and annealing temperatures of primers are summarized in Table 1. Expression of GAPDH mRNA was used as a reference (Table 1). PCR products were subjected to 1% agarose electrophoresis with ethidium bromide staining. PCR product bands were photographed under UV light. The intensities of the bands were densitometerically quantified using the NIH imageJ program (https://imagej.nih.gov/ij/).

Table 1. Primer sequence and PCR conditions used in this study.

Target Gene	Primer Sequence (5′–3′)	Annealing	Cycles	Product Size
GAPDH	F-AGATCCACAACGGATACATT	52 °C	25 cycles	309 bP
	R-TCCCTCAAGATTGTCAGCA			
SREP1-c	F-GGAGCCATGGATTGCACATT	58 °C	28 cycles	191 bP
	R-AGGAAGGCTTCCAGAGAGGA			
HSL	F-TGCCCAGGAGTGTGTCTGAG	61 °C	33 cycles	313 bP
	R-AGGACACCTTGGCTTGAGCG			
Leptin	F-CCTGTGGCTTTGGTCCTATCTG	59 °C	30 cycles	244 bP
	R-TATGCTTTGCTGGGGTTTTC			
Adiponectin	F-CTCCACCCAAGGAAACTTGT	52 °C	28 cycles	500 bP
	R-CTGGTCCACATTTTTTTCCT			
PK	F-ATTGCTGTGACTGGATCTGC	52 °C	28 cycles	229 bP
	R-CCCGCATGATGTTGGTATAG			
GLUT-2	F-AAGGATCAAAGCCATGTTGG	55 °C	28 cycles	330 bP
	R-GGAGACCTTCTGCTCAGTGG			
ACO	F-GCCCTCAGCTATGGTATTAC	53 °C	28 cycles	633 bP
	R-AGGAACTGCTCTCACAATGG			
CPT-1	F-TATGTGAGGATGCTGCTTCC	52 °C	28 cycles	628 bP
	R-CTCGGAGAGCTAAGCTTGCT			

2.8. Statistical Analysis

Results were analyzed statistically using one-way ANOVA and Scheffe's protected least significant difference test, by using SPSS software (SPSS version 13.0, IBM, Chicago, IL, USA) with $p < 0.05$. Results were expressed as means ± standard errors (SE).

3. Results

3.1. Chemical Composition of Ginger Water

HPLC analysis of the obtained ginger water revealed that, among the nine standards used in the HPLC analysis, only chrysin and galangin were detected in the ginger water, at concentrations of 0.24 µg/mL and 0.53 µg/mL, respectively (Figure 1).

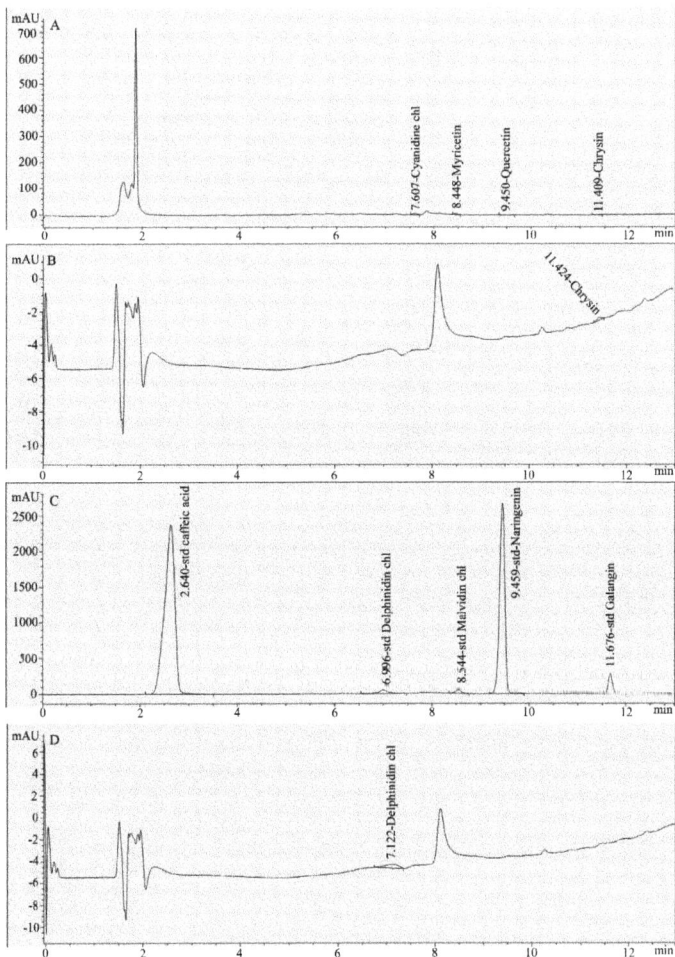

Figure 1. HPLC chromatograms of ginger water and reference standards. (**A**) Standard mix1, (**B**) ginger water, (**C**) standard mix2, and (**D**) ginger water.

3.2. Effect of Ginger Water on Food Consumption and Average Change of Body Weight

The obtained results indicated that there was no significant decrease in neither the food consumption nor the water intake in the groups that received ginger water compared to the control. On the other hand, the weekly average body weight exhibited significant differences in the groups that received 25% and 50% ginger water compared to the control group starting from the second week (Figure 2A). The difference was indicated in the lowering body weight gain in the 25% and 50% groups compared to the control. Meanwhile, there are no significant differences among groups that received ginger water at different dose rates.

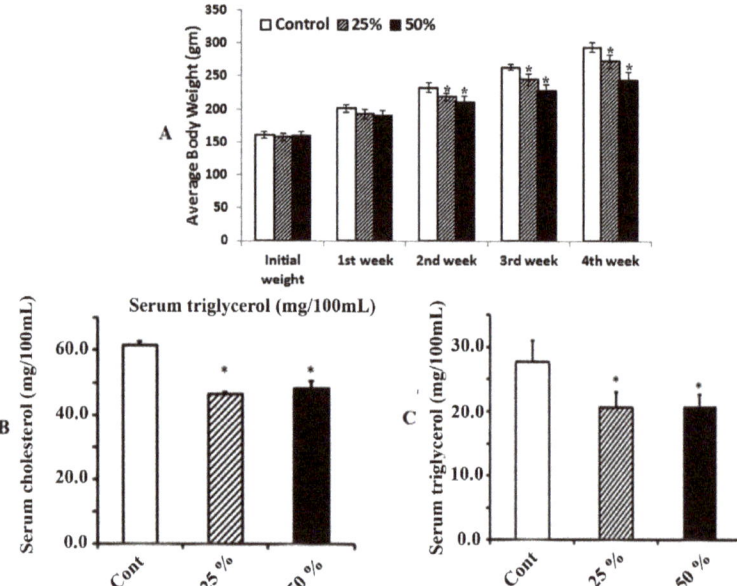

Figure 2. The effect of ginger water on body weight. Values are mean ± standard errors (SE) ($n = 5$). (**A**) Control, control group; 25%, 25% (v/v) ginger water-treated group; 50%, 50% (v/v) ginger water-treated group. The effect ginger water on serum level of (**B**) cholesterol and (**C**) triacylglycerol. Values are mean ± SE ($n = 5$). Cont: control, 25%:25% (v/v) ginger water-treated group, 50%:50% (v/v) ginger water-treated group. * $p < 0.05$ vs. the control.

3.3. Effect of Ginger Water on Serum Total Cholesterol and Triacylglycerol

Administration of ginger water significantly decreased both serum total cholesterol and serum triacylglycerol compared to the control group. Meanwhile, the difference between groups that received 25% and 50% ginger water is not significant (Figure 2B,C).

3.4. Effect of Ginger Water Treatment on HSL and SREBP-1c mRNA Expression

The obtained results showed that the ginger water-receiving groups did not show significant differences with the control group in hormone sensitive lipase (HSL) mRNA expression. On the other hand, ginger water treatment at 25% and 50% induced 50% and 60% downregulation in SREBP-1c mRNA expression, respectively (Figure 3A,B).

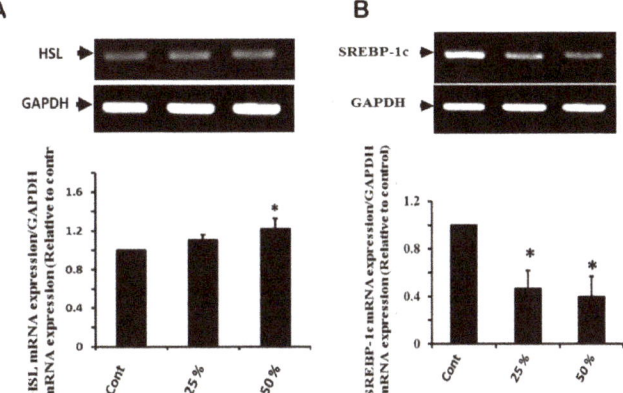

Figure 3. Effect of ginger water on HSL (**A**) SREBP-1c, (**B**) mRNA expressions in hepatic tissue of rats. Results of densitometric analyses and demonstrative blots of at least five independent experiments are displayed. Values are expressed as means ± SE. Cont: control, 25%:25% (v/v) ginger water-treated group, 50%:50% (v/v) ginger water-treated group. * $p < 0.05$ vs. the control.

3.5. Effect of Ginger Water Treatment on the Leptin, Adiponectine, and Resistin mRNA Expression in White Adipose Tissue

The expression of leptin mRNA was significantly downregulated (more than 3-fold) in response to receiving ginger water in both treated groups compared to the control one. Leptin mRNA expression did not show significant differences between 25% and 50% ginger water receiving groups (Figure 4A). Concerning adiponectin mRNA expression, the results showed a significant upregulation (about 2.5-fold) in groups that received ginger water compared to the control group, without significant differences between the two treated groups (Figure 4B). In the same context, ginger water treatment significantly suppressed resistin mRNA expression (Figure 4C).

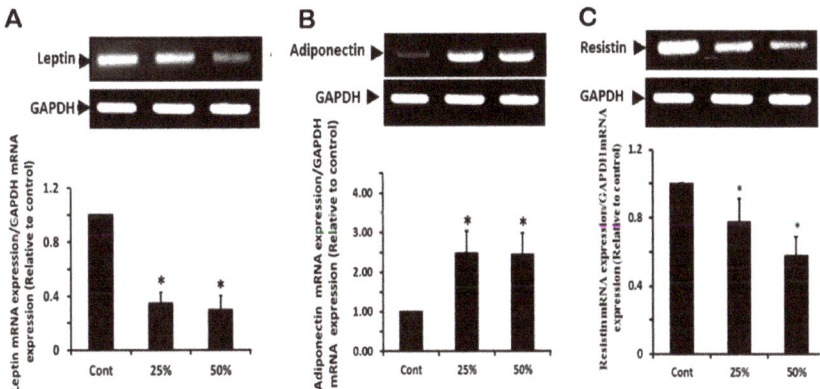

Figure 4. Effect of ginger water on leptin (**A**), adiponectin (**B**), and resistin (**C**), and expression of mRNA in white adipose tissue of rat. Results of densitometric analyses and demonstrative blots of at least five independent experiments are displayed. Values are expressed as means ± SE. Cont: control, 25%:25% (v/v) ginger water-treated group, 50%:50% (v/v) ginger water-treated group. * $p < 0.05$ vs. the control.

3.6. Effect of Ginger Water Treatment on the GLUT-2 and PK mRNA Expression

The expression of GLUT-2 mRNA showed a significant upregulation in groups that received 25% and 50% ginger water compared to the control group (Figure 5A). In a parallel manner to GLUT-2,

PK showed upregulation in groups that received ginger water that reached a significant degree in the group treated with 50% ginger water compared to the control group (Figure 5B).

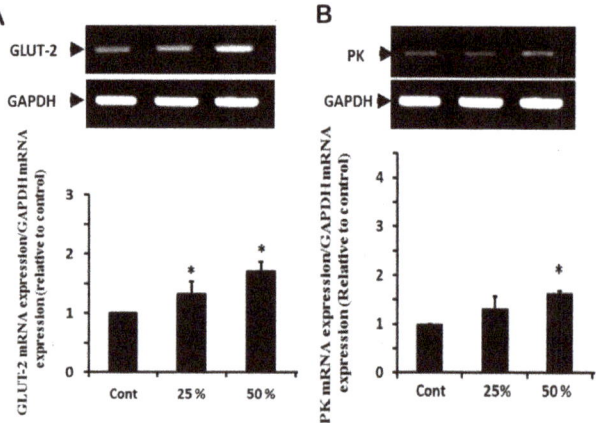

Figure 5. Effect of ginger water on GLUT-2 (**A**) and PK (**B**) mRNA expressions in the hepatic tissue of rats. Results of densitometric analyses and demonstrative blots of at least five independent experiments are displayed. Values are expressed as means ± SE. Cont: control, 25%:25% (v/v) ginger water-treated group, 50%:50% (v/v) ginger water-treated group. * $p < 0.05$ vs. the control.

3.7. Effect of Ginger Water Treatment on the CPT-1 and ACO mRNA Expression

The expression of CPT-1 mRNA showed upregulation in the groups that received ginger water with a significant degree in the 50% group compared to the control group (Figure 6A). Similarly, ACO mRNA showed significant upregulation in groups that received 25% and 50% ginger water compared to the control group (Figure 6B).

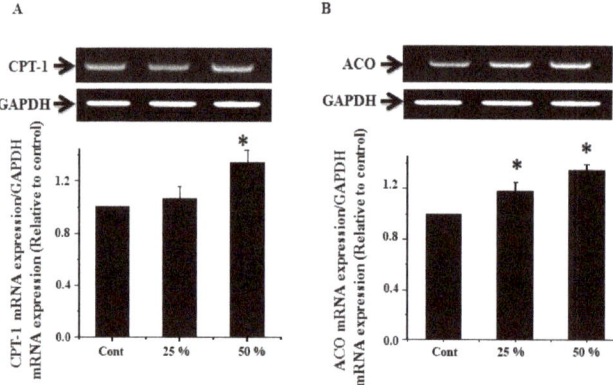

Figure 6. Effect of ginger water on CPT-1(**A**) and ACO (**B**) expression of mRNA in rat hepatic tissue. Results of densitometric analyses and demonstrative blots of at least five independent experiments are displayed. Values are expressed as means ± SE. Cont: control, 25%:25% (v/v) ginger water-treated group, 50%:50% (v/v) ginger water-treated group. * $p < 0.05$ vs. the control.

4. Discussion

The use of herbal medicines has increased over the last few years for treatment of obesity. This is due to the rise in population, high cost of medicinal treatment for common disorders, side effects of different current therapeutic drugs, and the appearance of drug resistance. Ginger is considered one of the most commonly used species worldwide [26]. It belongs to the plant family that includes turmeric and cardamom. It has a strong aroma due to its high content of the pungent ketones, including gingerol, which is used in research studies as an extract [27]. Beneficial effects of ginger on obesity and its associated metabolic disorders have been shown [28,29]. It was reported that ginger extract decreases aortic atherosclerotic lesion areas, plasma cholesterol, triacylglycerol, and low-density lipoprotein [30]. In addition, ginger powder strongly decreased serum lipid levels in volunteers [31]. Moreover, ginger meal (1%) significantly lowered cholesterol levels [32]. Our obtained results showed that administration of ginger water significantly reduces the serum triacylglycerol and total cholesterol compared to those of the control group, indicating the hypolipidemic effects of ginger water. Although gingerols constitute the main portion of fresh and dry ginger, many constituents have been detected using different analytical methods [33]. In the present study, two compounds (Chrysin, Galangin) were detected in the ginger water at concentrations of 0.24 µg/mL and 0.53 µg/mL, respectively, using HPLC analysis.

Galangin is a member of the flavonol class of flavonoids and chemically known as 3,5,7-trihydroxyflavone. It is the active constituent of the rhizome of the *Alpinia galanga* plant, which belongs to the Zingiberaceae family [34]. Galangin has been proven to have various pharmacological effects [35], such as antimicrobial activity [36], anticancer [37], anti-inflammatory [38], antioxidative [39], metabolic enzyme modulation [40], and antiobesity [41] effects. Moreover, galangin was found to produce a significant decrease in serum lipids [42]. Other recent studies have revealed that galangin significantly contributed to the protection against acetaminophen-induced acute injury in liver and kidney [43]. An earlier study has shown that galangin has antioxidant activity in vitro and in vivo, free radical scavenging activity, tweaks enzymatic activity, and suppresses genotoxicity of chemicals [39].

Chrysin ($C_{15}H_{10}O_4$) has been shown to be a very active flavonoid exerting some pharmacological properties, such as anti-inflammatory activity through blocking histamine release and expression of proinflammatory cytokines [44,45]. Antiasthmatic activity occurs via suppressing the nuclear factor-kB (NF-kB) and inducible nitric oxide synthase (iNOS) [46]. The anticancer activity of chrysin was also reported [47,48], as well antihypercholesterolemic and cardioprotective activities [49,50].

The antiobesity effect of plant preparations may act through inducing thermogenesis [51], stimulating lipolysis and decreasing lipogenesis [52], suppressing appetite [53], or decreasing lipid absorption [54]. In the current study, the administration of ginger water at a concentration of 25% and 50% showed a marked decrease in the lipogenesis process that was demonstrated by the inhibition of SEREP1c mRNA expression. The obtained data of body weights are parallel with that of leptin levels where nontreated controls showed higher body weights and leptin levels compared to the ginger water-treated groups. These results agree with that of previous studies [55].

On the contrary to leptin, adiponectin mRNA expression was higher in ginger water treated groups compared to the control group. Plasma adiponectin concentration and mRNA expression are decreased in obesity and insulin resistance [56]. Gingerol is well known to decrease serum adiponectin [57]. Therefore, this upregulated adiponectin expression could clarify the lowered blood glucose level. This might be caused by the reduced hepatic gluconeogesis and elevated insulin sensitivity [58].

Administration of ginger water apparently upregulated the hepatic mRNA expression of the lipid degradation gene, HSL, contrasted with the control. This suggested that the ginger water effects are partially caused by the downregulation of the mRNA expression of genes engaged with lipogenesis and upregulation of those concerned with lipolysis.

The lipogenic transcription factor, SREBP1c, regulates lipid metabolism via controlling the gene expression of enzymes for fatty acid synthesis, uptake, and triacylglycerol synthesis [59]. The obtained results showed a significant reduction in the mRNA expression of SREBP1c in groups that received ginger water compared to the control group. The ginger oil effectively suppressed the expression of PPARγ (Peroxisome proliferator-activated gamma), and SREBP1c [60]. Ethanolic extract of ginger reduces the levels of blood glucose in high fat diet-fed rats [15]. It has been also shown to have hypoglycemic and hypolipidemic effects in diabetic rats [16] and mice [61]. The current results showed that ginger water upregulated the expression of GLUT-2 mRNA, which plays a central role in glucose transportation from blood to liver. Moreover, Hepatic PK mRNA expression was upregulated by ginger water. PK is a key player in the glycolytic pathway. Thus, ginger water improves energy metabolism through enhancing glucose uptake via GLUT-2 mRNA expression upregulation, enhancing glucose oxidation via PK mRNA expression upregulation, and enhancing lipolysis and inhibiting lipogenesis via upregulating HSL and downregulating SREP1-c mRNA expressions, respectively. These findings could explain the obtained lipid profile in ginger water-treated groups. Moreover, ginger water could improve energy metabolism through enhancing insulin sensitivity via upregulation of adiponectin and/or downregulating both leptin and resistin expression [62,63]. These findings are in agreement with those of the previous study on the effect of vitamins A and E on lipid and carbohydrate metabolism in diet-induced obese rats [64].

The rate limiting enzyme, Acyl-CoA oxidase (ACO), catalyzes the first step in the peroxisomal β-oxidation [65]. The obtained results revealed that both 25% and 50% of ginger water resulted in upregulation of hepatic tissue ACO mRNA expression. These findings are in line with the previous work, which showed that the treatment with ginger extract led to upregulation of ACO mRNA expression, suggesting its ability to reduce liver fat accumulation through motivation of peroxisomal β-oxidation [66].

Carnitine palmitoyl transferase-I (CPT-I) is a regulatory enzyme of mitochondrial β-oxidation through controlling fatty acid transport to the mitochondrial matrix [18]. Our results revealed that ginger water administration led to upregulation of CPT-1 mRNA expression in hepatic tissue. Upregulation of cellular CPT-I expression motivated fatty acid oxidation and considerably decreased the hepatic triacylglycerol content in both high-fat diet or standard diet [67].

In conclusion, ginger water has a lowering body weight gain effect. It seems to show such activities by regulating the lipid metabolism through stimulation of lipolytic pathways and downregulation of lipogenic pathways. Additionally, ginger water may be helpful in insulin sensitization and facilitating glucose transportation to liver cells as well as improving glucose metabolism. Moreover, ginger water could have nutraceutical potential for controlling body weight, preventing obesity and obesity-associated diseases through its incorporation as food flavor, and in dietary supplements, especially for those going on a diet to lower body weight gain.

Author Contributions: Formal analysis, S.S.; Investigation, A.E.-S., H.E.-S. and S.E.-S.; Methodology, M.A. (Mohamed Alkafafy); Resources, S.A.-O., S.F.; Writing—original draft, M.A. (Mohamed Ahmed). All authors have read and agreed to the published version of the manuscript.

Funding: This research was funded by Taif University, Grant Number 1-440-6145.

Conflicts of Interest: The authors declare no conflict of interest.

References

1. WHO. *2000 Obesity: Preventing and Managing the Global Epidemic Report of a WHO Consultation*; WHO Technical Report Series No. 894; WHO: Geneva, Switzerland, 2000.
2. WHO 2013 Factson Obesity. Available online: http://www.who.int/features/factfiles/obesity/en/ (accessed on 24 February 2014).
3. Choquet, H.; Meyre, D. Molecular basis of obesity: Current status and future prospects. *Curr. Genom.* **2011**, *12*, 154–168. [CrossRef]
4. Nawrocki, A.R.; Scherer, P.E. Keynote review: The adipocyte as a drug discovery target. *Drug Discov. Today* **2005**, *10*, 1219–1230. [CrossRef]
5. Abdollahi, M.; Afshar-Imani, B. A review on obesity and weight loss measures. *Middle East Pharm.* **2003**, *11*, 6–10.
6. Hardy, G. Nutraceuticals and functional foods: Introduction and meaning. *Nutrition* **2000**, *16*, 688–689. [CrossRef]

7. Directive 2002/46/EC of the European Parliament and of the Council of 10 June 2002 on the Approximation of the Laws of the Member States Relating to Food Supplements. *Off. J. Eur. Communities* **2002**, L183/51–L183/57. Available online: http%3A%2F%2Feur-lex.europa.eu%2Flegal-content%2FEN%2FTXT%2FPDF%2F%3Furi%3DCELEX%3A32002L0046%26amp%3Bfrom%3DENhttp%3A%2F%2Feur-lex.europa.eu%2Flegal-content%2FEN%2FTXT%2FPDF%2F%3Furi%3DCELEX%3A32002L0046%26amp%3Bfrom%3DEN (accessed on 31 December 2019).
8. European Nutraceutical Association (ENA) (Ed.) *Science Behind Nutraceuticals*; European Nutraceutical Association: Basel, Switzerland, 2016; Volume 2016, p. 594.
9. Santini, A.; Cammarata, S.M.; Capone, G.; Ianaro, A.; Tenore, G.C.; Pani, L.; Novellino, E. Nutraceuticals: Opening the debate for a regulatory framework. *Br. J. Clin. Pharmacol.* **2018**, *84*, 659–672. [CrossRef]
10. Daliu, P.; Santini, A.; Novellino, E. A decade of nutraceutical patents: Where are we now in 2018? *Exp. Opin. Ther. Pat.* **2018**, *28*, 875–882. [CrossRef]
11. Chung, M.J.; Kang, A.Y.; Park, K.W.; Jun, H.J.; Lee, S.J. The effect of essential oil if dietary wormwood (Artemisia princeps), with and without added vitamin E, on oxidative stress and some genes involved in cholesterol metabolism. *Food Chem. Toxicol.* **2007**, *45*, 1400–1409. [CrossRef]
12. Hasani-Ranjbar, S.; Larijani, B.; Abdollahi, M. A systematic review of Iranian medicinal plants useful in diabetes mellitus. *Arch. Med. Sci.* **2008**, *4*, 285–292.
13. Moreno, D.A.; Ilic, N.; Poulev, A.; Raskin, I. Effects of Arachis hypogaea nutshell extract on lipid metabolic enzymes and obesity parameters. *Life Sci.* **2006**, *78*, 2797–2803. [CrossRef]
14. Ahmed, M.M.; Ibrahim, Z.S.; Alkafafy, M.; El-Shazly, S.A. L-Carnitine protects against testicular dysfunction caused by gamma irradiation in mice. *Acta Histochem.* **2014**, *116*, 1046–1055. [CrossRef] [PubMed]
15. Nammi, S.; Sreemantula, S.; Roufogalis, B.D. Protective effects of ethanolic extract of *Zingiber officinale* rhizome on the development of metabolic syndrome in high-fat diet-fed rats. *Basic Clin. Pharmacol. Toxicol.* **2009**, *104*, 366–373. [CrossRef] [PubMed]
16. Al-Amin, Z.M.; Thomson, M.; Al-Qattan, K.K. Antidiabetic and hypolipidaemic properties of ginger (Zingiber officinale) in streptozotocin-induced diabetic rats. *Br. J. Nutr.* **2006**, *96*, 660–666. [CrossRef] [PubMed]
17. Saravanan, G.; Ponmurugan, P.; Deepa, M.A.; Senthilkumar, B. Anti-obesity action of gingerol: Effect on lipid profile, insulin, leptin, amylase and lipase in male obese rats induced by a high-fat diet. *J. Sci. Food Agric.* **2014**, *94*, 2972–2977. [CrossRef]
18. Gao, H.; Guan, T.; Li, C.; Zuo, G.; Yamahara, J.; Wang, J.; Li, Y. Treatment with ginger ameliorates fructose-induced fatty liver and hypertriglyceridemia in rats: Modulation of the hepatic carbohydrate response element binding protein-mediated pathway. *Evid. Based Complement. Altern. Med.* **2012**, *2012*, 570948. [CrossRef]
19. Wang, J.; Gao, H.; Ke, D.; Zuo, G.; Yang, Y.; Yamahara, J.; Li, Y. Improvement of liquid fructose-induced adipose tissue insulin resistance by ginger treatment in rats is associated with suppression of adipose macrophage-related pro-inflammatory cytokines. *Evid. Based Complement. Altern. Med.* **2013**, *2013*, 590376. [CrossRef]
20. Yang, M.; Liu, C.; Jiang, J.; Zuo, G.; Lin, X.; Yamahara, J.; Wang, J.; Li, Y. Ginger extract diminishes chronic fructose consumption-induced kidney injury through suppression of renal overexpression of proinflammatory cytokines in rats. *BMC Complement. Altern. Med.* **2014**, *14*, 174. [CrossRef]
21. Latona, D.F.; Oyeleke, G.O.; Olayiwola, O.A. Chemical Analysis of Ginger Root. *IOSR J. Appl. Chem.* **2012**, *1*, 47–49.
22. Boissonneault, G.A. Obesity: The current treatment protocols. *JAAPA* **2009**, *22*, 18–19.
23. Thomson, M.; Al Qattan, K.K.; Al sawan, S.M. The use of ginger (Zingiber officinale rose) as a potential antiflammatory and antithrombotic agent. *Prostaglandins Leukot. Essent. Fatty Acids* **2002**, *67*, 475–478. [CrossRef]
24. Jung, H.A.; Kim, Y.S.; Choi, J.S. Quantitative HPLC analysis of two key flavonoids and inhibitory activities against aldose reductase from different parts of the Korean thistle, Cirsium maackii. *Food Chem. Toxicol.* **2009**, *47*, 2790–2797. [CrossRef] [PubMed]
25. Ahmed, M.M. Pineapple juice ameliorates the high fat diet-induced alterations in cardiac gene expression pattern in male rats. *Int. J. Biochem. Res. Rev.* **2016**, *15*, 1–11. [CrossRef]

26. Surh, Y.J. Molecular mechanisms of chemopreventive effects of selected dietary and medicinal phenolic substances. *Mutat. Res.* **1999**, *428*, 305–327. [CrossRef]
27. Brett, W. Ginger: An Overview. *Complement. Altern. Med.* **2007**, *75*, 1689–1691.
28. Choi, Y.Y.; Kim, M.H.; Hong, J.; Kim, S.H.; Yang, W.M. Dried ginger (*Zingiber officinalis*) inhibits inflammation in a lipopolysaccharide-induced mouse model. *Evid. Based Complement. Altern.* **2013**, *2013*, 914563. [CrossRef]
29. Misawa, K.; Hashizume, K.; Yamamoto, M.; Minegishi, Y.; Hase, T.; Shimotoyodome, A. Ginger extract prevents high-fat diet-induced obesity in mice via activation of the peroxisome proliferator-activated receptor δ pathway. *J. Nutr. Biochem.* **2015**, *26*, 1058–1067. [CrossRef]
30. Fuhrman, B.; Rosenblat, M.; Hayek, T.; Coleman, R.; Aviram, M. Ginger extract consumption reduces plasma cholesterol, inhibits LDL oxidation and attenuates development of atherosclerosis in atherosclerotic, apoliopoprotein E-deficient mice. *J. Nutr.* **2000**, *130*, 1124–1131. [CrossRef]
31. Alizadeh-Navaei, R.; Roozbeh, F.; Saravi, M.; Pouramir, M.; Jalali, F.; Moghadamnia, A.A. Investigation of the effect of ginger on the lipid levels. A double blind controlled clinical trial. *Saudi Med. J.* **2008**, *29*, 1280–1284.
32. Dias, M.C.; Spinardi-Barbisan, A.L.; Rodrigues, M.A.; de Camargo, J.L.; Teran, E.; Barbisan, L.F. Lack of chemopreventive effects of ginger on colon carcinogenesis induced by 1,2-dimethylhydrazine in rats. *Food Chem. Toxicol.* **2006**, *44*, 877–884. [CrossRef]
33. Jolad, S.D.; Lantz, R.C.; Chen, G.J.; Bates, R.B.; Timmermann, B.N. Commercially processed dry ginger (Zingiber officinale): Composition and effects on LPS-stimulated PGE2 production. *Phytochemistry* **2005**, *66*, 1614–1635. [CrossRef]
34. Kirtikar, K.R.; Basu, B.D. *Indian Medicinal Plants*; International Book Distributors Book Sellers and Publishers: Deheradun, India, 1999; Volume 3.
35. Patel, D.K.; Patel, K.; Gadewar, M.; Tahilyani, V. Pharmacological and bioanalytical aspects of galangin—A concise report. *Asian Pac. J. Trop. Biomed.* **2012**, *2*, 5449–5455. [CrossRef]
36. Campana, R.; Patrone, V.; Franzini, I.T.; Diamantini, G.; Vittoria, E.; Baffone, W. Antimicrobial activity of two propolis samples against human *Campylobacter jejuni*. *J. Med. Food* **2009**, *12*, 1050–1056. [CrossRef] [PubMed]
37. Zhu, L.; Luo, Q.; Bi, J.; Ding, J.; Ge, S.; Chen, F. Galangin inhibits growth of human head and neck squamous carcinoma cells in vitro and in vivo. *Chem. Biol. Interact.* **2014**, *224*, 149–156. [CrossRef] [PubMed]
38. Lee, J.; Kim, K.A.; Jeong, S.; Lee, S.; Park, H.J.; Kim, N.J.; Lim, S. Anti-inflammatory, anti-nociceptive, and anti-psychiatric effects by the rhizomes of Alpinia officinarum on complete Freund's adjuvant-induced arthritis in rats. *J. Ethnopharmacol.* **2009**, *126*, 258–264. [CrossRef]
39. Heo, M.Y.; Sohn, S.J.; Au, W.W. Anti-genotoxicity of galangin as a cancer chemoprotective agent candidate. *Mutat. Res.* **2001**, *488*, 135–150. [CrossRef]
40. Hamada, M.; Satsum, H.; Ashida, H.; Sugita-Konishi, Y.; Shimizu, M. Metabolites of Galangin by 2, 3, 7, 8-Tetrachlorodibenzo-*p*-dioxin-Inducible Cytochrome P450 1A1 in Human Intestinal Epithelial Caco-2 Cells and Their Antagonistic Activity toward Aryl Hydrocarbon Receptor. *J. Agric. Food Chem.* **2010**, *58*, 8111–8118. [CrossRef]
41. Jung, C.H.; Jang, S.J.; Ahn, J.; Gwon, S.Y.; Jeon, T.I.; Kim, T.W.; Ha, T.Y. *Alpinia officinarum* inhibits adipocyte differentiation and high-fat diet-induced obesity in mice through regulation of adipogenesis and lipogenesis. *J. Med. Food* **2012**, *15*, 959–967. [CrossRef]
42. Kumar, S.; Alagawadi, K.R. Anti-obesity effects of galangin, a pancreatic lipase inhibitor in cafeteria diet fed female rats. *Pharm. Biol.* **2013**, *151*, 607–613. [CrossRef]
43. Tsai, M.S.; Chien, C.C.; Lin, T.H.; Liu, C.C.; Liu, R.H.; Su, H.L.; Chiu, Y.T.; Wang, S.H. Galangin prevents acute hepatorenal toxicity in novel propacetamol-induced acetaminophen-overdosed mice. *J. Med. Food* **2015**, *18*, 1187–1197. [CrossRef]
44. Bae, Y.; Lee, S.; Kim, S.H. Chrysin suppresses mast cell-mediated allergic inflammation: Involvement of calcium, caspase-1 and nuclear factor-κB. *Toxicol. Appl. Pharmacol.* **2011**, *254*, 56–64. [CrossRef]
45. Bai, J.; Luo, Y.; Song, Z.; Fan, W.; Wang, Z.; Luan, T.; Jiang, J.; Zang, B. Effects and the mechanisms of chrysin on sepsis-associated acute lung injury of rats chrysin inhibits acute lung injury. *Life Sci. J.* **2013**, *10*, 1052–1058.
46. Wadibhasme, P.G.; Ghaisas, M.M.; Thakurdesai, P.A. Anti-asthmatic potential of chrysin on ovalbumin-induced bronchoalveolar hyperresponsiveness in rats. *Pharm. Biol.* **2011**, *49*, 508–515. [CrossRef] [PubMed]

47. Li, X.; Wang, J.N.; Huang, J.M.; Xiong, X.K.; Chen, M.F.; Ong, C.N.; Shen, H.M.; Yang, X.F. Chrysin promotes tumor necrosis factor (TNF)-related apoptosis-inducing ligand (TRAIL) induced apoptosis in human cancer cell lines. *Toxicol. In Vitro* **2011**, *25*, 630–635. [CrossRef] [PubMed]
48. Lirdprapamongkol, K.; Sakurai, H.; Abdelhamed, S.; Yokoyama, S.; Maruyama, T.; Athikomkulchai, S.; Viriyaroj, A.; Awale, S.; Yagita, H.; Ruchirawat, S. A flavonoid chrysin suppresses hypoxic survival and metastatic growth of mouse breast cancer cells. *Oncol. Rep.* **2013**, *30*, 2357–2364. [CrossRef] [PubMed]
49. Anandhi, R.; Annadurai, T.; Anitha, T.S.; Muralidharan, A.R.; Najmunnisha, K.; Nachiappan, V.; Thomas, P.A.; Geraldine, P. Antihypercholesterolemic and antioxidative effects of an extract of the Oyster mushroom, Pleurotus ostreatus, and its major constituent, chrysin, in triton WR-1339-induced hypercholesterolemic rats. *J. Physiol. Biochem.* **2013**, *69*, 313–323. [CrossRef]
50. Testai, L.; Martelli, A.; Cristofaro, M.; Breschi, M.C.; Calderone, V. Cardioprotective effects of different flavonoids against myocardial ischaemia/reperfusion injury in Langendorff-perfused rat hearts. *J. Pharm. Pharmacol.* **2013**, *65*, 750–756. [CrossRef]
51. Van Heerden, F.R. Hoodia gordonii: A natural appetite suppressant. *J. Ethnopharmacol.* **2008**, *119*, 434–437. [CrossRef]
52. Okuda, H.; Han, L.; Kimura, Y.; Saito, M.; Murata, T. Anti-Obesity Action of Herb Tea (Part 1). Effects or Various Herb Teas on Noradrenaline-Induced Lipolysis in Rat Fat Cells and Pancreatic Lipase Activity. *Jpn. J. Const. Med.* **2001**, *63*, 60–65.
53. Geoffroy, P.; Ressault, B.; Marchioni, E.; Miesch, M. Synthesis of Hoodigogenin A, aglycone of a natural appetite suppressant glycosteroid extracted from Hoodia gordonii. *Steroids* **2011**, *76*, 702–708. [CrossRef]
54. Haaz, S.; Fontaine, K.R.; Cutter, G.; Limdi, N.; Perumean-Chaney, S.; Allison, D.B. Citrus aurantium and synephrine alkaloids in the treatment of overweight and obesity: An update. *Obes. Rev.* **2006**, *7*, 79–88. [CrossRef]
55. Stefan, N.; Bunt, J.C.; Salbe, A.D.; Funahashi, T.; Matsuzawa, Y.; Tataranni, P.A. Plasma adiponectin concentrations in children: Relationships with obesity and insulinemia. *J. Clin. Endocrinol. Metab.* **2001**, *87*, 4652–4656. [CrossRef] [PubMed]
56. Weyer, C.; Funahashi, T.; Tanaka, S.; Hotta, K.; Matsuzawa, Y.; Pratley, R.E.; Tataranni, P.A. Hypoadiponectinemia in obesity and type 2 diabetes: Close association with insulin resistance and hyperinsulinemia. *J. Clin. Endocrinol. Metab.* **2001**, *86*, 1930–1935. [CrossRef] [PubMed]
57. Ebrahimzadeh Attari, V.; Ostadrahimi, A.; Asghari Jafarabadi, M.; Mehralizadeh, S.; Mahluji, S. Changes of serum adipocytokines and body weight following Zingiber officinale supplementation in obese women: A RCT. *Eur. J. Nutr.* **2016**, *55*, 2129–2136. [CrossRef] [PubMed]
58. Lihn, A.S.; Pedersen, S.B.; Richelsen, B. Adiponectin: Action, regulation and association to insulin sensitivity. *Obes. Rev.* **2005**, *6*, 13–21. [CrossRef]
59. Park, J.; Rho, H.K.; Kim, K.H.; Choe, S.S.; Lee, Y.S.; Kim, J.B. Overexpression of glucose-6-phosphate dehydrogenase is associated with lipid dysregulation and insulin resistance in obesity. *Mol. Cell Biol.* **2005**, *25*, 5146–5157. [CrossRef]
60. Thamilvaani, M.; Manaharan, T.; Kanthimathi, M.S. Ginger oil-mediated down-regulation of adipocyte specific genes inhibits adipogenesis and induces apoptosis in 3T3-L1 adipocytes. *Biochem. Biotechnol. Res.* **2016**, *4*, 38–47.
61. Ojewole, J.A. Analgesic, antiinflammatory and hypoglycaemic effects of ethanol extract of Zingiber officinale (Roscoe) rhizomes (Zingiberaceae) in mice and rats. *Phytother. Res.* **2006**, *20*, 764–772. [CrossRef]
62. Krskova-Tybitanclova, K.; Macejova, D.; Brtko, J.; Ba-culikova, M.; Krizanova, O.; Zorad, S. Short term 13-cis-retinoic acid treatment at therapeutic doses elevates expression of leptin, GLUT4, PPAR gamma and aP2 in rat adipose tissue. *J. Physiol. Pharmacol.* **2008**, *59*, 731–743.
63. Landrier, J.F.; Gouranton, E.; Yazidi, E.L.; Malezet, C.; Balaguer, P.; Borel, P.; Amiot, M.J. Adiponectin expression is induced by vitamin E via a peroxisome proliferator activated receptor gamma-dependent mechanism. *Endocrinology* **2009**, *150*, 5318–5325. [CrossRef]
64. Soliman, M.; Ahmed, M.; El-Shazly, S.; Ismail, T.; Attia, H.; Elkirdasy, A. Effect of vitamin A and E on carbohydrate and lipid metabolism in diet-induced obese wistar rats. *Adv. Biosci. Biotechnol.* **2014**, *5*, 4–11. [CrossRef]
65. Peluso, G.; Nicolai, R.; Reda, E.; Benatti, P.; Barbarisi, A.; .Calvani, M. Cancer and anticancer therapy-induced modifications on metabolism mediated by carnitine system. *J. Cell Physiol.* **2000**, *182*, 339–350. [CrossRef]

66. Soliman, M.M.; Ahmed, M.M.; El-Sawy, H.B.; Ibrahim, Z.S.; El-Shazly, S.A. Effect of ginger extract and L-carnitine on the expression of genes related to lipids and carbohydrates metabolism. *Biosci. Res.* **2018**, *15*, 4381–4389.
67. Hoehn, K.L.; Hohnen-Behrens, C.; Cederberg, A.; Wu, L.E.; Turner, N.; Yuasa, T.; Ebina, Y.; James, D.E. IRS1-independent defects define major nodes of insulin resistance. *Cell Metab.* **2008**, *7*, 421–433. [CrossRef] [PubMed]

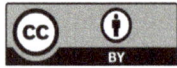

© 2020 by the authors. Licensee MDPI, Basel, Switzerland. This article is an open access article distributed under the terms and conditions of the Creative Commons Attribution (CC BY) license (http://creativecommons.org/licenses/by/4.0/).

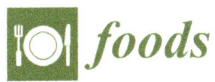

Article

Arthrospira Platensis (Spirulina) Supplementation on Laying Hens' Performance: Eggs Physical, Chemical, and Sensorial Qualities

Besma Omri [1,*], **Marwen Amraoui** [1], **Arbi Tarek** [1], **Massimo Lucarini** [2], **Alessandra Durazzo** [2], **Nicola Cicero** [3], **Antonello Santini** [4,*] **and Mounir Kamoun** [1]

1. Laboratory of improvement and integrated development of animal productivity and food resources, Department of animal production, Higher School of Agriculture of Mateur, University of Carthage, Carthage Avenue de la République, P.O. Box 77, Amilcar, Tunis 1054, Tunisia
2. CREA- Research Centre for Food and Nutrition, Via Ardeatina 546, 00178 Rome, Italy
3. Dipartimento di Scienze biomediche, odontoiatriche e delle immagini morfologiche e funzionali, Università degli Studi di Messina, Polo Universitario Annunziata, 98168 Messina, Italy
4. Department of Pharmacy, University of Napoli Federico II, Via D. Montesano, 49-80131 Napoli, Italy
* Correspondence: omribesma1@gmail.com (B.O.); asantini@unina.it (A.S.); Tel.: +216-27447098. (B.O.); +39-81-253-9317 (A.S.)

Received: 10 July 2019; Accepted: 28 August 2019; Published: 2 September 2019

Abstract: The present study evaluated the effects of dietary supplementation of spirulina on laying hens' performances: Eggs' physical, chemical, and sensorial qualities. A total of 45 Lohman White hens, 44 weeks of age, were randomized into 3 groups of 15 birds. Hens were given 120 g/d of a basal diet containing 0% (control), 1.5%, and 2.5% of spirulina for 6 weeks. Albumen height and consequently Haugh unit were significantly affected by dietary supplementation of spirulina ($p < 0.05$) and by weeks on diet ($p < 0.05$). This supplement did not affect ($p > 0.05$) egg yolk weight or height. However, spirulina increased egg yolk redness (a*) from 1.33 (C) to 12.67 (D1) and 16.19 (D2) and reduced ($p < 0.05$) the yellowness (b*) parameter from 62.1(C) to 58.17 (D1) and 55.87 (D2). Egg yolks from hens fed spirulina were darker, more red, and less yellow in color than egg yolks from hens fed the control-diet ($p < 0.0001$). However, spirulina did not affect ($p > 0.05$) egg yolks' total cholesterol concentration. In conclusion, a significant enhancement of egg yolk color was found in response to spirulina supplementation. Further investigations are needed to evaluate the impact of spirulina on egg yolks' fatty acids profile.

Keywords: cholesterol; egg quality; Haugh unit; spirulina; yolk color

1. Introduction

Arthrospira platensis (spirulina) is a filamentous spiral-shaped blue-green algae [1,2]. It has been recognized as a genus of photosynthetic bacteria (*Arthrospira*). This microorganism belongs to the class of Cyanophyta/Cyanobacteria that grow naturally in warm and alkaline aquatic media. From the perspective of a nutraceutical view [3–8], spirulina is considered as a functional food due to its high protein content (65% to 70% dry matter), high amount of vitamin and mineral content, and wide variety of natural carotene and xanthophyll phytopigments [9,10], and it is generally regarded as safe (GRAS) by the European Food Safety Authority (EFSA) [11]. Spirulina is a source of other nutritionally beneficial organic molecules, such as gamma linoleic acid, phenolic acids, and chlorophyll [12,13]. Deng et al. [14] and Bashandy et al. [15] reported that spirulina has many health benefits, including antioxidant properties, hypolipidemic action, and immunostimulating or anti-inflammatory effects [16,17]. These properties have been verified using laboratory animals [18,19]. Spirulina was used as alternative dietary sources in poultry diets [20]. In these diets, spirulina can be used up to 10% as a partial replacement of conventional proteins without any adverse effects [21]. Dietary vitamin and mineral premixes can be omitted when spirulina algae are included in chicken rations [22], due to its nutrient-rich composition. Zeweil et al. [23] reported that dietary supplementation of spirulina in chickens under heat stress conditions could decrease adverse effects of chronic heat stress on growth performance and immunity of a Gimmizah local strain of chicken. Spirulina could also be used as an effective way to improve the poultry product quality to meet consumer preferences [24], owing to its high concentration of carotenoids [25]. Zahroojian et al. [26] and Mariey et al. [12] found that dietary inclusion of spirulina at a concentration of 2% to 2.5% in laying hens' feed intensified egg yolk color to make it more aesthetically pleasing for consumers. This coloration intensification is thought to be due to spirulina's high concentration of β-carotene [27]. Dietary incorporation of spirulina can also reduce egg yolk total cholesterol and saturated fatty acid content and increase its omega-3 polyunsaturated fatty acids levels [28,29]. According to Zahroojian et al. [26], it has been shown that addition of spirulina at a level of 2% to 2.5% in the laying hen diet was associated with a significant increase of egg yolk color determined by comparison with the BASF Ovo-Color Fan, an Ovo-Color Yolk Fan supplied by BASF (Florham Park, NJ, USA). However, egg yolk color estimation using the color measuring device, Chroma Meter, was not reported. Therefore, the objective of the present study was to evaluate the effect of dietary incorporation of spirulina on laying hens' performances, egg physical characteristics, egg yolk color, and total cholesterol concentration.

2. Materials and Methods

2.1. Diet Preparation

Two kilos of spirulina (*Spirulina platensis*) were purchased from a regional producer located in the region of Gabes (Tunisia). A standard diet (control diet) (C) for laying hens based on corn and soybean meal and 2 supplemented diets, designated as follows: 1.5% of spirulina-supplemented diet (D1) and 2.5% of spirulina-supplemented diet (D2) were individually prepared by mixing the control diet (C) thoroughly with the designated supplements at the required incorporation levels as shown in Table 1.

Table 1. Ingredients and chemical composition of diets.

	Treatment		
Ingredients, %	C	D1 (1.5% spirulina)	D2 (2.5% spirulina)
Yellow corn	66.5	65.5	65.5
Soybean meal	25.5	25	24
Calcium carbonate, Mineral and Vitamin mixtureα	8	8	8
spirulina	0	1.5	2.5
Chemical Composition			
Dry Matter (%)	90.63	89.73	90.73
Organic Matter (% DM)	80.54	79.49	80.73
Crude Protein (% DM)	16.0	16.19	17.3
Ether Extract (% DM)	3.2	3.4	3.2
NDF (% DM)	10.15	10.5	11
¥ Metabolizable Energy, kcal/kg DM	2732.32	2738.42	2718.67

αControl (C) provided following nutrients per 100 g: Ca, 4.3 g; P, 0.6 g; Na, 0.14 g; Cl, 0.23 g; Fe, 4 mg; Zn, 40 mg; Mn, 7 mg; Cu, 0.3 mg; I, 0.08 mg; Se, 0.01 mg; Co, 0.02; methionine, 0.39 g; methionine + cysteine, 0.69 g; lysine, 0.89 g; Retinol, 800 IU; Cholecalciferol, 220 IU; α-tocopherol, 1.1 IU; Thiamin, 0.33 IU; Nicotinic acid, 909 IU. ¥ Metabolizable Energy = 2707.71 + 58.63 * EE−16.06 * NDF [30].

2.2. Ethical Considerations

All procedures related to animals' care, handling, and sampling were conducted under the approval of the Official Animal Care and Use Committee of the Higher School of Agriculture of Mateur (protocol N°05/15) before the initiation of the study and followed the Tunisian guidelines.

2.3. Experimental Design

Forty-five 44-week-old *Lohman White* laying hens were divided randomly into 3 groups of 15 birds. Each group was allocated to one of the three following dietary treatments: (1) Control diet (C), (2) 1.5% of spirulina-supplemented diet (D1), and (3) 2.5% of spirulina-supplemented diet (D2). Each hen was fed daily 120 g of a basal diet containing 0% (control), basal diet plus 1.5% g of spirulina, or basal diet plus 2.5% g of spirulina. The ingredients and chemical composition of the diets are shown in Table 1. Hens were housed in cages with individual feed troughs and common water troughs in a room with ambient temperature of about 20 °C and a photoperiod of 16 h light:8 h darkness cycle. Water was provided ad libitum throughout the trial period, which lasted 42 days.

2.4. Data Collection

All the birds were weighed individually at the beginning and the end of the experiment to determine the live weight changes. Feed was offered once daily at 7:30 a.m. and refusal was measured weekly. Egg production and weight were recorded daily. Daily feed consumption, laying rate (number of laid eggs × 100/number of feeding days), and feed conversion ratio (feed consumption/number of eggs × egg weight) were calculated per week.

Eggs laid during the 1st, 14th, 21st, 28th, 35th, and 42nd days were used for egg physical characteristics measurements (egg albumen, yolk and shell weights, albumen and yolk heights, Haugh unit, yolk diameter, yolk index, and shell thickness) and egg yolk color using the color measuring device Konica Minolta Chroma Meter CR- 400/410 (Minolta Corp.) according to the CIE (Commission Internationale de L'Eclairage) L * (lightness: negative towards black, positive towards white), a * (redness: negative towards green, positive towards red), and b * (yellowness: negative towards blue, positive towards yellow) color system and colorimetric interval, dL * (Lightness interval), da * (Red/Green interval), and db * (Yellow/Blue interval), between the spirulina-supplemented diet (D1 and D2) and control diet (C). The instrument was set perpendicular to the egg yolk surface in a Petri dish. The parameters, L *, a *, and b *, were measured three times and the final values were calculated as the averages of the three corresponding values measured.

Haugh unit (UH) was calculated according to the formula [31]:

$$\text{Haugh unit} = 100 \times \log (HA - 1.7 \times W0.37 + 7.6),$$

where: HA = albumen height (mm) and W = egg weight (g).

Yolk index was calculated according to the formula:

$$\text{Yolk index} = \text{Yolk height (mm)}/\text{Yolk diameter (mm)}.$$

Shell thickness, albumen and yolk heights, and yolk diameter were measured using a caliper.

Eggs laid during days 1 and 28 of the experimental period were pooled per hen and used for egg yolk total cholesterol determination.

2.5. Chemical Analysis

The dry matter of diets (DM) was determined at 105 °C for 24 h. All other analyses were done on samples dried at 65 °C and ground in a mill to pass through a 0.5-mm screen. Ash content was determined by igniting the ground sample at 550 °C in a muffle furnace for 10 h. The Association of Official Analytical Chemists method [32] was used for crude protein (CP) determination.

Egg yolk samples pooled per hen were solubilized in 2% (w/v) NaCl solution [33] and used for cholesterol determination using standard enzymatic-colorimetric methods (cholesterol enzymatic colorimetric test, CHOD-PAP Biomaghreb, Tunisia).

2.6. Statistical Analysis

Data of repeated measurements (feed refusal and intake, laying rate, egg mass, feed conversion ratio, egg physical characteristics, yolk total cholesterol, and yolk color traits) were tested for diet, week on diet effects, and their interaction using mixed models with compound symmetry covariance structures of SAS (Statistical Analysis System) [34].

Data of the hens' live weight change were tested for diet effect using the general linear model (GLM) procedure of the Statistical Analysis System (SAS) [34] according to the following model:

$$Y_{ij} = u + A_i + e_{ij},$$

where:

Y_{ij} = represents the jth observation on the ith treatment;
μ = overall mean;
A_i = main effect of the ith treatment;
e_{ij} = random error present in the jth observation on the ith treatment.

3. Results

3.1. Laying Performance

Laying hens' performances are shown in Table 2. All hens showed a loss of body weight at the end of the experimental period, but this weight loss was not affected ($p > 0.05$) by dietary treatment. Feed refusal and consumption was not affected ($p > 0.05$) by dietary addition of spirulina and did not change ($p > 0.05$) over the weeks on the diet. In parallel, the laying rate and consequently daily egg mass production were not affected ($p > 0.05$) by dietary treatment and weeks on the diet and their interaction. Only egg weight was affected ($p < 0.05$) by dietary treatment. Supplementation of 2.5% spirulina (D2) increased ($p < 0.05$) egg weight from 62.76 ± 1.53 g to 64.33 ± 1.83 g. The feed conversion ratio (FCR) was not affected ($p > 0.05$) by dietary treatment, weeks on diet, and their interaction.

Table 2. Effect of spirulina on hens' live weight changes and laying performances.

	Treatment			SEM [&]	p-value		
	C [α]	D1 [α]	D2 [α]		Trt [β]	W [β]	Trt * W [β]
LW change, (g/42 days)	−56.00 ± 101.05	−19.33 ± 120.9	−30.00 ± 139.01	31.30	NS	–	–
Feed intake, g DM/hen/day	105.11 ± 3.89	106.79 ± 0.71	105.43 ± 4.09	0.66	NS	NS	NS
Feed Refusal, g DM/hen/day	3.65 ± 3.89	2.88 ± 0.71	3.44 ± 4.09	0.66	NS	NS	NS
Laying rate, %	96.38 ± 4.18	94.67 ± 4.19	92.19 ± 9.41	1.28	NS	NS	NS
Egg weight, g	62.76 b ± 1.53	63.18b ± 1.47	64.33a ± 1.83	0.32	*	NS	NS
Egg mass, g/hen/day	60.47 ± 2.57	59.80 ± 2.83	59.34 ± 6.58	0.88	NS	NS	NS
Feed conversion ratio	1.74 ± 0.089	1.78 ± 0.082	1.79 ± 0.23	0.03	NS	NS	NS

[α] C = control diet with 0% of spirulina; [α] D1 = control diet supplemented with 1.5% of spirulina; [α] D2 = control diet supplemented with 2.5% of spirulina; and SEM = standard error of the mean; [β] trt = treatment; [β] W = week; [β] trt * W = treatment − week interaction; * = $p < 0.05$; NS = $p \geq 0.05$; [ab]: Mean in the same row with different superscripts are significantly different ($p < 0.05$).

3.2. Egg Physical Characteristics

The determined physical characteristics of eggs (egg, yolk, albumen and shell weights, yolk and albumen heights, yolk diameter, UH (Haugh Unit), and yolk index) are shown in Table 3.

Ours results showed that egg and albumen weights were affected ($p < 0.05$) by dietary inclusion of spirulina. Mean egg weight varied from 62.22 ± 2.98 g (C) to 64.43 ± 3.04 g (D2). Albumen weight of hens fed on 2.5% spirulina was the highest, with mean values of 36.20 ± 2.1 g vs. 35.08 ± 2.5 g (D1) and 34.41 ± 1.81 g (C). Shell thickness was affected by dietary treatment ($p < 0.05$), weeks on diet ($p < 0.0001$), and their interaction ($p < 0.0001$).

Albumen height and consequently Haugh unit were significantly affected by dietary supplementation of spirulina ($p < 0.05$) and by weeks on diet ($p < 0.05$). Dietary incorporation of spirulina did not affect ($p > 0.05$) egg yolk weight and height. However, these parameters were influenced ($p < 0.05$) by weeks on diet. Egg yolk diameter and index were affected by weeks on diet ($p < 0.0001$) and the interaction, treatment*week on diet.

Concerning albumen height, UH, and shell thickness, for each diet, differences between parameters at week 1 and their average mean at week 3 and week 6, as well as differences between means at week 3 and week 6, were compared (Table 4). Tested differences of albumen height were significant ($p < 0.05$) for the control diet, indicating an increase of albumen height at week 1. For each of the D1- and D2-diets, only differences between heights at week 3 and week 6 were significant ($p < 0.05$), indicating an increase of albumen height at week 6. UH did not change ($p < 0.05$) over time for the control, decreased ($p > 0.05$) at week 3 for the D1-diet, and increased ($p > 0.05$) for the D1-diet and D2-diet at week 6. Shell thickness increased ($p > 0.05$) for the D2-diet at week 1, week 3, and week 2 and for the D2-diet at week 6.

Table 3. Effect of spirulina on egg physical characteristics.

	Treatment			SEM [&]	p-value		
	C [α]	D1 [α]	D2 [α]		Trt [β]	W [β]	Trt * W [β]
Egg weight, g	$62.22^b \pm 2.98$	$62.98^{ab} \pm 3.54$	$64.43^a \pm 3.04$	0.54	*	NS	NS
Yolk weight, g	$17.92^a \pm 1.41$	$18.1^a \pm 1.17$	$18.22^a \pm 1.23$	0.22	NS	*	NS
Albumen weight, g	$34.41^b \pm 1.81$	$35.08^{ab} \pm 2.5$	$36.20^a \pm 2.71$	0.4	*	NS	NS
Shell weight, g	$6.63^a \pm 0.41$	$6.55^a \pm 0.41$	$6.75^a \pm 0.46$	0.07	NS	*	*
Shell thickness, mm	$0.39^{ab} \pm 0.05$	$0.41^a \pm 0.06$	$0.38^b \pm 0.04$	0.008	*	***	***
Yolk height, mm	$18.10^a \pm 0.97$	$18.59^a \pm 1.14$	$18.50^a \pm 1.08$	0.18	NS	***	NS
Albumen height, mm	$8.64^b \pm 0.79$	$9.51^a \pm 0.94$	$9.24^a \pm 0.93$	0.15	*	***	NS
Yolk diameter, mm	$42.15^a \pm 1.55$	$42.55^a \pm 1.52$	$42.39^a \pm 1.68$	0.27	NS	***	***
UH	$93.22^b \pm 3.92$	$97.28^a \pm 4.39$	$95.99^a \pm 4.32$	0.71	**	*	NS
Yolk index	$0.43^a \pm 0.025$	$0.43^a \pm 0.027$	$0.44^a \pm 0.031$	0.005	NS	***	*

[α] C = control diet with 0% of spirulina; [α] D1 = control diet supplemented with 1.5% spirulina; [α] D2 = control diet supplemented with 2.5% spirulina; SEM [&] = standard error of the mean; [β] trt = treatment; [β] W = week; [β] trt * W = treatment–week interaction; *** = $p < 0.0001$; ** = $p < 0.001$; * = $p < 0.05$; NS = $p \geq 0.05$; [a,b]: Mean in the same row with different superscripts are significantly different ($p < 0.05$).

Table 4. Week effect of the diet's distribution on albumen height, UH (Haugh Unit), and shell thickness.

	Diets	Actual Mean at Week 1	Mean of Difference		
			Week 1 and Subsequent Weeks	Week 3 and Subsequent Weeks	Week 3 and Week 6
Albumen height, mm	α C	8.02	1.49 *	0.56 NS	−0.09 NS
	α D1	8.67	0.66 NS	−0.25 NS	0.44 **
	α D2	8.83	0.45 NS	0.5 NS	0.73 ***
UH	α C	90.90	−2.1 NS	1.6 NS	6.7 NS
	α D1	93.19	−3.76 NS	−1.65 *	5.17 *
	α D2	93.91	−1.03 NS	0.7 *	6.1 ***
Shell thickness, mm	α C	0.46	0.03 NS	−0.016 NS	−0.006 NS
	α D1	0.42	0.008 NS	0.016 NS	0.11 *
	α D2	0.42	0.01 *	0.1 **	0.3 ***

α C = control diet with 0% spirulina; α D1 = control diet supplemented with 1.5% spirulina; α D2 = control diet supplemented with 2.5% spirulina; *** = $p < 0.0001$; ** = $p < 0.001$; * = $p < 0.05$; NS = $p \geq 0.05$.

3.3. Egg Yolk Color

Egg yolk color traits determined by a Konica Minolta Chroma Meter CR-410 were affected by dietary treatment ($p < 0.0001$), weeks on diet ($p < 0.0001$), and their interaction ($p < 0.0001$) (Table 5). Hens fed the control diet had the highest ($p < 0.0001$) lightness L*, with a mean value of 70.55 vs. 65.98 and 63.74 corresponding to hens fed with 1.5% and 2.5% spirulina, respectively. These values showed that the egg yolk of the control group was characterized by an intense yellow color.

Dietary supplementation of spirulina increased egg yolk redness, a*, from 1.33 ± 2.34 (C) to 12.67 ± 8.94 (D1) and 16.19 ± 9.85 (D2). The redness mean value (a*) corresponding to the control group indicated that this group had a weak red hue. Concerning the yellowness (b*), hens fed the diet without spirulina supplementation had the highest mean value (62.1 ± 2.66), which indicated that egg yolk color was sufficiently intense. Dietary inclusion of spirulina resulted in a significant decrease ($p < 0.0001$) of the egg yolk yellowness (b*). In fact, hens fed 2.5% and 1.5% spirulina had a yellowness mean value of 55.87 ± 3.93 and 58.17 ± 3.41, respectively.

The colorimetric interval between the spirulina-supplemented diet and control diet are represented in Table 6. These colorimetric intervals, dL*(lightness interval), da*(red/green interval), and db*(yellow/blue interval), between the spirulina-supplemented diet and control diet (C), determined by a Chroma Meter, showed that egg yolks from hens fed spirulina were darker, more red and, less yellow in color than egg yolks from hens fed the C-diet ($p < 0.0001$). It was found that egg yolk color parameters (L*, a *, and b*) changed over time for all diets (Table 7). L* decreased ($p < 0.0001$) in the C-diet, D1-diet, and D2-diet after the first week and increased ($p < 0.0001$) at week 3 and 6 for the D1-diet and D2-diet. However, egg yolk lightness decreased ($p < 0.001$) at the sixth week for the control diet. Concerning egg yolk redness (a*), a significant increase ($p < 0.0001$) was found at week 1 for the three diets. This increase was recorded during the experimental period for the D1 and D2 differences between the mean a* values at week 3 and were significant ($p < 0.0001$), indicating a decrease of egg yolk redness. Egg yolk yellowness increased ($p < 0.0001$) at week 1, week 3, and week 6 for C-, D1-, and D2-diets. By contrast, differences between the mean b* values for D2 at week 3 and for C at week 6 were negative ($p < 0.0001$), indicating a decrease of egg yolk yellowness.

Table 5. Effect of spirulina on egg yolk color.

	Treatment			SEM $^{\&}$	p-value		
	C $^{\alpha}$	D1 $^{\alpha}$	D2 $^{\alpha}$		Trt $^{\beta}$	W $^{\beta}$	Trt *W $^{\beta}$
L*	70.55^{a} ± 1.17	65.98^{b} ± 4.42	63.74^{c} ± 5.07	0.67	***	***	***
a*	1.33^{b} ± 2.34	12.76^{a} ± 8.94	16.19^{a} ± 9.85	1.32	***	***	***
b*	62.10^{a} ± 2.66	58.17^{b} ± 3.41	55.87^{c} ± 3.93	0.57	***	***	***

$^{\alpha}$ C = control diet with 0% spirulina; $^{\alpha}$ D1 = control diet supplemented with 1.5% spirulina; $^{\alpha}$ D2 = control diet supplemented with 2.5% spirulina; SEM $^{\&}$ = standard error of the mean; $^{\beta}$ trt = treatment; $^{\beta}$ W = week; $^{\beta}$ trt * W = treatment–week interaction; *** = $p < 0.0001$; ^{a,b,c}: Means in the same row with different superscripts are significantly different ($p < 0.05$); L*: lightness, a*: redness and b*: yellowness.

Table 6. Colorimetric interval between the spirulina-supplemented diet and control diet.

	Treatment		SEM $^{\&}$	p-Value		
	C$^{\alpha}$ and D1 $^{\alpha}$	C $^{\alpha}$ and D2 $^{\alpha}$		Trt $^{\beta}$	W $^{\beta}$	Trt *W $^{\beta}$
ΔL*	−4.57 ^{a} ± 4.25	−6.81 ^{b} ± 5.07	0.65	***	***	***
Δa*	11.43 ^{b} ± 8.22	14.86 ^{a} ± 9.85	1.37	***	***	***
Δb*	−3.93 ^{a} ± 3.41	−6.23 ^{b} ± 3.94	0.57	***	***	*

$^{\alpha}$ C = control diet with 0% spirulina; $^{\alpha}$ D1 = control diet supplemented with 1.5% spirulina; $^{\alpha}$ D2 = control diet supplemented with 2.5% spirulina; SEM $^{\&}$ = standard error of the mean; $^{\beta}$ trt = treatment; $^{\beta}$ W = week; $^{\beta}$ trt*W = treatment–week interaction; *** = $p < 0.0001$; * = $p < 0.05$; ^{a,b}: Means in the same row with different superscripts are significantly different ($p < 0.05$).

Table 7. Week effect of the diet's distribution on egg yolk color.

	Diets	Mean of Difference			
		Actual Mean at Week 1	Week 1 and Subsequent Weeks	Week 3 and Subsequent Weeks	Week 3 and Week 6
L*	$^{\alpha}$ C	72.31	−2.1 ***	0.4 ***	−0.1***
	$^{\alpha}$ D1	73.80	−6.3 ***	2.41 ***	3.95 ***
	$^{\alpha}$ D2	72.55	−9.25 ***	2.79 ***	3.30 ***
a*	$^{\alpha}$ C	−2.79	4.5 ***	−0.4 ***	0.5 ***
	$^{\alpha}$ D1	−2.75	8.57 ***	7.64 ***	7.65 ***
	$^{\alpha}$ D2	−1.68	10.19 ***	7.08 ***	6.42 ***
b*	$^{\alpha}$ C	61.99	0.4 ***	0.4 ***	−1.0 ***
	$^{\alpha}$ D1	58.48	3.8 ***	−0.02 ***	4.97 ***
	$^{\alpha}$ D2	59.81	6.1 ***	4.98 ***	5.18 ***

$^{\alpha}$ C = control diet with 0% spirulina; $^{\alpha}$ D1 = control diet supplemented with 1.5% spirulina; $^{\alpha}$ D2 = control diet supplemented with 2.5% spirulina; *** = $p < 0.0001$.

3.4. Egg Yolk Cholesterol Concentration

The effect of dietary supplementation of 1.5% and 2.5% spirulina on egg yolk total cholesterol concentration is represented in Table 8.

Our data showed that egg yolk concentration of total cholesterol was only affected ($p < 0.05$) by the weeks on diet. However, egg yolk concentration of total cholesterol was 14.35 ± 0.88 mg/g for hens fed the C-diet vs. 13.89 ± 1.21 and 14.39 ± 1.23 mg/g for hens fed 1.5% and 2.5% spirulina, respectively.

Table 8. Effect of dietary incorporation of spirulina on egg yolk cholesterol concentration.

	Treatment			SEM	p-Value		
	C	D1	D2		Trt	W	Trt * W
Egg yolk total cholesterol, mg/g of yolk	14.35 ± 0.88	13.89 ± 1.21	14.39 ± 1.23	0.35	NS	*	NS

C = control diet with 0% spirulina; D1 = control diet supplemented with 1.5% spirulina; D2 = control diet supplemented with 2.5% spirulina; SEM = standard error of the mean; Trt = treatment; W = week; Trt * W = treatment–week interaction; * = $p < 0.05$; NS = $p \geq 0.05$; [a]: Means in the same row with the same superscripts are not significantly different ($p \geq 0.05$).

4. Discussion

4.1. Laying Performances

Spirulina inclusion was without impact on feed consumption. Our results are in agreement with those reported by Dogan et al. [35], who reported that dietary addition of 0.5%, 1%, and 2% of spirulina did not affect feed consumption of laying quails.

In the present study, hens' live body weight losses were 56.00 vs. 19.33 g/42 d and laying rates were high (92.19% vs. 96.38%) and not affected by spirulina inclusion. Hens were fed ad libitum before our experimental study and then feed was restricted to 120 g/d so that animals showed this loss of body weight throughout the experimental period. Furthermore, only egg weight was significantly increased from 62.76 (C) to 63.18 g (1.5% spirulina) and 64.33g (2.5% spirulina). This increase of egg weight could be attributed to the high protein content in spirulina. These results are partially in agreement with those reported by Mariey et al. [12], who found that hens' live weight of Sinai (S) and Gimmizah (G) was not affected by dietary supplementation of 0.1%, 0.15%, and 0.2% spirulina. However, this supplementation decreased the feed conversion ratio. The lowest value was attributed to hens fed 0.2% spirulina; 3.46 versus 4.54 for the control group. Dogan et al. [35] also reported that dietary inclusion of 0.5%, 1%, and 2% spirulina did not affect the laying rate, feed conversion ratio, and egg weight. By contrast, Selim et al. [36] found that inclusion of 0%, 0.1%, 0.2%, and 0.3% spirulina increased hens' final weight from 1222 g (0%) to 1227 (0.1%), 1238 (0.2%), and 1253 g (0.3%). However, Mariey et al. [12] reported that dietary incorporation of 0.1%, 0.15%, and 0.2% spirulina increased the laying rate, egg weight, and egg mass. Zahroojian et al. [26] showed that addition of 1.5%, 2%, and 2.5% spirulina in the diet of 128 Hy-line White hens did not affect the laying rate and egg weight. This absence of changes in laying hens' performances associated with the use of spirulina might be attributed to the rate of inclusion of this alga, the variety, cultural practices, and climate.

4.2. Egg Physical Characteristics

With the exception of egg and albumen weights, albumen height, UH, and shell thickness, egg characteristics were not affected ($p > 0.05$) by dietary treatment and observed changes over time were numerically small and, therefore, of little physiological significance. Selim et al. [36] reported that dietary addition of 0.1%, 0.2%, and 0.3% spirulina did not affect egg physical characteristics (albumen index, albumen, yolk and shell weights, yolk index, and Haugh unit) determined at the end of the fourth week of the experiment trial. However, hens fed 0.1%, 0.2%, and 0.3% spirulina had a thicker shell of 0.356, 0.401, and 0.423 mm compared to those fed the control diet (0.314 mm). This finding could be attributed to the high calcium content of spirulina. Concerning the Haugh unit, Parisse [37] reported that eggs with a Haugh unit higher than 70 are considered excellent eggs, eggs with 70 to 60 Haugh units are acceptable, while eggs with Haugh units below 60 are of poor quality. Our results showed that hens fed 1.5% spirulina had the highest Haugh unit, with a mean value of 97.28 versus 95.99 (2.5%) and 93.33 (0%). Mean values of the present study were higher than 70, thus our eggs may be considered as excellent eggs. This high Haugh unit could be attributed to the fact that this parameter was determined on each egg laid on the same day and not on stored eggs. The pigment content of the supplemented spirulina could be responsible for the observed difference between treatments.

Mariey et al. [12] reported that dietary supplementation of spirulina at 0.1%, 0.15%, and 0.2% did not affect shell weight, albumen percentage and index, and Haugh's unit. Our data showed that dietary inclusion of spirulina did not affect egg yolk weight, height, diameter, and index. These results were not in agreement with those reported by Dogan et al. [35], who found that incorporation of 2% spirulina increased the egg yolk index of laying quails from 47.48 to 48.45 mm, shell weight from 1.55 to 1.68 g, and shell thickness from 0.199 to 0.207 mm. Mariey et al. [12] also reported that dietary supplementation of 0.15% spirulina increased egg yolk weight from 31.10 to 32.90 g.

By contrast, Zahroojian et al. [26] reported that incorporation of 1.5%, 2%, and 2.5% spirulina did not affect eggs' physical qualities (yolk index, Haugh unit, shell thickness, shell weight, and specific gravity)

4.3. Egg Yolk Color

Egg choice by consumers is no longer only based on yolk cholesterol content or fatty acids profile but also on its color [38]. The required degree of pigmentation varies among and within countries, but golden to yellow colors are usually considered more attractive [39]. Egg yolk color intensification can be achieved by dietary supplementation of carotenoids. However, laying hens are unable to synthesize these pigments. They need to be provided in their diet's ingredients [40]. Carotenoids are synthesized by algae, plants, fungi, and some bacteria. In the present study, egg yolk color intensification was achieved with dietary incorporation of spirulina. Concerning egg yolk color evaluation, it was estimated by colorimetric determination of lightness (L *), redness (a *), and yellowness (b*) indexes and colorimetric intervals (ΔL *, Δa *, Δb *).

Our results showed dietary supplementation of spirulina increased egg yolk redness and reduced yolk yellowness. Studies on the effect of spirulina on egg yolk color traits measured by a Chroma Meter are lacking. However, Mariey et al. [12] reported that dietary incorporation of 0.1%, 0.15%, and 0.2% spirulina increased the egg yolk color score (RYCF) from 6.3 (0.1%) and 6.7 (0.15%) to 7.6 (0.2%). Zahroojian et al. [26] also found that supplementation of 1.5%, 2%, and 2.5% spirulina increased the egg yolk color score from 10.55 (1.5%) and 11.43 (2%) to 11.66 (2.5%) compared to the control. Dietary inclusion of 0.1%, 0.2%, and 0.3% spirulina increased the egg yolk color score from 6.11 (0.1%) to 6.89 (0.2%) and 7.33 (0.3%) [36]. Anderson et al. [27] also evaluated the effect of dietary addition of 0.25%, 0.5%, 1.2%, and 4% spirulina, which increased quail egg yolk color measured at the 2nd and 23rd day of treatment. Park et al. [41] reported that incorporation of marine microalgae (*schizochytrium*) at 0.5% and 1% in laying hens' diet increased the egg yolk color score after 6 weeks of treatment, with a mean value of 9 and 8.8 compared to 8.7 corresponding to the control group.

4.4. Egg Yolk Cholesterol Concentration

Dietary supplementation of spirulina did not affect the egg yolks' total cholesterol concentration. The absence of the effect of spirulina on egg yolk total cholesterol was in agreement with the results reported by Zahroojian et al. [26], who reported that dietary addition of 1.5%, 2%, and 2.5% spirulina did not affect the egg yolk concentration of cholesterol, with mean values of 10 (1.5%), 10.59 (2%), and 11.81 mg/g (2.5%). By contrast, Dogan et al. [35] reported a reduction in egg yolk cholesterol concentration per gram of yolk from 19.65 to 18.93 when laying hens' diet were supplemented with 1% and 2% spirulina. Mariey et al. [12] also reported that egg yolk concentration of cholesterol decreased from 13.50 to 10.20 mg/g with dietary addition of 0.2% spirulina. Total egg cholesterol also decreased from 12.9 to 9.9 mg/g when spirulina was supplemented at a level of 0.3% [28].

Selim et al. [36] reported that dietary incorporation of 0.1%, 0.2%, and 0.3% spirulina reduced egg yolk cholesterol concentration from 13.6 mg/g (control) to 13.1 (0.1%), 12.4 (0.2%), and 11.7 mg/g (0.3%). Park et al. [41] also found that incorporation of *schizochytrium*, a marine microalgae, in laying hens' diets at a level of 0.5% and 1% reduced serum cholesterol from 133.8 to 118.5 mg/dl. These authors attributed this reduction to the high contents of polyunsaturated fatty acids in spirulina. In fact, omega-3 fatty acids stimulate the activity of LCAT (lecithin cholesterol acyltransferase) [42], an enzyme responsible for the serum cholesterol esterification [43], so that most newly formed cholesterol esters are initially incorporated in HDL (High-Density Lipoprotein) [44].

Chen et al. [45] also reported that the docosahexanoic acid (DHA) of microalgae may inhibit the activity of 3-hydroxy-3-methylglutaryl-coenzyme A (HMG-CoA) reductase by reducing cholesterol synthesis so that the serum cholesterol concentration decreases.

It can be concluded that incorporation of spirulina in 44-week-old Lohman White laying hens' diets was without effects on laying hens' performances and increased egg weight, shell thickness, albumen weight and height, and Haugh unit. The use of *Spirulina platensis* as a laying hens' feed additive increased egg yolk color, as measured by a chromameter, and did not affect the total cholesterol concentration. Further investigations are needed to evaluate the impact of spirulina on egg yolk

Author Contributions: B.O., M. K., and A.S., have conceived the work. B.O., M.A., A.T. and M.K. have carried out the experimental study and analyzed the data. B.O., M.A., A.T., M.K., M.L., A.D., N.C. and A.S. wrote the manuscript. All authors have made a substantial contribution to revise the work, and approved it for publication.

Funding: This research received no external funding.

Conflicts of Interest: The authors declare no conflict of interest.

References

1. Wu, Q.; Liu, L.; Miron, A.; Klímová, B.; Wan, D.; Kuča, K. The antioxidant, immunomodulatory, and anti-inflammatory activities of Spirulina: An overview. *Arch. Toxicol.* **2016**, *90*, 1817–1840. [CrossRef]
2. Finamore, A.; Palmery, M.; Bensehaila, S.; Peluso, I. Antioxidant, immunomodulating, and microbial-modulating activities of the sustainable and ecofriendly Spirulina. *Oxid. Med. Cell. Longev.* **2017**, *2017*, 3247528. [CrossRef]
3. Santini, A.; Tenore, G.C.; Novellino, E. Nutraceuticals: A paradigm of proactive medicine. *Eur. J. Pharm. Sci.* **2017**, *96*, 53–61. [CrossRef]
4. Daliu, P.; Santini, A.; Novellino, E. A decade of nutraceutical patents: Where are we now in 2018? *Expert Opin. Ther. Pat.* **2018**, *28*, 875–882. [CrossRef]
5. Durazzo, A.; D'Addezio, L.; Camilli, E.; Piccinelli, R.; Turrini, A.; Marletta, L.; Marconi, S.; Lucarini, M.; Lisciani, S.; Gabrielli, P.; et al. From plant compounds to botanicals and back: A current snapshot. *Molecules* **2018**, *23*, 1844. [CrossRef]
6. Di Lena, G.; Casini, I.; Lucarini, M.; Lombardi-Boccia, G. Carotenoid profiling of five microalgae species from large-scale production. *Food Res. Int.* **2019**, *120*, 810–818. [CrossRef]
7. Durazzo, A.; Lucarini, M. Extractable and non-extractable antioxidants. *Molecules* **2019**, *24*, 1933. [CrossRef]
8. Durazzo, A.; Lucarini, M.; Souto, E.B.; Cicala, C.; Caiazzo, E.; Izzo, A.A.; Novellino, E.; Santini, A. Polyphenols: A concise overview on the chemistry, occurrence and human health. *Phytother. Res* **2019**. [CrossRef]
9. Farag, M.R.; Alagawany, M.; Abd El-Hack, M.E.; Dhama, K. Nutritional and healthical aspects of Spirulina (*Arthrospira*) for poultry, animals and human. *Int. J. Pharm.* **2016**, *12*, 36–51. [CrossRef]
10. Lupatini, A.L.; Colla, L.M.; Canan, C.; Colla, E. Potential application of microalga Spirulina platensis as a protein source. *J. Sci. Food Agric.* **2017**, *97*, 724–732. [CrossRef]
11. Chacon-Lee, T.; Gonzàlez-Marino, G. Microalgae for "healthy" foods—Possibilities and challenges. *Compr. Rev. Food Sci. Food Saf.* **2010**, *9*, 655–675. [CrossRef]
12. Mariey, Y.; Samak, A.H.R.; Ibrahem, M.A. Effect of using spirulina platensis algae as a feed additive for poultry diets: Productive and reproductive performances of local laying hens. *Egypt. Poult. Sci.* **2012**, *32*, 201–215.
13. Al-Dhabi, N.A.; Valan Arasu, M. Quantification of phytochemicals from commercial spirulina products and their antioxidant activities. *Evid. Based Complement. Altern. Med.* **2016**, *2016*, 7631864. [CrossRef]
14. Deng, R.; Chow, T.J. Hypolipidemic, antioxidant, and antiinflammatory activities of microalgae Spirulina. *Cardiovsac. Ther.* **2010**, *28*, 33–45. [CrossRef]
15. Bashandry, S.A.; Alhazza, I.M.; El-Desoky, G.E.; Al-Othman, ZA. Hepatoprotective and hypolipidemic effects of Spirulina platensis in rats administered mercuric chloride. *Afr. J. Pharm.* **2011**, *5*, 175–182.

16. Abu-Taweel, G.M.; Mohsen, G.A.M.; Antonisamy, P.; Arokiyaraj, S.; Kim, H.J.; Kim, S.J.; Park, K.H.; Kim, Y.O. Spirulina consumption effectively reduces anti-inflammatory and pain related infectious diseases. *J. Infect. Public Health* **2019**, in press. [CrossRef]
17. Hamed, M.; Soliman, H.A.M.; Sayed, A.E.H. Ameliorative effect of Spirulina platensis against lead nitrate-induced cytotoxicity and genotoxicity in catfish Clarias gariepinus. *Environ. Sci. Pollut. Res. Int.* **2019**, *26*, 20610–20618. [CrossRef]
18. Li, T.T.; Tong, A.J.; Liu, Y.Y.; Huang, Z.R.; Wan, X.Z.; Pan, Y.Y.; Jia, R.B.; Liu, B.; Chen, X.H.; Zhao, C. Polyunsaturated fatty acids from microalgae Spirulina platensis modulates lipid metabolism disorders and gut microbiota in high-fat diet rats. *Food Chem. Toxicol.* **2019**, *131*, 110558. [CrossRef]
19. Zhao, B.; Cui, Y.; Fan, X.; Qi, P.; Liu, C.; Zhou, X.; Zhang, X. Anti-obesity effects of Spirulina platensis protein hydrolysate by modulating brain-liver axis in high-fat diet fed mice. *PLoS ONE* **2019**, *14*, e0218543. [CrossRef]
20. Altmann, B.A.; Neumann, C.; Velten, S.; Liebert, F.; Mörlein, D. Meat quality derived from high inclusion of a micro-alga or insect meal as an alternative protein source in poultry diets: A pilot study. *Foods* **2018**, *7*, 34. [CrossRef]
21. Spolaore, P.; Joannis-Cassan, C.; Duran, E.; Isambert, A. Commercial applications of microalgae. *J. Biosci. Bioeng.* **2006**, *101*, 87–96. [CrossRef]
22. Venkataraman, L.V.; Somasekaran, T.; Becker, E.W. Replacement value of blue-green alga (*Spirulina platensis*) for fishmeal and a vitamin-mineral premix for broiler chicks. *Br. Poult. Sci.* **1994**, *35*, 373–381. [CrossRef]
23. Zeweil, H.; Abaza, I.M.; Zahran, S.M. Effect of *Spirulina platensis* as dietary supplement on some biological traits for chickens under heat stress condition. *Asian J. Biomed. Pharm. Sci.* **2016**, *6*, 8–12.
24. Dismukes, G.C.; Carrieri, D.; Bennette, N.; Aanyev, G.M.; Poswitz, MC. Aquatic phototrophs: Efficient alternatives to land-based crops for biofuels. *Curr. Opin. Biotechnol.* **2008**, *19*, 235–240. [CrossRef]
25. Takashi, S. Effect of administration of Spirulina on egg quality and egg components. *Anim. Husb.* **2003**, *57*, 191–195.
26. Zahroojian, N.; Morave, H.; Shivazad, M. Effects of dietary marine algae (*Spirulina platensis*) on egg quality and production performance of laying hens. *J. Agric. Sci. Technol.* **2013**, *15*, 1353–1360.
27. Anderson, D.W.; Chung-Shih, T.; Ross, E. The Xanthophylls of Spirulina and their effect on egg yolk pigmentation. *Poult. Sci.* **1991**, *70*, 115–119. [CrossRef]
28. Sujatha, T.; Narahari, D. Effect of designer diets on egg yolk composition of 'White Leghorn' hens. *J. Food Sci. Technol.* **2011**, *48*, 494–497. [CrossRef]
29. Ginzberg, A.; Cohen, M.; Sod-Moriah, U.A.; Shany, S.; Rosenshtrauch, A.; Arad, S.M. Chickens fed with biomass of the red microalga *Porphyridium* sp. Have reduced blood cholesterol level and modified fatty acid composition in egg yolk. *J. Appl. Phycol.* **2000**, *12*, 325–330. [CrossRef]
30. Nascimento, G.A.J. Prediction Equations of the Energetic Values of Poultry Feedstuffs for Utilizing the Meta-Analysis Principle. Ph.D. Thesis, University Lavras, Minas Gerais, Brazil, 2007.
31. Haugh, R.R. The Haugh unit for measuring egg quality. *U. S. Egg Poult. Mag.* **1973**, *43*, 552–555.
32. Association of Official Analytical Chemists. *Official Methods of Analysis*, 10th ed.; Association of Official Analytical Chemists: Washington, DC, USA, 1984.
33. Pasin, G.; Smith, G.M.; O'mahony, M. Rapid determination of total cholesterol in egg yolk using commercial diagnostic cholesterol reagent. *Food Chem.* **1998**, *61*, 255–259. [CrossRef]
34. SAS. *SAS: Statistical Analysis System, Version 6*; SAS Inst. Inco: Raleigh, NC, USA, 1989.
35. Dogan, S.C.; Baylan, M.; Erdogan, Z.; Akpinar, G.C.; Kucukgul, A.; Duzguner, V. Performance, egg quality and serum parameters of japanese quails fed diet supplemented with spirulinaplatensis. *Fresenius Environ. Bull.* **2016**, *25*, 5857–5862.
36. Selim, S.; Hussein, E.; Abou Elkhar, R. Effect of *Spirulina platensis* as a feed additive on laying performance, egg quality and hepatoprotective activity of laying hens. *Eur. Poult. Sci.* **2018**, *82*, 1–14.
37. Parisse, A. Évolution qualitative et quantitative des composantes de l'oeuf pendant les trois phases de ponte chez la poule. *J. Appl. Biosci.* **2014**, *74*, 6080–6085.
38. Englmairova, M.; Skriva, M.; Bubancova, A. A comparaison of lutein spray dreid *Chlorella* and synthetic carotenooids effects on yolk, oxidative stability and reproductive performance of laying hens. *Czech J. Anim. Sci.* **2013**, *58*, 412–419. [CrossRef]

39. Baiao, N.C.; Mendez, J.; Mateos, J.; Garcia, M.; Matoes, G.G. Pigmeting efficacy of several oxycarotenoids on egg yolk. *J. Appl. Poult. Res.* **1999**, *8*, 472–479. [CrossRef]
40. Adams, C.A. Pigmenters & poultry feeds. *Feed Compd.* **1985**, *5*, 12–14.
41. Park, J.H.; Upadhaya, S.D.; Kim, I.H. Effect of dietary marine microalgae (*schizochytrium*) powder on egg production, blood lipid profiles, egg quality, and fatty acid composition of egg yolk in layers. Asian-Austra. *J. Anim. Sci.* **2015**, *28*, 391–397. [CrossRef]
42. Vaysse-Boue, C.; Dabadie, H.; Peuchant, E.; Le Ruvet, P. Moderate dietry intake of myristic and alpha-linolenic acids increases lecithin-cholesterol acyltransferase activity in humans. *Lipids* **2007**, *42*, 717–722. [CrossRef]
43. Ferchaud-Roucher, V.; Croyal, M.; Krempf, M.; Ouguerram, K. Les acides gras polyinsaturés oméga 3 augmentent l'activité de la lécithine cholestérol acyltransférase. *Nutr. Clin. Métabolisme* **2014**, *28*, S133. [CrossRef]
44. Rajaram, O.V.; Barter, P.J. Increase in the particle size of high- density lipoproteins induced by purified lecithin: Cholesterol acyltransferase: Effect of low density 46 lipoproteins. *Biochim. Biophys. Acta* **1986**, *877*, 406–414. [CrossRef]
45. Chen, J.; Jiang, Y.; Ma, K.Y.; Chen, F.; Chen, Z.Y. Microalga decreases plasma cholesterol by down-regulation of intestinal NPC1L1, hepatic LDL receptor, and 42 HMG-CoA reductase. *J. Agric. Food Chem.* **2011**, *59*, 6790–6797. [CrossRef]

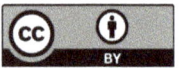

© 2019 by the authors. Licensee MDPI, Basel, Switzerland. This article is an open access article distributed under the terms and conditions of the Creative Commons Attribution (CC BY) license (http://creativecommons.org/licenses/by/4.0/).

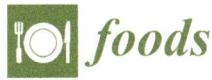

Article

Egg Yolk Antioxidants Profiles: Effect of Diet Supplementation with Linseeds and Tomato-Red Pepper Mixture before and after Storage

Besma Omri [1,2], Nadir Alloui [3], Alessandra Durazzo [4], Massimo Lucarini [4], Alessandra Aiello [5], Raffaele Romano [5], Antonello Santini [6,*] and Hedi Abdouli [1]

1. Laboratory of Improvement & Integrated Development of Animal Productivity & Food Resources, Higher School of Agriculture of Mateur, University of Carthage, Avenue de la République P.O. Box 77, Amilcar 1054, Tunisia
2. National Agronomy Institute, Tunis, University of Carthage, Avenue de la République P.O. Box 77, Amilcar 1054, Tunisia
3. Department of Veterinary Sciences, University of Batna, Batna 05000, Algeria
4. CREA—Research Centre for Food and Nutrition, Via Ardeatina 546, 00178 Roma, Italy
5. Department of Agriculture, University of Napoli Federico II, 80138 Napoli, Italy
6. Department of Pharmacy, University of Napoli Federico II, Via D. Montesano 49, 80131 Napoli, Italy
* Correspondence: asantini@unina.it; Tel.: +39-81-253-9317

Received: 24 June 2019; Accepted: 30 July 2019; Published: 7 August 2019

Abstract: This study evaluated the effect of dietary incorporation of linseed alone or along with dried tomato paste-pepper powder mix on egg physical characteristics, antioxidant profiles, lipid oxidative status, and yolk coloration before and after storage at 4 °C for one month. Sixty Novogen White laying hens, 27 weeks-old, were divided into three groups and given 100 g/hen/day of a standard diet (C), standard diet containing 4.5% of ground linseed (L), linseed diet containing 1% of dried tomato paste and 1% of sweet red pepper (LTP). Linseeds increased ($p < 0.05$) egg yolk antioxidant capacity but not lipid oxidative stability ($p > 0.05$). However, dietary inclusion of LTP did not improve fresh egg yolk antioxidant activity and lipid oxidation stability ($p > 0.05$). With reference to the stored eggs, only antioxidant activity measured by phosphomolybdenum reduction and lipid oxidative stability were influenced ($p < 0.05$) by the dietary treatment. Fresh egg yolk of hens fed on linseeds tended to have a slightly more yellow, redder, and less light color than the eggs of hens fed with the control diet. Dietary supplementation of LTP increased ($p < 0.05$) the Roche yolk color fan (RYCF) score and redness (a*) and decreased ($p < 0.05$) lightness (L*) without affecting ($p > 0.05$) saturation (C*). Storage of hens' eggs fed on the control diet did not influence ($p > 0.05$) yolk color.

Keywords: carotenoid; flavonoids; oxidative status; polyphenols; yolk color

1. Introduction

The hen's egg is considered as a functional food, since it represents a valuable source of high quality proteins, minerals, vitamins, and lipids, i.e., polyunsaturated fatty acids (PUFA) and phospholipids [1–6]. Beside their nutritional value, eggs represent a good source of antioxidants [6]: egg proteins (i.e., ovalbumin, ovotransferrin, phosvitin), phospholipids, and vitamin A, vitamin E, selenium, carotenoid, show antioxidant [7–16] and nutraceuticals properties [13–27].

Moreover, eggs can be also enriched with antioxidants by manipulation of poultry feed [28–32]. Omega-3 fatty acids and carotenoids are biologically active compounds utilized for egg biofortification [33,34] also using by-products of agro system chain in an environmentally friendly way [34–40].

Carotenoid [41] can be supplemented as dried synthetic pigments or as natural pigments from red pepper [42], tomato powder [36,37,43–45] and colored carrot [46]. They cannot be produced by hens de novo. Carotenoid must be provided in their diet's ingredients [47]. These compounds were used as pigments for many years so as to obtain a desired color of egg yolk [48]. Egg choice by consumers is no longer only based on yolk cholesterol content or fatty acids profile, but also on its color [49] due to the health benefits associated with the pigment source [50–52]. As antioxidants [53], carotenoids, were used to neutralize the excess of free radicals, to protect the cell against their toxic effects and to contribute to disease prevention such as arthrosclerosis, cardiac hypertrophy, congestive heart failure and Alzheimer [54–57]. For example, according to Willcox et al. [54] beta-carotene is a strong antioxidant and is the best quencher of singlet oxygen. Lycopene, a carotenoid, has been found to be very protective, particularly for prostate cancer [55]. The current review of Bohn [56] well summarizes human observational studies/intervention trials targeting carotenoids in relation to chronic diseases characterized by oxidative stress and markers thereof: the author underlines, that, even if different markers of oxidative stress were studied, no single one gives a complete shot of oxidative stress homeostasis, related to the involvement of many body compartments, mechanisms and the type/number of bioactive compounds.

It is worth mentioning the review of Pham-Huy et al. [57] on the role of antioxidants in the prevention of chronic diseases such as cancer, autoimmune disorders, aging, cataract, rheumatoid arthritis, cardiovascular and neurodegenerative disease; antioxidants present different physiological properties, i.e., anti-allergic, antimicrobial, anti-inflammatory, anti-atherogenic, vasodilatory effects [58–64].

Also, the current work of Yeung et al. [65] reported, by means of a scientific literature analysis of works since 1991, that there has been a transition of scientific interest from vitamins and minerals to antioxidant phytochemicals.

Red pepper, the source of red and yellow carotenoid [66,67], used at 0.8%, increased egg yolk color scores [42]. However, dried tomato contained lycopene, the main red carotenoid responsible for egg yolk red color. The combination of red and yellow carotenoid has been found to be effective for yolk pigmentation [68]. Yellow carotenoid deposition creates a yellow base, which is necessary for the saturation of the final color. When the saturated phase was established, red carotenoid addition increased the orange-red yolk color. Furthermore, feeding hens with linseed, sunflower and palm oil accelerated egg yolk lipid oxidation, related to long chain polyunsaturated fatty acids [69].

Lipid oxidation is a process that affects egg yolk lipid stability during storage. It can alter egg nutritional quality and may lead to taste, flavor, odor and color depreciation and to toxic substances production [70,71]. Prevention of cholesterol oxidation and PUFA auto-oxidation could be reached by carotenoid supplementation, tomatoes or sweet red pepper, as sources of antioxidants into hens' feed.

The use of linseeds, tomato by-products or red pepper as natural or biological feed additives has been done to supplement laying hens' feeds, and consequently, the egg industry, with essential micro-ingredients (polyunsaturated fatty acids (ω-3 and ω-6) and antioxidant (α-carotene, β-carotene, β-cryptoxanthine, lycopene, zeaxanthin, total phenols and flavonoids), as well as for animal wellbeing purposes and improved efficiency. As far as red pepper is concerned, Li et al. [41] reported that the development of an environmental friendly technique which would allow the egg yolk coloring ability of red peppers to be obtained at a lower cost with enhanced efficiency could be extremely beneficial to the poultry industry; moreover, this result has led to an increase of interest of consumers.

Dietary supplementation of tomato by-products or red pepper was also a new solution to optimize livestock economic (reducing the prices of feed ingredients) and environmental performance at the industry level. This supplementation may reduce the need for synthetic antioxidants at industry level through advanced knowledge of the impact of these ingredients and their composition on animal and human health and the use of natural antioxidant to optimize the safety, sustainability and nutritional value of feed ingredients; moreover this result has led to an increase of interest from consumer.

In view of the above, the present study aims at evaluating the effect of dietary incorporation of linseed alone or along with a dried tomato paste-pepper powder mix on egg physical characteristics, egg yolk antioxidant profile, lipid oxidative status and coloration before and after storage at 4 °C for one month.

2. Materials and Methods

2.1. Ethical Considerations

All procedures concerning animals' care, handling, and sampling were conducted under the approval of the Official Animal Care and Use Committee of the Higher School of Agriculture of Mateur (protocol N°05/15) before the initiation of the study and followed the Tunisian guidelines.

2.2. Experimental Design

A total of sixty, *Novogen* White laying hens (initial live weight = 1449.95 g ± 71.99 g) of 27 weeks-old were randomly regrouped into 3 homogeneous groups of 20 hens each. Corn and soybean-meal were used as a standard mash diet (C) for laying hens. Two supplemented diets were designated as follows: (1) linseed (L) and (2) linseed–tomato–pepper (LTP), which were individually prepared by mixing the control diet thoroughly with the designated supplements at the required incorporation levels, as described by Omri et al. [72] (Table 1).

Table 1. Ingredients, chemical and antioxidants composition of the experimental diet (g/Kg) *.

	Diets		
	Control (C)	Linseeds (L)	Linseeds–Tomato–Pepper (LTP)
Ingredients (%)			
Linseed	0	4.5	4.5
Dried Tomato	0	0	1
Sweet red pepper	0	0	1
Yellow corn	66.5	63.5	61.5
Soybean meal	25.5	24.0	24.0
Calcium carbonate, Mineral and Vitamin mixture	8.0	8.0	8.0
Chemical Composition			
Crude protein, (%, dry matter (DM))	18.1	18	18
Ether extract (%, DM)	3.56	5.6	5.27
Metabolizable energy (Kcal/Kg DM)	2750	2850	2830
Antioxidants			
α-carotene, * (10^{-9}) g/kg DM	3.41	5.1	21.7
β-carotene, * (10^{-9}) g/kg DM	3.37	5.36	23.2
β-cryptoxanthine,* (10^{-9}) g/kg DM	3.84	5.50	25.3
Lycopene, * (10^{-9}) g/kg DM	1.77	3.48	15.7
Zeaxanthine, * (10^{-9}) g/kg DM	3.90	5.59	25.7
£ Flavonoids, g CE/kg DM	2.26	1.59	2.03
¥ Total phenols, g GAE/kg DM	3.02	3.53	2.98

* Note: C = Control diet; L = diet supplemented with ground linseed at 4.5%, LTP = diet supplemented with ground linseed (4.5%), dried tomato paste (1%) and sweet pepper powder (1%) mix; ¥ Total phenols expressed in g gallic acid equivalent, g GAE/kg DM; £ Flavonoids expressed in g catechin equivalent, g CE/kg DM. Control (C) provided following nutrients per 100 g: Ca, 4.3 g; P, 0.6 g; Na, 0.14 g; Cl, 0.23 g; Fe, 4 mg; Zn, 40 mg; Mn, 7 mg; Cu, 0.3 mg; I, 0.08 mg; Se, 0.01 mg; Co, 0.02; methionine, 0.39 g; methionine + cysteine, 0.69 g; lysine, 0.89 g; Retinol, 800 IU; Cholecalciferol, 220 IU; α-tocopherol, 1.1 IU; Thiamin, 0.33 IU; Nicotinic acid, 909 IU.

To reduce the feed-selection behavior typically observed in laying hens diets were restricted to 100 g/hen/d. Feed was offered once daily at 7:30 AM. Hens were allocated individually in standard pens with individual feed-trough and common water-trough in an ambient temperature of about

20 ± 4 °C. A lighting schedule of 16 h light and 8 h dark was followed. Water was offered *ad libitum.* during the experimental period, which lasted 47 days.

2.3. Data Collection and Chemical Analyses

Eggs laid from the 26th to the 30th days of the experimental period were weighed and used for egg physical characteristics measurements (egg albumen, yolk and shell weights). Egg yolks were pooled per two hens belonging to the same dietary treatment group so that 10 yolk samples per group were obtained instead of 20. Yolk samples were then used for analyses: antioxidant profile, oxidative status and egg yolk color. Eggs laid during the 31st day of the experimental trial were weighted and stored at 4 °C for one month. After storage, the eggs were used for the same analyses as those conducted prior to storage.

2.4. Egg Yolk Color

Egg yolk color was determined using the Yolk Color Fan® Scale DSM Yolk Color Fan (DSM Nutritional Products Europe, Wurmisweg 576, CH-4303 Kaiseraugst, Switzerland) (1 for light yellow and 15 for orange) and the color measuring device Konica Minolta Chroma Meter CR- 400/410 (Minolta, Tokyo, Japan) following the CIE (Commission Internationale de L'Eclairage) color system, L* (lightness: negative towards black, positive towards white) a* (redness: negative towards green, positive towards red) and b* (yellowness: negative towards blue, positive towards yellow). Chroma Meter was set up perpendicularly to the egg yolk surface in a Petri dish. L*, a* and b* parameters were measured three times. Final values were calculated as the averages of the three corresponding values measured.

Egg chroma was calculated according to the formula:

$$C^* = (a^{*2} + b^{*2})^{1/2}$$

2.5. Antioxidant Profile Determination

2.5.1. Total Carotenoid Determination

Total carotenoid of fresh, stored egg yolk and diets were determined in accordance with Amaya, [73]. Samples of 0.5 g were extracted in 5 mL of Butylated Hydroxy Toluene (BHT) (0.05%) in cold acetone (4 °C) and stirred for 1 h 30 min. After 15 min of centrifugation at 3000 rpm, the supernatant was transferred to another tube containing 7 mL of petroleum ether.

Then 20 mL of distilled water was slowly added along the tube. After separation of two phases for 1 h, 10 mL of distilled water was added. The aqueous phase was discarded. The ether phase was transferred to another tube and absorbance was measured.

2.5.2. Total Phenol Determination

The Folin–Ciocalteu method following the procedure of Makkar et al. [74] was used for total phenol content of acetone extracts evaluation. A total of 1 mL of acetone extract was mixed with 0.5 mL of Folin–Ciocalteu reagent, then 2.5 mL of Na_2CO_3 solution (20% w/v) were added. The solution was incubated for 40 min at 60 °C after vortexing and absorbance was measured at 750 nm against a blank (distilled water). Total phenolics content was expressed as mg equivalents gallic acid (EGA) (standard) per g of sample.

2.5.3. Flavonoid Determination

Flavonoid content was determined by the aluminum chloride method as reported by Patel et al. [75]. Fresh, stored egg yolk or diet samples (100 mg) were extracted in 5 mL of diethyl. After centrifugation for 15 min at 2000 rpm, the precipitate was extracted in 5 mL of 80% methanol for 5 h and filtered using Wathman filter paper. The filtrate was adjusted to 50 mL with distilled water. An Aliquot of 2.5 mL was mixed with 0.15 mL $NaNO_2$ (5%). After 5 min, 0.15 mL of aluminum chloride (10%) was added. Six minutes later, 1 mL of NaOH (1N) and 1.2 mL of distilled water were added. The solution was vortexed and absorbance was measured at 510 nm against distilled water (blank). The flavonoid content was expressed as mg equivalents catechin (standard) per g of sample.

2.5.4. Oxidative Status Determination

Antioxidant activity [76,77] of fresh and stored egg yolk was measured by the phosphomolybdenum method according to the procedure described by Prieto et al. [78]. A total of 0.5 g of fresh egg yolk was diluted in 10 mL of NaCl (2%). A total of 100 µL of the suspension was adjusted to 2 mL with distilled water. Then, 2 mL of phosphomolybdenum reagent (2.8 mM of sodium phosphate and 4 mM ammonium molybdate in 0.6 M sulphuric acid) was added. After incubation at 95 °C for 90 min., the mixture was cooled at room temperature and the absorbance was measured at 695 nm ($A_{695\ nm}$) using a UV-visible spectrophotometer (CECIL Auruis series CE 2041 UV/Vis) against 2% NaCl (blank). Antioxidant capacity is expressed as mg equivalents of ascorbic acid (EAA) (standard) per g of sample.

Total antioxidant activity was also evaluated by ferric reducing antioxidant power assay, according to Benzie and Szeto [79], with slight modifications. Aqueous solutions of egg yolk prepared as reported above were used for this assay. A total of 150 µL of solution was mixed with 2.4 mL of distilled water, 0.45 mL of ethanol, 0.75 mL of HCl, 0.75 mL of 1% potassium ferricyanide, 0.25 mL of 1% SDS and 0.25 mL of 0.2% ferric chloride. The solution was left in a water bath at 50 °C for 20 min then cooled at room temperature and absorbance was measured at 750 nm. Antioxidant capacity is expressed as mg Equivalents Gallic Acid (EGA) (standard) per g of sample.

The malondialdehyde (MDA) measurement method described by Draper and Hadeley [80] was used for lipid oxidation of fresh and stored egg yolk estimation. A total of 0.5 g of egg yolk was diluted in 5 mL of TCA (20%) with 0.5 mL of BHT (1%) in absolute ethanol. After stirring for 1 h at room temperature, samples were centrifuged for 15 min at 3000 rpm. A total of 2.95 mL of thiobarbituric acid (TBA) (50 mM) were added to 1.5 mL of solution. After incubation at 100 °C for 10 min, the samples were cooled at room temperature and centrifuged at 3500 rpm for 10 min. Absorbance was measured at 532 nm using an UV-visible spectrophotometer against 2% NaCl (blank). Thiobarbituric acid was used as a standard. The thiobarbituric acid reactive substances (TBARS) are expressed as µg of MDA per g of sample.

2.6. Statistical Analysis

Data were tested for 'diet' (C, L and LTP) and 'type of eggs' (fresh or stored) effects and their interaction using mixed models with compound symmetry covariance structures of SAS [81]. Interaction 'diet × type of eggs' effects were not so significant for all parameters that comparisons of intra-diet means/egg type (C versus L and L vs. LTP for fresh and stored eggs separately) and intra-type of eggs/diet (fresh versus stored eggs for each diet) were not possible. Eggs were also stored without separation between yolk, albumen and shell so that all parameters were not determined on the same eggs before and after storage, but separately, on representative samples of eggs laid/diet.

Data were tested for 'diet' (C, L and LTP) using the GLM procedure (General Linear Model) of SAS according to the following model:

$$Y_{ij} = \mu + T_i + e_{ij}$$

where:

Y_{ij} = represents the jth observation on the ith treatment
μ = overall mean
T_i = the main effect of the ith treatment
e_{ij} = random error present in the jth observation on the ith treatment

When diet and/or egg type effects were significant at α < 0.05, means comparisons were tested using the CONTRAST statement of SAS [82]. The effect of storage on eggs/diet was tested using the Student T-test. Correlations between egg yolk color traits and carotenoid concentration were tested using the procedure CORR of SAS [81]. All statistical procedures were tested using SAS [81].

3. Results and Discussion

3.1. Egg Physical Characteristics

Egg physical characteristics before and after storage at 4 °C for 30 days are reported in Table 2.

Table 2. Physical characteristics of eggs before and after storage at 4 °C for one month.

Parameters	Eggs	Diets			p-Value
		C $^\alpha$	L $^\alpha$	LTP $^\alpha$	
Egg weight, g	Fresh	55.48 ^{aA}	57.67 ^{aA}	57.09 ^{aA}	0.07
	Stored	54.08 ^{cA}	56.87 ^{aA}	56.21 ^{abA}	0.024
Yolk weight, g	Fresh	13.79 ^{aA}	13.84 ^{aA}	13.86 ^{aA}	0.99
	Stored	14.54 ^{aA}	14.69 ^{aB}	14.48 ^{aB}	0.92
Albumen weight, g	Fresh	33.95 ^{aA}	35.53 ^{aA}	34.73 ^{aA}	0.13
	Stored	31.88 ^{bB}	34.00 ^{aA}	33.68 ^{aA}	0.046
Shell weight, g	Fresh	5.4 ^{aA}	6.15 ^{aA}	5.89 ^{aA}	0.16
	Stored	5.2 ^{cA}	5.65 ^{aA}	5.58 ^{abB}	0.004
Shell thickness, mm	Fresh	0.39 ^{aA}	0.4 ^{aA}	0.42 ^{aA}	0.15
	Stored	0.4 ^{aA}	0.42 ^{aA}	0.41 ^{aA}	0.41

Note: $^\alpha$ C = Control diet; L = diet supplemented with ground linseed at 4.5%, LTP = diet supplemented with ground linseed (4.5%), dried tomato paste (1%) and sweet pepper powder (1%) mix; ^{a,b,c}: Means within the same row with no different superscripts letters are not significantly different (p > 0.05); ^{A,B}: Means of the same parameters within the same column with no different superscripts letters are not significantly different (p > 0.05); Data for fresh eggs from Omri et al. [72].

As reported in our previous research study [72], dietary supplementation of 4.5% of linseeds increased (p > 0.05) fresh egg weight, and compared to the linseeds (L), tomato-sweet pepper mixture was without effect (p > 0.05). However, stored egg weight was influenced (p < 0.05) with dietary treatment and, for each of the four treatments, there was a slight loss of egg weight after storage at 4 °C. Fresh and stored egg yolk weights were not influenced (p > 0.05) by dietary treatment. Dietary treatment did not affect (p > 0.05) the fresh eggs' albumen weight. However, LTP increased (p < 0.05) the stored eggs' albumen weight. Storage decreased (p < 0.05) albumen weight of hens fed with the control diet. The shell weight of fresh eggs was not affected (p > 0.05) by dietary treatment, but increased (p < 0.05) by L and LTP addition for stored eggs. Storage decreased (p < 0.05) egg shell weight of hens fed on the LTP diet. Shell thickness was affected (p > 0.05) neither by dietary treatment nor by storage. In this regard, Yassein et al. [83] showed that dietary addition of 5% of linseeds did not affect egg weight and albumen, yolk and shell percentages. Ahmad et al. [84] found that feeding hens with 5% of linseed did not affect egg weight (59.93 g vs. 60.47 g), yolk weight (15.15 g vs. 14.81 g), albumen weight (9.05 g vs. 10.51 g), shell weight (8.13 g vs. 8.48 g) and shell thickness (0.39 g vs. 0.38 mm).

Concerning tomato, Akdemir et al. [43] reported that the dietary supplementation of 0.5% and 1% of tomato powder did not influence yolk weight (16.59 g vs. 17.11 g), shell weight (6.79 g vs. 6.97 g) and shell thickness (0.399 mm vs. 0.393 mm).

Studies on the effect of egg storage on its physical characteristics are lacking. However, Niemiec et al. [85] reported that the dietary addition of primrose, linseeds and rapeseeds at, respectively, 2.88%, 3.66% and 5%, with or without supplementation of 200 mg vitamin E/kg, did not affect egg weight after 20 days of storage at 12 °C. A significant reduction in the egg yolk weight after storage was found, from 24.23% (control group) to 23.35% (primrose, linseeds and rapeseeds) and 23.18% (primrose, linseeds, rapeseeds and vitamin E).

3.2. Egg Yolk Antioxidant Profile

Egg yolk antioxidants [86] (α-carotene, β-carotene, β-cryptoxanthine, lycopene, zeaxanthine, total phenols and flavonoids) concentrations before and after storage at 4 °C for 30 days are reported in Table 3.

Table 3. Egg yolk antioxidants profile before and after storage at 4 °C for one month.

Parameters	Eggs	Diets			p-Value
		C $^\alpha$	L $^\alpha$	LTP $^\alpha$	
α-carotene, µg/g	Fresh	11.0 ^{bA}	12.26 ^{aA}	12.7 ^{aA}	0.0002
	Stored	11.47 ^{abA}	11.66 ^{aA}	12.03 ^{aA}	0.033
β-carotene, µg/g	Fresh	11.2 ^{bA}	12.3 ^{aA}	12.9 ^{aA}	0.0001
	Stored	11.53 ^{aA}	11.71 ^{aA}	12.18 ^{aA}	0.06
β-Cryptoxanthine, µg/g	Fresh	12.4 ^{bA}	13.81 ^{aA}	14.42 ^{aA}	0.0001
	Stored	12.59 ^{aA}	13.11 ^{aA}	13.45 ^{aA}	0.089
Lycopene, µg/g	Fresh	7.67 ^{bA}	8.42 ^{aA}	8.90 ^{aA}	<0.0001
	Stored	7.98 ^{bA}	8.09 ^{aA}	8.37 ^{aA}	0.034
Zeaxanthine, µg/g	Fresh	12.4 ^{bA}	13.81 ^{aA}	14.42 ^{aA}	0.0001
	Stored	12.59 ^{aA}	13.11 ^{aA}	13.45 ^{aA}	0.089
Total phenols, mg GAE/g $^¥$	Fresh	1.86 ^{bA}	2.17 ^{aA}	2.16 ^{aA}	0.0034
	Stored	1.57 ^{aB}	1.74 ^{aB}	1.64 ^{aB}	0.69
Flavonoids, mg CE/g $^£$	Fresh	1.92 ^{bA}	1.53 ^{bA}	2.96 ^{aA}	0.0009
	Stored	1.50 ^{aA}	1.39 ^{aA}	2.17 ^{aA}	0.38

Note: $^\alpha$ C = Control diet; L = diet supplemented with ground linseed at 4.5%, LTP = diet supplemented with ground linseed (4.5%), dried tomato paste (1%) and sweet pepper powder (1%) mix; $^¥$: Total phenols expressed in mg gallic acid equivalent, mg GAE/g; $^£$: Flavonoids expressed in mg catechin equivalent, mg CE/g; ^{a,b,c}: Means within the same row with no different superscripts letters are not significantly different ($p > 0.05$); ^{A,B}: Means of the same parameters within the same column with no different superscripts letters are not significantly different ($p > 0.05$); data for fresh eggs from Omri et al. [72].

Fresh eggs concentrations of all antioxidants were affected ($p < 0.05$) by dietary treatment. Carotenoid concentrations of fresh eggs of hens fed with control diet (C) varied from 7.7 to 12.4 µg/g of yolk, respectively, for lycopene and zeaxanthine [72]. These levels were in agreement with those (12.8 and 9.2 µg/g DM, respectively, for luteine and zeaxanthine) reported by Englmaierovà et al. [49] of eggs from hens fed with corn, wheat, soybean meal and alfalfa meal. Our results, were higher than those reported by Hammershøj et al. [46] who found that eggs of hens fed on a standard organic food (wheat, oats, peas, sunflower meal, fish meal) contained: 7.46 µg/g of lutein, 2.6 µg/g of zeaxanthine, 0.01 µg/g of α-carotene/g and 0.03 µg/g of β-carotene. Our results were also higher than those (7.09 µg/g of luteine, 0.85 µg/g of cis-luteine, 7.09 µg/g of zeaxanthine, 0.69 µg/g of cis-zeaxanthine and 1.07 µg/g of β-carotene) reported by Kotrbáček et al. [87] for a diet containing 33% of wheat, 30% of corn and 24% of soybean meal. Studies in the literature with regard to this aspect are lacking. However, a total phenol content equal to 0.54 mg GAE/g DM was reported by Amar et al. [88] and equal to 0.72 mg GAE/g (diet based on yellow corn) and 0.66 mg GAE/g DM (diet based on wheat) were found by Nimalaratne et al. [14]. Dietary incorporation of linseeds increased ($p < 0.05$) fresh egg yolk concentrations of carotenoid and total phenols and did not affect ($p > 0.05$) egg yolk concentration of flavonoids.

Diet with dried tomato (1%) and sweet red pepper (1%) mix contained four times more carotenoid than diet with linseeds (L). However, fresh egg yolk carotenoid concentrations of hens fed with L and LTP were not different ($p > 0.05$). Studies on the effects of linseeds on the egg yolk antioxidants profile are lacking. Concerning tomato, Habanabashaka et al. [89] reported that dietary incorporation of 0, 3, 6 or 9% of tomato by-products increased egg yolk concentration of lycopene from 0.01 to 0.95 µg/g, lutein from 10.1 to 13.9 µg/g and of zeaxanthine from 9.4 to 12.9µg/g. However, Amar et al. [88] reported that dietary incorporation of 0, 4, 7, 10 and 13% of tomato peel increased egg yolk concentration of lycopene from 26.5 µg/g DM (4%) to 42.8 µg/g DM (7%); 37.6 µg/g DM (10%) and 41.8 µg/g DM (13%) and of β-carotene from 6.5 µg/g DM (0%); 11.3 (4%) µg/g DM; 17.6 (7%) µg/g DM; 12.3 (10%) µg/g DM to 16.7 µg/g DM (13%). Akdemir et al. [43] evaluated the effect of the dietary addition of 0.5%, 1% of tomato powder reported that an increase in egg yolk concentration of lycopene from 6.53 (0.5%) to 8.05 µg/g (1%), of β- carotene form 172 µg/g (0%) to 331 µg/g (0.5%) and 551 µg/g (1%) and of lutein from 6.85 µg/g (0%) to 7.23 µg/g (0.5%) and 9.03 µg/g (1%). Dietary incorporation of 0.1%, 0.2%, 0.4%, 0.8% of paprika extract increased egg yolk concentration of total carotenoid from 3.43 µg/g (0%) to 7.7 µg/g (0.1%), 10.86 µg/g (0.2%), 14.60 µg/g (0.4%) and 16.83 µg/g (0.8%) [90]. Egg storage for one month did not affect ($p > 0.05$) the egg yolk concentrations of all carotenoids (α-carotene, β-carotene, cryptoxanthin, lycopene and zeaxanthin) and decreased ($p < 0.05$) the total phenol concentrations of each treatment.

Reports on the effect of storage of eggs of hens fed with similar treatments to ours diets are lacking. However, Barbarosa et al. [91] reported that egg storage for 35 days at room temperature (26.5 °C) reduced egg yolk total carotenoid concentration from 28.55 to 22.09 µg/g. By contrast, egg storage for 35 days at 7.9 °C reduced total carotenoid egg yolk concentration from 28.55 to 23.57 µg/g. Gawecki et al. [92] also reported that egg storage for 8 weeks at 2 °C did not reduce egg yolk total carotenoid concentration. However, after 15 weeks of storage, the total carotenoid concentration in the egg yolk decreased from 28.55 µg/g to 27.03 µg/g.

In the present study, egg yolk antioxidant capacity was evaluated by determining egg yolk capacity to reduce MO^{6+} to MO^{5+} and Fe^{3+} to Fe^{2+}. Lipid oxidative stability determined by thiobarbituric acid reactive substances (TBARS) was even higher than the concentration of MDA, which was low.

Only fresh egg antioxidant activity determined by the reduction of MO^{6+} to MO^{5+} was influenced ($p < 0.05$) by dietary treatment. Fresh egg antioxidant activity of the control group was equal to 4.48 mg AAE/g. Reports in the literature concerning egg yolk antioxidant activity expressed as AAE and as GAE are lacking. Fresh egg yolk concentration of MDA was not affected ($p > 0.05$) by dietary treatment. Fresh egg yolk concentration of MDA of the control treatment was equal to 0.11 µg/g [72]. This value was lower than the 1.17 µg/g reported by Englmaierovà et al. [49] and the 0.7 µg/g reported by Venglovská et al. [93] for fresh eggs of hens fed on corn, wheat and soybean meal. Our results were similar to those reported by Hayat et al. [94] with a mean value of 0.1 µg/g for fresh eggs of hens fed on corn meal and soybean meal.

The dietary addition of 4.5% of linseeds increased ($p < 0.05$) the egg yolk antioxidant capacity, but not its lipids oxidative stability ($p > 0.05$). Thus, egg enrichment with fatty acids (polyunsaturated and polyunsaturated ω-3) through the dietary supplementation of linseeds did not reduce egg yolk lipid oxidative stability. This lipid protection against oxidation may be attributed to the increase of fresh egg yolk pigments and total phenol concentrations (Table 3). In this regard, Hayat et al. [94] reported that egg yolk MDA concentration increased from 0.1 to 0.23 µg/g (10% of linseeds flaxseed), 0.32 µg/g (10% of linseeds plus 50 IU of α-tocopherol) and 0.28 µg/g (10% of linseeds plus 150 mg of BHT). However, Boruta and Niemiec [95] reported that the dietary addition of 3% of linseeds with or without supplementation of 200 mg/kg of vitamin E did not affect fresh egg yolk concentration of thiobarbituric acid-reactive substances (TBARS). The dietary inclusion of 1% of dried tomato and 1% of sweet red pepper in addition to the linseeds did not improve fresh egg yolk antioxidant activity and its lipid oxidative stability ($p > 0.05$). This inefficiency of dried tomato and sweet red pepper mixture could be due to its low level of incorporation (2%) that did not affect egg yolk concentrations of pigments, total phenols and flavonoids when compared to diet with linseeds (Table 4).

Table 4. Egg yolk lipid oxidative status before and after storage at 4 °C for one month.

Parameters	Eggs	Diets			p-Value
		C [α]	L [α]	LTP [α]	
Antioxidant activity, mg AAE/g [§]	Fresh	4.48 [bA]	5.07 [aA]	5.16 [aA]	0.0009
	Stored	3.68 [aB]	3.89 [aB]	3.99 [aB]	0.0004
Antioxidant activity, mg GAE/g [¥]	Fresh	3.14 [aA]	4.38 [aA]	4.14 [aA]	0.11
	Stored	1.16 [aB]	1.40 [aB]	1.58 [aB]	0.16
Thiobarbituric acid reactive substances (TBARS), µg MDA/g	Fresh	0.11 [aA]	0.14 [aA]	0.15 [aA]	0.28
	Stored	0.14 [bA]	0.24 [aA]	0.16 [bA]	0.01

Note: [α] C = Control diet; L = diet supplemented with ground linseed at 4.5%, LTP = diet supplemented with ground linseed (4.5%), dried tomato paste (1%) and sweet pepper powder (1%) mix; [§]: Antioxidant activity evaluated as phosphomolybdenum reducing power and expressed in ascorbic acid equivalent (AAE); [¥]: Antioxidant activity evaluated as ferric reducing power and expressed in gallic acid equivalent (GAE); [a,b,c]: Means within the same row with no different superscripts letters are not significantly different ($p > 0.05$); [A,B]: Means of the same parameters within the same column with no different superscripts letters are not significantly different ($p > 0.05$); data for fresh eggs from Omri et al. [72].

Akdemir et al. [43] showed that the dietary addition of 0.5% and 1% tomato powder reduced egg yolk concentration of MDA from 0.33 µg/g (control) to 0.25 µg/g (0.5%) and 0.21 µg/g (1%). Sahin et al. [96] also reported the dietary addition of 100 and 200 mg of lycopene/kg in Japanese quail diet reduced the egg yolk concentration of MDA from 0.86 (control) to 0.79 µg/g (100 mg of lycopene/kg) and 0.74 µg/g (200 mg of lycopene/kg). Dietary addition of carophyll, lutein or algae (chlorella) improved egg yolk the oxidative stability from 1.17 µg/g (control) to 1 µg/g (carophyll), 0.87 µg/g (lutein) and 0.90 mg/kg (algae) [49].

Concerning stored eggs, only antioxidant activity measured by phosphomolybdenum reduction and lipid oxidative stability were influenced ($p < 0.05$) by dietary treatment. Diet with linseeds (4.5%) plus sweet red pepper and tomato mix (2%) was associated with higher ($p < 0.05$) lipid oxidative stability than diet with linseeds. However, egg storage decreased ($p < 0.05$) yolk antioxidant activity but not lipid stability to the oxidation of the four treatments. In this regard, Pereira [97] reported that MDA egg yolk concentration increased from 0.52 to 0.71 and 0.90 µg/g after storage at 4 °C for, respectively, 60 and 90 j. By contrast, Hayat et al. [94] reported that egg storage at 4 °C for 20, 40 and 60 days did not affect MDA concentration. Shahryar et al. [70] reported that ω-3 and ω-6 enriched eggs stored at 4 °C for 30 and 60 days increased MDA concentrations. Boruta and Niemiec [95] evaluated the effect of dietary addition of 4% rapeseed, 3% linseeds and 2% primrose, with or without supplementation of 200 mg/kg of vitamin E, on egg antioxidant status and reported that egg storage for 3 and 6 months increased yolk MDA concentration. However, vitamin E supplementation decreased egg yolk MDA concentration after 6 months of storage.

3.3. Egg Yolk Coloration

Egg yolk coloration before and after storage at 4 °C for one month are represented in Table 5.

Color scores determined by the Yolk Color Fan® scale (RYCF) were affected by dietary treatment ($p < 0.0001$). Fresh egg yolk score of the control group was the lowest with a mean value of 4.67 [72]. Our values were not in agreement with 6.65 reported by Abdouli et al. [98] and 8.64 found by Lokaewmanee et al. [99] for eggs of hens fed with a similar diet to our control treatment. b* mean value showed that egg yolk yellow color was sufficiently intense. Our results were lower than 32.5 and 48.2 reported, respectively by, Abdouli et al. [98] and Dvorak et al. [100]. Negative mean value of a* indicated an absence of the red hue. Higher mean values ranging from 0.05 to 13.5 were reported by Dvorak et al. [100]. L* and C* mean values showed that the egg yolks of hens fed with control treatment were characterized by an intense, light yellow color. Dietary incorporation of 4.5% of linseeds increased ($p < 0.05$) the egg yolk color score (RYCF). The fresh egg yolk of hens fed with linseeds tended to have a slightly more yellow, redder and less light color than the eggs of the control group.

Correlations between the yolk color scores (RYCF), parameters determined by Chroma Meter and pigments concentrations (Table 6), showed that the yolk color scores (RYCF) and redness (a *) were positively correlated with all the determined pigments.

Table 5. Egg yolk coloration before and after storage at 4 °C for one month.

Parameters	Eggs	Diets			p-Value
		C [α]	L [α]	LTP [α]	
RYCF	Fresh	4.67 [cA]	5.65 [bA]	8.2 [aA]	<0.0001
	Stored	4.7 [cA]	5.4 [bA]	7.53 [aA]	<0.0001
L*	Fresh	72.65 [aA]	71.63 [aA]	69.42 [bA]	<0.0001
	Stored	73.32 [aA]	72.84 [aB]	70.47 [bB]	0.003
a*	Fresh	−0.59 [bA]	1.19 [bA]	6.59 [aA]	<0.0001
	Stored	0.59 [bA]	0.53 [bB]	6.44 [aA]	<0.0001
b*	Fresh	62.81 [aA]	64.91 [aA]	60.28 [aA]	0.1
	Stored	64.59 [aA]	64.06 [aA]	61.22 [bA]	0.003
C*	Fresh	62.85 [aA]	64.95 [aA]	60.70 [aA]	0.15
	Stored	64.46 [aA]	64.07 [aA]	61.58 [aA]	0.06

Note: [α] C= Control diet; L = diet supplemented with ground linseed at 4.5%, LTP = diet supplemented with ground linseed (4.5%), dried tomato paste (1%) and sweet pepper powder (1%) mix; RYCF: Roche Yolk Color Fan; [a,b,c] Means within the same row with no different superscripts letters are not significantly different ($p > 0.05$); [A,B] Means of the same parameters within the same column with no different superscripts letters are not significantly different ($p > 0.05$); data on fresh eggs from Omri et al. [72].

Table 6. Correlation between fresh and stored egg yolk coloration and carotenoid concentration.

Parameters	Eggs	α-Carotene	β-Carotene	β-Cryptoxanthine	Lycopene	Zeaxanthine
RYCF	Fresh	0.53 **	0.55 **	0.52 **	0.57 ***	0.52 **
	Stored	0.41 *	0.39 *	0.34 *	0.40 *	0.34 *
L*	Fresh	−0.56 **	−0.54 **	−0.47 *	−0.58 ***	−0.47 *
	Stored	−0.09	−0.29	−0.24	−0.09	−0.24
a*	Fresh	0.54 **	0.52 **	0.47 *	0.57 ***	0.47 *
	Stored	0.38 *	0.37 *	0.30	0.38 *	0.30
b*	Fresh	−0.12	−0.17	−0.018	−0.13	0.018
	Stored	0.13	0.07	0.02	0.12	0.02
C*	Fresh	−0.10	−0.15	0.003	−0.115	0.003
	Stored	0.15	0.09	0.04	0.14	0.04

*** = $p < 0.0001$, ** = $p < 0.001$, * = $p < 0.05$.

However, lightness (L*) and yellowness (b*) were negatively correlated with all the determined pigments. Dietary supplementation of the tomato and the red pepper mixture (2%) increased ($p < 0.05$) the RYCF score and the red hue (a*), and decreased ($p < 0.05$) the lightness (L*) without affecting ($p > 0.05$) the saturation (C*). These results are in agreement with those reported by Akdemir et al. [43] who found that dietary supplementation of 0.5% or 1% of dried tomato increased egg yolk color from 11.25 (control) to 13.08 (0.5%) and 13.58 (1%). The dietary addition of 130 g of dried tomato peel/kg DM increased the egg yolk color index from 8.5 to 14.6 [88]. Habanabashaka et al. [89] reported that the supplementation of 6% of tomato waste meal increased egg yolk scores from 4.66 (control) to 9.15 (6%). Salajedheh et al. [101] found that dietary incorporation of 19% of dried tomato pomace had a significant effect on egg yolk color scores which increased from 7.25 to 9.38. Dietary addition of 50 and 100 g/kg of dried tomato powder increased egg yolk color from 6.7 (control) to 9.7 and 10.3 for respectively, 50 and 100 g/kg of dried tomato powder [102]. Salajedheh et al. [101], also reported that the dietary supplementation of 150 and 190 g/kg of dried tomato powder increased egg yolk color from 7.25 (control) to, respectively, 8.50 (150 g/kg) and 9.83 (190 g/kg). Studies on the effect of red pepper powder on the egg yolk color are lacking. However, Niu et al. [90] showed that the dietary addition of 0.8% of paprika increased egg yolk color from 1.7 to 9.9. Li et al. [42] also reported that dietary supplementation of 0.3 to 4.8 or 9.6 ppm and 0.8% of red pepper powder increased egg yolk color from 7.7 to 12.7.

Studies on the effect of linseeds on egg yolk color are lacking. However, Yassein et al. [83] showed a decrease in yolk color related to linseed supplementation at a level of 5%. Reports on L*a*b* color space in response to dietary supplementation of carotenoid are also lacking.

Concerning stored eggs, with the exception of saturation (C*), all other parameters were influenced ($p < 0.05$) by dietary treatment. Storage of eggs of hens fed with the control diet (C) did not affect ($p > 0.05$) the yolk score and color parameters determined by colorimetry. By contrast, the storage increased ($p < 0.05$) yolk lightness (L*) and decreased redness (a*) of eggs corresponding to linseeds treatment (L). However, stored eggs corresponding to the LTP- treatment were found to be less colorful (lower RYCF score) and lighter (higher L*) than fresh eggs. Studies on the effect of the storage on egg yolk color are lacking. However, Barbarosa et al. [91] reported that storage of ω-3 enriched eggs for 35 days with or without refrigeration decreased the yolk color. This decrease became significant from the 28th day of storage for eggs stored at room temperature (26.5°). For eggs stored at 7.9 °C, egg yolk color reduction was not significant during the 35 days.

The use of dried tomato and red pepper as natural or biological antioxidants has been a new solution to reduce the supplementation of synthetic pigments as feed additives in laying hens' diets. However, the stability of these antioxidants may be affected over a long period of storage. In fact, degradation reactions (chemical, enzymatic and physical) can cause undesirable changes in the appearance, color and texture as well as in the nutrient content of the laying hens' diets. These reactions can be responsible for pigment losses during storage. These losses must be considered when formulating feed in order to avoid complaints. Also, the quality of these supplements may be affected by several factors such as tomato and pepper variety, soil, cultural practices and climate.

4. Conclusions

The results of this study clearly show how dietary inclusion of 4.5% of linseed significantly increased egg yolk concentrations of antioxidants profile. This dietary supplementation did not increase yolk concentration of MDA before and after storage at 4 °C for one month. Enriching linseed-supplemented feed with 1% tomato and 1% sweet red pepper did not enhance egg physical characteristics, yolk color, antioxidants profile and its lipid oxidative stability.

Author Contributions: B.O., A.S., N.A., H.A., A.D., M.L., R.R. have conceived the work. B.O., A.S., N.A., H.A., A.D., M.L. wrote the manuscript., B.O., N.A., H.A., R.R. have carried out the experimental study and analyzed the data. All authors have made a substantial contribution to revising the work, and approved it for publication.

Funding: This research received no external funding.

Conflicts of Interest: The authors declare no conflict of interest.

References

1. Anton, M.; Nau, F.; Nys, Y. Bioactive egg components and their potential uses. *World's Poult. Sci. J.* **2006**, *62*, 429–438. [CrossRef]
2. Nau, F.; Yamakawa, Y.N.Y.; Réhault-Godbert, S. Nutritional value of the hen egg for humans. *Prod. Anim. Paris Inst. Natl. Rech. Agron.* **2010**, *23*, 225–236.
3. Ruxton, C. Recommendations for the use of eggs in the diet. *Nurs. Stand.* **2010**, *24*, 47–55. [CrossRef] [PubMed]
4. Zdrojewicz, Z.; Herman, M.; Starostecka, E. Hen's egg as a source of valuable biologically active substances. *Postępy Hig. Med. Doświadczalnej* **2016**, *70*, 751–759. [CrossRef] [PubMed]
5. Heflin, L.E.; Malheiros, R.; Anderson, K.E.; Johnson, L.K.; Raatz, S.K. Mineral content of eggs differs with hen strain, age, and rearing environment. *Poult. Sci.* **2018**, *97*, 1605–1613. [CrossRef] [PubMed]

6. Abeyrathne, E.D.N.S.; Lee, H.Y.; Ahn, D.U. Egg white proteins and their potential use in food processing or as nutraceutical and pharmaceutical agents—A review. *Poult. Sci.* **2013**, *92*, 3292–3299. [CrossRef] [PubMed]
7. Nimalaratne, C.; Schieber, A.; Wu, J. Effects of storage and cooking on the antioxidant capacity of laying hen eggs. *Food Chem.* **2016**, *194*, 111–116. [CrossRef] [PubMed]
8. Liu, H.; Zheng, F.; Cao, Q.; Ren, B.; Zhu, L.; Striker, G.; Vlassara, H. Amelioration of oxidant stress by the defensin lysozyme. *Am. J. Physiol. Metab.* **2006**, *290*, E824–E832. [CrossRef]
9. Ibrahim, H.R.; Hoq, M.I.; Aoki, T. Ovotransferrin possesses SOD-like superoxide anion scavenging activity that is promoted by copper and manganese binding. *Int. J. Biol. Macromol.* **2007**, *41*, 631–640. [CrossRef]
10. Nimalaratne, C.; Lopes-Lutz, D.; Schieber, A.; Wu, J. Free aromatic amino acids in egg yolk show antioxidant properties. *Food Chem.* **2011**, *129*, 155–161. [CrossRef]
11. Young, D.; Nau, F.; Pasco, M.; Mine, Y. Identification of hen egg yolk-derived phosvitin phosphopeptides and their effects on gene expression profiling against oxidative stress-induced Caco-2 cells. *J. Agric. Food Chem.* **2011**, *59*, 9207–9218. [CrossRef] [PubMed]
12. Lin, S.; Jin, Y.; Liu, M.; Yang, Y.; Zhang, M.; Guo, Y. Research on the preparation of antioxidant peptides derived from egg white with assisting of high-intensity pulsed electric field. *Food Chem.* **2013**, *139*, 300–306. [CrossRef] [PubMed]
13. Liu, J.; Jin, Y.; Lin, S.; Jones, G.S.; Chen, F. Purification and identification of novel antioxidant peptides from egg white protein and their antioxidant activities. *Food Chem.* **2015**, *175*, 258–266. [CrossRef] [PubMed]
14. Nimalaratne, C.; Bandara, N.; Wu, J. Purification and characterization of antioxidant peptides from enzymatically hydrolyzed chicken egg white. *Food Chem.* **2015**, *188*, 467–472. [CrossRef]
15. Lee, J.H.; Moon, S.H.; Kim, H.S.; Park, E.; Ahn, D.U.; Paik, H.-D.; Paik, H. Antioxidant and anticancer effects of functional peptides from ovotransferrin hydrolysates. *J. Sci. Food Agric.* **2017**, *97*, 4857–4864. [CrossRef]
16. Yoo, H.; Bamdad, F.; Gujral, N.; Suh, J.-W.; Sunwoo, H. High Hydrostatic Pressure-Assisted Enzymatic Treatment Improves Antioxidant and Anti-inflammatory Properties of Phosvitin. *Curr. Pharm. Biotechnol.* **2017**, *18*, 158–167. [CrossRef]
17. Abeyrathne, E.D.N.S.; Huang, X.; Ahn, D.U. Antioxidant, angiotensin-converting enzyme inhibitory activity and other functional properties of egg white proteins and their derived peptides—A review. *Poult. Sci.* **2018**, *97*, 1462–1468. [CrossRef]
18. Santini, A.; Novellino, E.; Armini, V.; Ritieni, A. State of the art of Ready-to-Use Therapeutic Food: A tool for nutraceuticals addition to foodstuff. *Food Chem.* **2013**, *140*, 843–849. [CrossRef]
19. Santini, A.; Novellino, E. To Nutraceuticals and Back: Rethinking a Concept. *Foods* **2017**, *6*, 74. [CrossRef]
20. Santini, A.; Tenore, G.C.; Novellino, E. Nutraceuticals: A paradigm of proactive medicine. *Eur. J. Pharm. Sci.* **2017**, *96*, 53–61. [CrossRef]
21. Santini, A.; Novellino, E. Nutraceuticals—Shedding light on the grey area between pharmaceuticals and food. *Expert Rev. Clin. Pharmacol.* **2018**, *11*, 545–547. [CrossRef]
22. Santini, A.; Cammarata, S.M.; Capone, G.; Ianaro, A.; Tenore, G.C.; Pani, L.; Novellino, E. Nutraceuticals: Opening the debate for a regulatory framework. *Br. J. Clin. Pharmacol.* **2018**, *84*, 659–672. [CrossRef]
23. Daliu, P.; Santini, A.; Novellino, E. From pharmaceuticals to nutraceuticals: Bridging disease prevention and management. *Expert Rev. Clin. Pharmacol.* **2018**, *12*, 1–7. [CrossRef]
24. Daliu, P.; Santini, A.; Novellino, E. A decade of nutraceutical patents: Where are we now in 2018? *Expert Opin. Ther. Pat.* **2018**, *28*, 875–882. [CrossRef]
25. Durazzo, A.; D'Addezio, L.; Camilli, E.; Piccinelli, R.; Turrini, A.; Marletta, L.; Marconi, S.; Lucarini, M.; Lisciani, S.; Gabrielli, P.; et al. From Plant Compounds to Botanicals and Back: A Current Snapshot. *Molecules* **2018**, *23*, 1844. [CrossRef]
26. Durazzo, A. Study Approach of Antioxidant Properties in Foods: Update and Considerations. *Foods* **2017**, *6*, 17. [CrossRef]
27. Durazzo, A.; Lucarini, M. A Current shot and re-thinking of antioxidant research strategy. *Braz. J. Anal. Chem.* **2018**, *5*, 9–11. [CrossRef]
28. Ngo, D.-H.; Wijesekara, I.; Vo, T.-S.; Van Ta, Q.; Kim, S.-K. Marine food-derived functional ingredients as potential antioxidants in the food industry: An overview. *Food Res. Int.* **2011**, *44*, 523–529. [CrossRef]
29. Walker, L.A.; Wang, T.; Xin, H.; Dolde, D. Supplementation of Laying-Hen Feed with Palm Tocos and Algae Astaxanthin for Egg Yolk Nutrient Enrichment. *J. Agric. Food Chem.* **2012**, *60*, 1989–1999. [CrossRef]

30. Iskender, H.; Yenice, G.; Dokumacioglu, E.; Kaynar, O.; Hayirli, A.; Kaya, A. Comparison of the effects of dietary supplementation of flavonoids on laying hen performance, egg quality and egg nutrient profile. *Br. Poult. Sci.* **2017**, *58*, 550–556. [CrossRef]
31. Damaziak, K.; Marzec, A.; Riedel, J.; Szeliga, J.; Koczywąs, E.; Cisneros, F.; Michalczuk, M.; Łukasiewicz, M.; Gozdowski, D.; Siennicka, A.; et al. Effect of dietary canthaxanthin and iodine on the production performance and egg quality of laying hens. *Poult. Sci.* **2018**, *97*, 4008–4019. [CrossRef]
32. Surai, P.F.; Kochish, I.I. Nutritional modulation of the antioxidant capacities in poultry: The case of selenium. *Poult. Sci.* **2018**. [CrossRef]
33. Campos, J.; Severino, P.; Ferreira, C.; Zielinska, A.; Santini, A.; Souto, S.; Souto, E.B. Linseed essential oil-Source of Lipids as Active Ingredients for Pharmaceuticals and Nutraceuticals. *Curr. Med. Chem.* **2018**. [CrossRef]
34. Naviglio, D.; Romano, R.; Pizzolongo, F.; Santini, A.; De Vito, A.; Schiavo, L.; Nota, G.; Musso, S.S. Rapid determination of esterified glycerol and glycerides in triglyceride fats and oils by means of periodate method after transesterification. *Food Chem.* **2007**, *102*, 399–405. [CrossRef]
35. Naviglio, D.; Pizzolongo, F.; Ferrara, L.; Aragón, A.; Santini, A. Extraction of pure lycopene from industrial tomato by-products in water using a new high-pressure process. *J. Sci. Food Agric.* **2008**, *88*, 2414–2420. [CrossRef]
36. Naviglio, D.; Caruso, T.; Iannece, P.; Aragòn, A.; Santini, A. Characterization of high purity lycopene from tomato wastes using a new pressurized extraction approach. *J. Agric. Food Chem.* **2008**, *56*, 6227–6231. [CrossRef]
37. Romano, R.; Masucci, F.; Giordano, A.; Musso, S.S.; Naviglio, D.; Santini, A. Effect of tomato by-products in the diet of Comisana sheep on composition and conjugated linoleic acid content of milk fat. *Int. Dairy J.* **2010**, *20*, 858–862. [CrossRef]
38. Santini, A.; Graziani, G.; Ritieni, A. Nutraceuticals Recovery from Tomato Processing Waste and By-Products: Lycopene. In *Tomatoes: Cultivation, Varieties and Nutrition*; Chapter 17; (NARO Institute of Vegetables and Tea Science, National Agriculture and Food Research Organization, Ibaraki, Japan) ; Series: Food Science and Technology; Higashide, T., Ed.; Nova Science Publishers Inc.: Hauppauge, NY, USA, 2013; pp. 313–322, ISBN 978-1-62417-915-0.
39. Gervasi, T.; Pellizzeri, V.; Benameur, Q.; Gervasi, C.; Santini, A.; Cicero, N.; Dugo, G. Valorization of raw materials from agricultural industry for astaxanthin and beta-carotene production by Xanthophyllomyces dendrorhous. *Nat. Prod. Res.* **2017**, *32*, 1554–1561. [CrossRef]
40. Lucarini, M.; Durazzo, A.; Romani, A.; Campo, M.; Lombardi-Boccia, G.; Cecchini, F. Bio-Based Compounds from Grape Seeds: A Biorefinery Approach. *Molecules* **2018**, *23*, 1888. [CrossRef]
41. Goodwin, T.W. *The Biochemistry of Carotenoids: Volume II, Animals*, 2nd ed.; Chapman and Hall: New York, NY, USA, 1984.
42. Li, H.; Jin, L.; Wu, F.; Thacker, P.H.; Li, X.; Wang, X.; Liu, S.I.; Li, S.H.; Xu, Y. Effect of Red Pepper (Capsicum frutescens) Powder or Red Pepper Pigment on the Performance and Egg Yolk Color of Laying Hens Asian-Aust. *J. Anim. Sci.* **2012**, *25*, 1605–1610. [CrossRef]
43. Akdemir, F.; Orhan, C.; Sahin, N.; Sahin, K.; Hayirli, A. Tomato powder in laying hen diets: Effects on concentrations of yolk carotenoids and lipid peroxidation. *Br. Poult. Sci.* **2012**, *53*, 675–680. [CrossRef]
44. D'Evoli, L.; Lombardi-Boccia, G.; Lucarini, M. Influence of Heat Treatments on Carotenoid Content of Cherry Tomatoes. *Foods* **2013**, *2*, 352–363. [CrossRef]
45. Manzo, N.; Santini, A.; Pizzolongo, F.; Aiello, A.; Romano, R. Degradation kinetic (D100) of lycopene during the thermal treatment of concentrated tomato paste. *Nat. Prod. Res.* **2018**, *21*, 1–7. [CrossRef]
46. Hammershøj, M.; Kidmose, U.; Steenfeldt, S. Deposition of carotenoids in egg yolk by short-term supplement of coloured carrot (Daucus carota) varieties as forage material for egg-laying hens. *J. Sci. Food Agric.* **2010**, *90*, 1163–1171. [CrossRef]
47. Lucarini, M.; Lanzi, S.; D'Evoli, L.; Aguzzi, A.; Lombardi-Boccia, G. Intake of vitamin A and carotenoids from the Italian population-results of an Italian total diet study. *Int. J. Vitam. Nutr. Res.* **2006**, *76*, 103–109. [CrossRef]
48. Adams, C.A. Pigmenters & poultry feeds. *Feed Compd.* **1985**, *5*, 12–14.

49. Englmaierová, M.; Skřivan, M.; Bubancová, I. A comparison of lutein, spray-dried Chlorella, and synthetic carotenoids effects on yolk colour, oxidative stability, and reproductive performance of laying hens. *Czech J. Anim. Sci.* **2013**, *58*, 412–419. [CrossRef]
50. Leesson, S.; Caston, L. Enrichment of eggs with lutein. *Poult. Sci.* **2004**, *83*, 1709–1712. [CrossRef]
51. Fredriksson, S.; Elwinger, K.; Pickova, J. Fatty acid and carotenoid composition of egg yolk as an effect of microalgae addition to feed formula for laying hens. *Food Chem.* **2006**, *99*, 530–537. [CrossRef]
52. Karadas, F.; Grammenidis, E.; Surai, P.F.; Acamovic, T.; Sparks, N. Effects of carotenoids from lucerne, marigold and tomato on egg yolk pigmentation and carotenoid composition. *Br. Poult. Sci.* **2006**, *47*, 561–566. [CrossRef]
53. Surai, P.F.; Kochish, I.I.; Fisinin, V.I.; Kidd, M.T. Antioxidant Defence Systems and Oxidative Stress in Poultry Biology: An Update. *Antioxidants* **2019**, *8*, 235. [CrossRef]
54. Willcox, J.K.; Ash, S.L.; Catignani, G.L. Antioxidants and Prevention of Chronic Disease. *Crit. Rev. Food Sci. Nutr.* **2004**, *44*, 275–295. [CrossRef]
55. Dahan, K.; Fennal, M.; Kumar, N.B. Lycopene in the prevention of prostate cancer. *J. Soc. Integr. Oncol.* **2008**, *6*, 29–36.
56. Bohn, T. Carotenoids and Markers of Oxidative Stress in Human Observational Studies and Intervention Trials: Implications for Chronic Diseases. *Antioxidants* **2019**, *8*, 179. [CrossRef]
57. Pham-Huy, L.A.; He, H.; Pham-Huy, C. Free Radicals, Antioxidants in Disease and Health. *Int. J. Biomed. Sci.* **2008**, *4*, 89–96.
58. Andrew, R.; Izzo, A.A. Principles of pharmacological research of nutraceuticals. *Br. J. Pharmacol.* **2017**, *174*, 1177–1194. [CrossRef]
59. Jain, A.K.; Mehra, N.K.; Swarnakar, N.K. Role of Antioxidants for the Treatment of Cardiovascular Diseases: Challenges and Opportunities. *Curr. Pharm. Des.* **2015**, *21*, 4441–4455. [CrossRef]
60. Athreya, K.; Xavier, M.F. Antioxidants in the Treatment of Cancer. *Nutr. Cancer* **2017**, *69*, 1099–1104. [CrossRef]
61. Costantini, D. Understanding diversity in oxidative status and oxidative stress: The opportunities and challenges ahead. *J. Exp. Biol.* **2019**, *222*, jeb194688. [CrossRef]
62. Shafi, S.; Ansari, H.R.; Bahitham, W.; Aouabdi, S. The Impact of Natural Antioxidants on the Regenerative Potential of Vascular Cells. *Front. Cardiovasc. Med.* **2019**, *6*, 28. [CrossRef]
63. Durazzo, A.; Lucarini, M.; Souto, E.B.; Cicala, C.; Caiazzo, E.; Izzo, A.A.; Novellino, E.; Santini, A. Polyphenols: A concise overview on the chemistry, occurrence and human health. *Phyt. Res.* **2019**. [CrossRef]
64. Miller, E.D.; Dziedzic, A.; Saluk-Bijak, J.; Bijak, M. A Review of Various Antioxidant Compounds and their Potential Utility as Complementary Therapy in Multiple Sclerosis. *Nutrients* **2019**, *11*, 1528. [CrossRef]
65. Yeung, A.W.K.; Tzvetkov, N.T.; El-Tawil, O.S.; Bungău, S.G.; Abdel-Daim, M.M.; Atanasov, A.G. Antioxidants: Scientific Literature Landscape Analysis. *Oxidative Med. Cell. Longev.* **2019**, *2019*, 8278454. [CrossRef]
66. Hamilton, P.B.; Tirado, J.F.; Garcia-Hernandz, F. Deposition in egg yolks of the carotenoids from saponified and unsaponified oleoresin of red pepper (Capsicum annuum). *Poult. Sci.* **1999**, *69*, 462–470. [CrossRef]
67. Gonzalez, M.; Castaño, E.; Avila, E.; De Mejia, E.G. Effect of capsaicin from red pepper (Capsicum sp) on the deposition of carotenoids in egg yolk. *J. Sci. Food Agric.* **1999**, *79*, 1904–1908. [CrossRef]
68. Amaya, E.; Becquet, P.; Carné, S.; Peris, S.; Miralles, P. *Carotenoids in Animal Nutrition*; Fefana Publications: Bruxelles, Belgium, 2014; ISBN 978-2-9601289-4-9.
69. Sim, J.S.; Sunwoo, H.H. Designer eggs: Nutritional and functional significance. In *Eggs and Health Nutrition*; Watson, R.R., Ed.; John Wiley & Sons: Hoboken, NJ, USA, 2002.
70. Shahryar, H.A.; Salamatdoust, R.; Chekani-Azar, S.; Ahadi, F.; Vahdatpour, T. Lipid oxidation in fresh and stored eggs enriched with dietary ω3 and ω6 polyunsaturated fatty acids and vitamin E and A dosages. *Afr. J. Biotechnol.* **2010**, *9*, 1827–1832.
71. Wang, Q.; Jin, G.; Wang, N.; Guo, X.; Jin, Y.; Ma, M. Lipolysis and oxidation of lipids during egg storage at different temperatures. *Czech J. Food Sci.* **2017**, *35*, 229–235.
72. Omri, B.; Chalghoumi, R.; Abdouli, H. Study of the Effects of Dietary Supplementation of Linseed, Fenugreek Seeds and Tomato-Pepper Mix on Laying Hen's Performances, Egg Yolk Lipids and Antioxidants Profiles and Lipid Oxidation Status. *J. Anim. Sci. Livest. Prod.* **2017**, *1*, 2. [CrossRef]
73. Amaya, D.B. *Harvestplus Handbook for Carotenoids Analysis*; International Food Policy Research Institute (IFPRI) and International Center for Tropical Agriculture (CIAT): Washington, DC, USA, 2004.

74. Makkar, H.P.S. Antinutritional factors in foods for livestock. *BSAP Occas. Publ.* **1993**, *16*, 69–85. [CrossRef]
75. Patel, A.; Patel, A.; Patel, N.M. Estimation of flavonoid, polyphenolic content and In vitro antioxidant capacity of leaves of Tephrosiapurpurea Linn. (Leguminosae). *Int. J. Pharm. Sci. Res.* **2010**, *1*, 66–77.
76. Gutteridge, J.M. Biological origin of free radicals, and mechanisms of antioxidant protection. *Chem. Interact.* **1994**, *91*, 133–140. [CrossRef]
77. Durazzo, A. Extractable and Non-extractable Polyphenols: An Overview. In *Non-extractable Polyphenols and Carotenoids: Importance in Human Nutrition and Health*; Saura-Calixto, F., Pérez-Jiménez, J., Eds.; Food Chemistry, Function and Analysis No. 5; Royal Society of Chemistry: London, UK, 2018; p. 3761.
78. Prieto, P.; Pineda, M.; Aguilar, M. Spectrophotometric Quantitation of Antioxidant Capacity through the Formation of a Phosphomolybdenum Complex: Specific Application to the Determination of Vitamin E. *Anal. Biochem.* **1999**, *269*, 337–341. [CrossRef]
79. Benzie, I.F.F.; Szeto, Y.T. Total antioxidant capacity of teas by the ferric reducing/antioxidant power (FRAP) assay. *J. Agric. Food Chem.* **1999**, *47*, 633–636. [CrossRef]
80. Draper, H.H.; Hadeley, M. Malondialdehyde determination as Index of lipid peroxidation. *Methods Enzym.* **1990**, *186*, 421–431.
81. SAS: Statistical Analysis System. *User's Guide Version*; SAS Institute: Raleigh, NC, USA, 1989.
82. Cox, C. Delta Method. In *Encyclopedia of Biostatistics*; Armitage, P., Colton, T., Eds.; John Wiley & Sons: New York, NY, USA, 1998; pp. 1125–1127.
83. Yassein, S.A.; El-Mallah, G.M.; Sawsan, M.A.; El-Ghamry, A.A.; Abdel-Fattah, M.M.; El-Harriry, D.M. Response of laying hens to dietary flaxseed levels on performance, egg quality criteria, fatty acid composition of egg and some blood parameters. *Int. J. Res. Stud. Biosci.* **2015**, *3*, 27–34.
84. Ahmad, S.; Ahsan-Ul-Haq, Y.; Kamran, M.; Ata-Ur-Rehman, Z.; Sahail, M.U.; Shahid-Ur-Rahman. Effect of feeding whole linseed as a source of polyunsaturated fatty acids on performance and egg characteristics of laying hens kept at high ambient temperature. *Braz. J. Poult. Sci.* **2010**, *15*, 21–26. [CrossRef]
85. Niemiec, J.; Stępińska, M.; Świerczewska, E.; Riedel, J.; Boruta, A. The effect of storage on egg quality and fatty acid content in PUFA-enriched eggs. *J. Anim. Feed. Sci.* **2001**, *10*, 267–272. [CrossRef]
86. Nimalaratne, C.; Wu, J. Hen Egg as an Antioxidant Food Commodity: A Review. *Nutrients* **2015**, *7*, 8274–8293. [CrossRef]
87. Kotrbáček, V.; Skřivan, M.; Kopecký, J.; Pěnkava, O.; Hudečková, P.; Uhríková, L.; Doubek, J. Retention of carotenoids in egg yolks of laying hens supplemented with heterotrophic Chlorella. *Czech J. Anim. Sci.* **2013**, *58*, 193–200. [CrossRef]
88. Amar, B.K.; Larid, R.; Zidaini, S. Enriching Egg Yolk with Carotenoids & Phenols. *Int. J. Agric. Biol. Sci. Eng.* **2013**, *7*, 489–493.
89. Habanabashaka, M.; Sengabo, M.; Oladunjoye, I.O. Effect of Tomato Waste Meal on Lay Performance, Egg Quality, Lipid Profile and Carotene Content of Eggs in Laying Hens. *Iran. J. Appl. Anim. Sci.* **2014**, *4*, 555–559.
90. Niu, Z.; Gao, Y.; Liu, F.; Fu, J. Influence of Paprika Extract Supplement on Egg Quality of Laying Hens Fed Wheat-Based Diet. *Int. J. Poult. Sci.* **2008**, *7*, 887–889.
91. Barbosa, V.C.; Gaspar, A.; Calixto, L.F.L.; Agostinho, T.S.P. Stability of the pigmentation of egg yolks enriched with omega-3 and carophyll stored at room temperature and under refrigeration. *Rev. Bras. Zootec.* **2011**, *40*, 1540–1544. [CrossRef]
92. Gawecki, K.; Awecki, K.; Potkanmski, A.; Lipinska, H. Effect of carophyll yellow and carophyll red added to comercial feeds for laying hens on yolk colour and its stability during short-term refrigeration. *Rocz. Akad. Rol. W Pozn.* **1977**, *94*, 85–93.
93. Venglovská, K.; Grešáková, Ľ.; Placha, I.; Ryzner, M.; Cobanova, K. Effects of feed supplementation with manganese from its different sources on performance and egg parameters of laying hens. *Czech J. Anim. Sci.* **2014**, *59*, 147–155. [CrossRef]
94. Hayat, Z.; Gherian, G.; Pasha, T.N.; Khatak, F.M.; Jabbar, M.A. Effect of feeding flax and two types of antioxidants on egg production egg quality and lipid composition of eggs. *J. Appl. Poult. Res.* **2010**, *18*, 541–551. [CrossRef]
95. Boruta, A.; Niemiec, J. The effect of diet composition and length of storing eggs on changes in the fatty acid profile of egg yolk. *J. Anim. Feed. Sci.* **2005**, *14*, 427–430. [CrossRef]
96. Sahin, N.; Akdemir, F.; Orhan, C.; Kucuk, O.; Hayirli, A.; Sahin, K. Lycopene-enriched quail egg as functional food for humans. *Food Res. Int.* **2004**, *41*, 295–300. [CrossRef]

97. Pereira, G.V.N. Inheritance of Acyl-Sugar Contents in Tomato Genotypes and Its Relationship to Foliar Trichomes and Repellence to Spider Mites Tetrancychus Evani. Ph.D. Thesis, Université de Lovaras, Minas Gerais, Brasil, 2005.
98. Abdouli, H.; Belhouane, S.; Hcini, E. Effect of fenugreek seeds on hens' egg yolk color and sensory quality. *J. New Sci.* **2014**, *5*, 20–24.
99. Lokaewmanee, K.; Komori, T.; Yamauchi, K.-E.; Saito, K. Effects on egg yolk colour of paprika or paprika combined with marigold flower extract. *Ital. J. Anim. Sci.* **2010**, *9*, 67. [CrossRef]
100. Dvorak, P.; Dolezalova, J.; Suchy, P. Photocolorimetric determination of yolk colour in relation to selected quality parameters of eggs. *J. Sci. Food Agric.* **2009**, *89*, 1886–1889. [CrossRef]
101. Salajedheh, M.H.; Ghazi, S.; Mahdavi, R.; Mozafari, O. Effects of different levels of dried tomato pomace on performance, egg quality and serum metabolites of laying hens. *Afr. J. Biotechnol.* **2012**, *11*, 15373–15379.
102. Mansoori, B.; Modirsanei, M.; Kiaei, M.M. Influence of dried tomato pomace as an alternative to wheat bran in maize or wheat based diets, on the performance of laying hens and traits of produced eggs. *Iran. J. Veter. Res.* **2008**, *9*, 341–346.

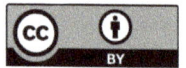

© 2019 by the authors. Licensee MDPI, Basel, Switzerland. This article is an open access article distributed under the terms and conditions of the Creative Commons Attribution (CC BY) license (http://creativecommons.org/licenses/by/4.0/).

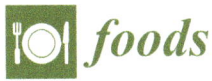

Article

Effect of a Combination of Fenugreek Seeds, Linseeds, Garlic and Copper Sulfate on Laying Hens Performances, Egg Physical and Chemical Qualities

Besma Omri [1,2], Ben Larbi Manel [3,*], Zemzmi Jihed [1], Alessandra Durazzo [4], Massimo Lucarini [4], Raffaele Romano [5], Antonello Santini [6,*] and Hédi Abdouli [1]

[1] Laboratory of improvement and integrated development of animal productivity and food resources, Department of animal production, Higher School of Agriculture of Mateur, University of Carthage, 1054 Carthage, Tunisia
[2] National Agronomy Institute-Tunis, University of Carthage, 1054 Carthage, Tunisia
[3] Research Unit of biodiversity and resource development in mountain areas of Tunisia (UR17AGR14), Higher School of Agriculture of Mateur, University of Carthage, 1054 Carthage, Tunisia
[4] CREA—Research Centre for Food and Nutrition, Via Ardeatina 546, 00178 Rome, Italy
[5] Department of Agriculture, University of Napoli Federico II, Via Università 100, 80055 Portici (NA), Italy
[6] Department of Pharmacy, University of Napoli Federico II, Via D. Montesano 49, 80131 Napoli, Italy
* Correspondence: arbi_mana@yahoo.fr (B.L.M.); asantini@unina.it (A.S.)

Received: 10 July 2019; Accepted: 29 July 2019; Published: 2 August 2019

Abstract: Several investigations have suggested that fenugreek seeds may have a hypocholesterolemic activity, and thus be efficient in the treatment of egg yolk cholesterol. The objective of the current study was to evaluate the effect of dietary incorporation of 3% of fenugreek seed combined with 3% of linseed, 1% of garlic paste, and 0.078% of copper sulfate on laying performance, egg quality and lipids profile. Forty four, 41 weeks old, Novogen White laying hens received for 42 days 100 g/d of basal diet (control) or experimental diet (CFSGLSCS). With the exception of egg weight, which showed a significant increase for hens fed on CFSGLSCS with 57.99 g compared to 56.34 g for the control group, egg production (90.84% for control compared to 87.89% for experimental diet), egg mass (50.95 g/d for control compared to 50.87 g/d for CFSGLSCS), feed efficiency (1.94 for control compared to 1.98 for CFSGLSCS) were not affected by dietary treatments. The addition of CFSGLSCS reduced ($p < 0.05$) egg yolk cholesterol by 5.4% and blood cholesterol from 158.42 mg/dL to 122.82 mg/dL for control and CFSGLSCS, respectively. The dietary addition of CFSGLSCS increased ($p < 0.05$) total lipids from 4.5 g/egg to 5.23 g/egg and didn't affect ($p > 0.05$) yolk triglycerides.

Keywords: fenugreek seed; garlic; linseed; copper sulfate; yolk; cholesterol

1. Introduction

In the perspective of functional foods and nutraceuticals [1–5], many researchers and egg producers are actually working together to produce a designer or multi-enriched egg. This egg is a source of high quality proteins, vitamins, and lipids, such as phospholipids and polyunsaturated fatty acids (PUFA) [6,7]. In fact, compared to the multi-enriched or designer egg, the standard egg contains from 183 mg/egg [8] to 386 mg/egg [9,10] of cholesterol and around 150 mg/egg of saturated fatty acids [11–13]. In this field, many studies have been made to decrease egg yolk cholesterol concentration [9,10,14] using natural plant products like garlic [15], fenugreek seeds [9,10,16] and copper [17,18]. Egg yolk polyunsaturated fatty acids enhancement using linseeds [19–21]. The effect of dietary incorporation of fenugreek seeds on egg cholesterol content has been inconsistent and the reduction was low not exceeding 1 mg/g egg yolk [16,20]. Dietary garlic paste (38 g/kg) reduced serum cholesterol by 23% in 12 weeks-old Leghorn pullets, when diets were fed for four weeks [22]. Egg yolk cholesterol was reduced by feeding of 10 or 30 g/kg garlic powder to laying hens for three weeks [23]. Concerning linseed, it is a very rich source of n-3 polyunsaturated fatty acids (PUFA) among many vegetable sources [24]. It is well documented that n-3 PUFA bring potential benefits for the human health. That is why, many researchers have focused on linseeds inclusion in the diets of layers to enhance the egg n-3 PUFA content [25–28]. In view of the above, the objective of the present study was to evaluate the effect of the dietary incorporation of fenugreek seeds combined with linseeds, garlic paste, and of copper sulfate on laying performance, egg quality, and lipids profile.

2. Materials and Methods

2.1. Dish Preparation

Three kg of fresh fenugreek seeds were offered from the Higher School of Agriculture of Mateur, north of Tunisia and carefully cleaned from foreign matter. Three kg of linseed were purchased from a regional producer located at Mateur and cleaned from foreign matter. One kg of garlic was pelt, cut in a little fragment and mixed with distilled water. The composition of the basal diet was: 95 kg of basal diet were mixed with 5 kg of vegetable oil. The experimental diet contained: 2.9 kg of fenugreek seed, 2.9 kg of linseed, 76 g of $CuSO_4$ and 970 g of garlic mixed with 92 kg of basal diet (CFSGLSCS).

2.2. Ethical Considerations

The experimental protocol was approved by the Official Animal Care and Use Committee of the Higher School of Agriculture of Mateur (protocol N° 05/15) before the initiation of research and followed the Tunisian guidelines approved by the committee on care, handling, and sampling of the animals.

2.3. Experimental Design

Forty-four Novogen White laying hens aged 41 weeks were divided randomly into two treatment groups with 22 birds each. They were allocated each group to one of two dietary treatments: Basal diet and experimental diet. Each hen was daily fed 100 g of diet. The composition of the diets is shown in Table 1. Authors model some ingredients on other studies as follows:

Whole Fenugreek seeds at 2.9 kg equivalent to 3%. Fenugreek seed has been used in many previous researches to reduce egg cholesterol content [10,12,29,30]. However, it contains many bioactive compounds including powerful antioxidants that could prevent lipids oxidation, particularly in eggs enriched with polyunsaturated fatty acids. In this study, in order to reevaluate its effect on egg cholesterol content and fenugreek seed was included at 3% (2.9 kg) into the linseed supplemented diet.

Garlic at 970 g equivalent to 1%. Many animal studies have suggested that garlic supplemented diets may inhibit the synthesis of cholesterol and fatty acids in the liver [31–33]. For example, Motamedi et al. [32] reported that dietary supplementation of 1% of garlic powder and of 1% of fenugreek powder reduced laying hens' serum cholesterol from 242.00 mg/dL to 175 mg/dL.

CuSO4 at 76 g equivalent to 0.078%. Copper supplementation to laying hen diets at pharmacological concentrations (>250 mg/kg) has been demonstrated to cause a reduction in egg yolk cholesterol content [34,35].

Linseeds at 2.9 kg equivalent to 3% [36,37]. Linseed is often used in the production of ω3-enriched eggs and some reports indicated that there was an increase in egg yolk unsaturated fatty acids concentrations when hens were fed yellow corn-soybean meal diets containing linseed at an incorporation rate of 5% [38]. It was found that the long-term use of linseed at an incorporation level of 10% increased the incidence of liver hemorrhages [21] presumably due to the oxidative rancidity of the accumulated long chain unsaturated fatty acids.

Table 1. Ingredients and calculated offered components of experimental diets.

Ingredients	Diets	
	Control (C)	Experimental (CGFSLSSC)
Yellow corn	61	59.92
Soybean meal	22	21
Calcium carbonate	8	8
Mineral and vitamin mixture [§]	4	4
Basal Diet, kg	95	92.92
Whole fenugreek seeds(WFS), kg	0	2.9
Garlic paste, g	0	970
Whole Linseeds (WLS), kg	0	2.9
CuSO4, g	0	76
Vegetable Oil, kg	5	0
Total	100	100
Chemical Composition, % Dry Matter		
Dry Matter	91.56	90.35
Ash	21.76	23.62
Crude Protein	16.54	17.27
Ether Extract	3.35	7.91
NDF	10.15	13.00
Hemi-cellulose	6.98	8.92
[¥] Metabolizable Energy, kcal/kg DM	2741.1	2962.7

Note: [§] Control provided following nutrients per 100 g: Ca, 4.3 g; P, 0.6 g; Na, 0.14 g; Cl, 0.23 g; Fe, 4 mg; Zn, 40 mg; Mn, 7 mg; Cu, 0.3 mg; I, 0.08 mg; Se, 0.01 mg; Co, 0.02; methionine,0.39 g; methionine + cysteine, 0.69 g; lysine, 0.89 g; Retinol, 800 IU; Cholecalciferol, 220 IU; α-tocopherol, 1.1 IU; Thiamin, 0.33 IU; Nicotinic acid, 909 IU. NDF: Neutral detergent fiber. [¥] Metabolizable Energy = 2707.71 + 58.63*EE 16.06*NDF [39].

Hens were housed in individual cages with individual feed-trough and common water-trough in a room with an ambient temperature of about 20 °C and a photoperiod of 16 h light: 8 h darkness cycle. Water was provided ad libitum intake throughout the trial period which lasted 42 days.

2.4. Data Collection

All birds were weighed individually at the beginning and the end of the experiment trial to determine the hens live weight changes. The feed was offered daily at 7:30 a.m. and refusal was measured on days 7, 14, 21, 28, 35 and 42 of the experiment assay. Egg production and weight were recorded daily. Daily feed consumption, hen-day laying rate (number of laid eggs ×100/number of feeding days) and feed efficiency (feed consumption/(number of eggs × egg weight)) were calculated per period (P1–P6) corresponding to the days 1–7, 8–14, 15–21, 22–28, 29–35 and 36–42. Two yolks of each egg laid during the 33rd and 34th days of the experiment assay were mixed (11 yolks/lots) and were used for the analysis of egg qualities (egg weight, shell weight, egg shell thickness, yolk weight and yolk cholesterol, triglycerides and total lipids).

Blood samples of nine hens/lot were collected at the end of the experiment (the 42nd day) from the brachial wing vein using sterilized syringes and needles and used for serum cholesterol determination after centrifugation at 3000 rpm for 15 min.

2.5. Chemical Analysis

The dry matter of the diets (DM) was determined at 105 °C for 24 h while all other analyses were done on samples dried at 65 °C and ground in a mill to pass through a 0.5 mm screen. Ash content was determined by igniting the ground sample at 550 °C in a muffle furnace for 12 h. The Association of Official Analytical Chemists method [40] was used for crude proteins (CP) determination. Neutral detergent fiber (NDF) was determined as described by Van Soest et al. [41], but sodium sulphite and alpha amylase were omitted from the NDF procedure.

An enzymatic method (cholesterol enzymatic colorimetric test, CHOD-PAP, triglycerides enzymatic colorimetric GPO-PAP Biomaghreb, Ariana, Tunisia) were used for cholesterol in the serum and in egg yolk solubilized in 2% (w/v) NaCl solution [42].

Total lipids of the homogenized egg yolk was determined by extraction with isopropanol: hexane (30:70) (v/v) and then gravimetrically estimated.

2.6. Statistical Analysis

Collected data were subjected to the analysis of variance using the General Linear Model (GLM) procedure of the Statistical Analysis System SAS [43]. Daily feed consumption, hen-daily laying rate, egg weight and mass and feed efficiency data were first tested for the diet, period and diet x period effects. Period and treatment x period effects were found to be not significant ($\alpha = 0.05$) and, therefore, only treatment (diets) effect was retained. Multiple comparison tests were subjected to the Duncan test.

3. Results and Discussion

3.1. Laying Performance

Body weight changes, daily refusal, hen-day laying rate, egg mass and feed efficiency during the experimental assay are shown in Table 2.

Table 2. Effects of various diets on the laying hen performances.

Parameters	Diets		Statistics	
	Control (C)	CFSGLSCS	SEM	p-Value
Daily refusal (g DM/d)	2.46 [a] ± 3.97	0.62 [b] ± 1.33	0.26	<0.0001
Feed consumption (g DM/d)	97.54 [b] ± 3.97	99.37 [a] ± 1.34	0.25	<0.0001
Hen-day laying rate (%)	90.84 [a] ± 11.89	87.89 [b] ± 10.95	0.99	<0.036
Body weight change (g)	−71.41 ± 109.23	−120.86 ± 112.23	23.61	0.146
Egg mass (g/hen/d)	50.95 ± 3.61	50.87 ± 6.19	0.53	0.92
Feed efficiency	1.94 ± 0.27	1.98 ± 0.3	0.02	0.19

Note: C = control; CFSGLSCS = diet contained: 2.9 kg of fenugreek seed, 2.9 kg of linseed, 76 g of $CuSO_4$ and 970 g of garlic mixed with 92 kg of basal diet; SEM = Standard Error of the mean; [a,b]: Mean in the same row having different superscripts are significantly different ($p < 0.05$).

Although the feed was restricted to 100 g/hen/day, daily refusal and feed consumption, were both affected by dietary treatment ($p < 0.05$). Daily refusal was reduced ($p < 0.05$) for the experimental group from 0.62 g DM/day to 2.46 g DM/day for the control group. Consequently, daily consumption of the control group was the lowest with a mean value of 97.54 g DM/d compared to 99.37 g DM/d for the CFSGLSCS group. To begin with the dietary effect of the whole fenugreek seed, Mustafa [44] reported that the dietary addition of the fenugreek seed at a level of 0.05%, 0.1% and 0.15% didn't affect feed consumption of Hy-Line White layers during a 40–59 week of age. A similar finding to the previous was reported by Abdouli et al. [9] who showed that the ground fenugreek at two to six levels didn't affect feed intake of 69 wk-old Lohman White laying hens. A study conducted by Nasra et al. [20] reported that the supplementation of 0.5% ground fenugreek on local Mandarah strain hens diets during their 16–28 weeks of age decreased feed consumption after eight weeks. By contrast, feed consumption increased after 12 weeks of treatment. Our data are in accordance with those reported by Ademola et al. [45] who found that garlic oil and cholestyramine increased feed intake of Black Harco laying hens. By contrast, Olobatoke and Mulugeta [46] showed that garlic powder at 3% or 4% reduced feed consumption of 30 weeks old Dekalb White laying birds. Sibel et al. [47] showed that feed consumption was not affected by the dietary supplementation of garlic powder during a 12-week period. Similar results have been reported by Safaa [16] who showed that the dietary incorporation of 2% of garlic powder or fenugreek seed did not affect the daily feed intake. Chowdhury et al. [48] showed that the dietary addition of 0% to 10% of garlic paste during a six week-period did not affect feed consumption. Concerning the linseed effect, Ahmad et al. [49] reported that feed intake of White Leghorn laying hens decreased with the increase of linseed level from 0% to 15%. However, Criste-Rodica et al. [50] found that feed intake was not affected by the dietary addition of 5% linseed from the 35th to 42nd week-old of Lohman Brown layers. The dietary effect of copper has been investigated by several studies. Idowu et al. [51] demonstrated that feed intake of 30 week-aged Black Harco layer strain increased when inorganic Cu ($CuSO_4.5H_2O$) was added for 10 weeks compared with Cu Proteinate. By contrast, Kaya et al. [52] showed that the dietary supplementation of 200 ppm of copper didn't affect the feed intake of 38 week-old Lohman White layers.

Similar results have been reported by Rahimi et al. [53] who found that the dietary addition of 15 g/kg of sun dried garlic powder, 200 mg/kg of cupric sulfate pentahydrate alone or together for 40 week-aged Single Comb White Leghorn (SCWL) laying hens didn't affect feed consumption. Pekel et al. [34] showed that the Lohman Brown laying hens receiving 250 ppm of Cu decreased their feed consumption. Hens' body weight loss was not affected ($p > 0.05$) by the dietary restriction. Body weight losses varied from 71.41 g to 120.86 g during the 42nd day. Similar data were found by Abdouli et al. [9] who reported that the Lohman White laying hens received 100 g of basal diet/d without or with fenugreek seed addition during 49 days had a body loss with a mean value of −115.3 g. In the present study, egg production and egg mass decreased for the laying hens fed on the experimental diet when compared to the control group. However, these changes were not statistically significant ($p > 0.05$) for egg mass. Feed efficiency increased ($p > 0.05$) for CFSGLSCS with a mean value of 1.98 compared to 1.94 for control. Our data were partially in accord with these of Aderemi et al. [54] who reported that the laying production and egg weight increased when garlic powder was incorporated at 4% garlic powder. Sibel et al. [47] showed that an increase of egg production was found when 0.5% and 1% of garlic powder was supplemented compared to the 2% garlic powder supplemented group. Hens receiving 1% of garlic powder had the highest egg production and egg weight when compared to those fed on 0%, 0.5%, and 2% of garlic powder. The previous author had attributed the negative effect of the 2% of garlic powder on feed consumption to the strong odor of garlic acting as a deterrent. According to Safaa [16], the dietary incorporation of 2% garlic or fenugreek did not affect egg rate, egg weight, egg mass and feed conversion. In agreement with the previous study, Chowdhury et al. [48] showed that egg production and feed efficiency was not affected by the dietary addition of 0% to 10% of garlic paste. The effect of linseed on laying performance has been reported by Ahmad et al. [49], Al-Nasser et al. [55] and Criste-Rodica et al. [50] who showed that the dietary addition of flaxseed didn't affect egg production rate and weight. By contrast Krawczyk et al. [56] reported that the dietary supplementation of 10% of linseed increased egg weight. Pekel et al. [34] showed that laying hens fed on 250 ppm of Cu from Cu sulfate had the highest egg production mean value with the lowest egg weight. However Attia et al. [57] reported that 60 ppm of inorganic Cu increased egg weight and egg mass of laying hens. Rahimi et al. [53] reported that the dietary incorporation of garlic powder, Cu sulfate together or alone did not affect laying production, egg weight, egg mass and feed conversion ratio.

3.2. Egg Physical Characteristics

Egg weight and physical characteristics are shown in Table 3. It seems clear that the dietary addition of CFSGLSCS increased ($p < 0.05$) egg and shell weight. This combination didn't affect ($p > 0.05$) albumen weight, yolk weight and shell thickness. Our data were in agreement with these reported by Abdouli et al. [9] who showed that egg and shell weights of hens fed on water and hexane insoluble fraction of whole fenugreek seed were the highest when compared to the group fed on whole fenugreek seed. The effect of feeding garlic on the egg physical characteristics has been treated by Safaa [16] who found an increase of egg yolk percentages and a decrease of albumen weight percentages. According to Ahmad et al. [49], the dietary incorporation of linseed at a level of 0% to 15% did not affect egg quality characteristics. However, Pekel et al. [34] reported a decrease of egg shell thickness of laying hens fed on 250 mg/kg of Cu lysine.

Table 3. Effects of various diets on egg characteristics.

	Diets		Statistics	
	Control (C)	CFSGLSCS	SEM	p-Value
Egg weight (g)	55.18 [b] ± 3.99	61.09 [a] ± 3.36	0.62	0.0058
Shell weight (g)	6.12 [b] ± 0.56	6.58 [a] ± 0.44	0.08	0.0001
Shell thickness (mm)	0.39 ± 0.035	0.4 ± 0.04	0.0058	0.32
Albumen weight (g)	32.83 [b] ± 3.11	34.12 [a] ± 2.9	0.48	0.058
Yolk weight (g)	14.74 [b] ± 0.93	15.24 [a] ± 1.32	0.18	0.056

Note: C = control; CFSGLSCS = diet contained: 2.9 kg of fenugreek seed, 2.9 kg of linseed, 76 g of CuSO$_4$ and 970 g of garlic mixed with 92 kg of basal diet; SEM = Standard Error of the mean; [a,b]: Mean in the same row having different superscripts are significantly different ($p < 0.05$).

3.3. Lipid Profile

Egg yolk cholesterol concentration reduction may be achieved by feeding laying hens with a diet containing special mixtures of fenugreek seeds, garlic and CuSO4. In fact, many medicinal properties attributed to fenugreek seed (*Trigonella foenum graecum* L.) [58–60], but there is scanty documented literature on its use to lower egg yolk cholesterol. However, Abdouli et al. [9], showed that the positive effect of ground fenugreek seeds on serum cholesterol concentrations would be due the particular composition of the saponins in fenugreek seed, or to an unknown synergetic effect of saponins and other bioactive compounds in fenugreek seed. Concerning copper, it is an essential mineral with a regulating activity of cholesterol biosynthesis by reducing the glutathione concentration. This co-enzyme decreases the mevalonate activity so that cholesterol one [61]. Two components of garlic, S-allylcysteine sulfoxide (alliin) and diallyl disulfide-oxide (allicin) were shown to lower cholesterol levels [62,63]. The overall effects of these constituents on lipid metabolism in chickens have not been described. Data of egg yolk triglycerides, lipids, total cholesterol and serum cholesterol are summarized in Table 4. Dietary treatment reduced egg yolk cholesterol ($p < 0.05$). Laying hens fed on CAFSLSSC had the lowest egg yolk cholesterol concentration with a mean value of 16.09 mg/g compared to 17.01 mg/g for the control group. However, the egg yolk cholesterol concentration decreased ($p < 0.05$) by 5.4% and egg weight increased ($p < 0.05$) from 55.18 g to 61.09 g. Consequently, the total egg cholesterol content was 240.98 mg/egg for the control group compared to 236.25 mg/egg for the experimental. These differences were not statistically significant ($p > 0.05$). Our results were in accordance with those reported by Safaa [16] who showed that the dietary supplementation of 2% of garlic or fenugreek decreased egg yolk cholesterol concentration to 7%. Ademola et al. [45] reported that garlic oil supplementation at 100 mg/kg reduced egg yolk cholesterol concentration when compared with hens' given 200 mg/kg of garlic powder. A statistically significant decrease of egg yolk cholesterol concentration was also reported by Sibel et al. [47] who reported that the dietary addition of 0.5%, 1%, and 2% of garlic powder reduced egg yolk cholesterol concentration from 20.27 mg/g (control) to 13.21 mg/g (0.5%), 12.89 mg/g (1%) and 13.20 mg/g (2%). Dietary supplementation of garlic powder, copper sulfate or both decreased the egg yolk cholesterol concentration [53]. The latter reported that the hypocholesterolomic effect of 200 mg/kg of copper sulfate was more effective than 15 g/kg of garlic powder. According to Attia et al. [57], the dietary addition of Cu at 16 ppm and 120 ppm decreased egg yolk cholesterol with 9% and 13%, respectively. As well as the yolk cholesterol serum cholesterol decreased from 158.42 (C) mg/dL to 122.88 mg/dL (CFSGLSCS). A similar finding has been reported by Abdouli et al. [9] who showed that ground fenugreek seed at levels ranging from zero to six g/hen/d decreased serum cholesterol concentration from 106.4 mg/dL (control) to 85.8

mg/dL, 92.7 mg/dL, and 86.2 mg/dL for respectively, 2 g, 4 g, and 6 g. This decrease in the serum cholesterol concentration would be attributable to phenols, saponins and other bioactive compounds of the fenugreek seed. Saponins content of fenugreek seeds was 2.4%. According to Sauvaire et al. [64] diosgenin, the principal furostanol of fenugreek seeds may have a hypocholesterolemic effect on plasma cholesterol concentration. The mechanism of these reductions had been demonstrated that diosgenin is responsible for cholesterol absorption inhibition and thus reduces liver cholesterol concentration and consequently increases the cholesterol secretion of bile and the fecal excretion of neutral sterols. Chowdhury et al. [48] showed that garlic paste at 2%, 4%, 6%, 8% or 10% in laying hens diet reduced egg yolk cholesterol by 5%, 9%, 14%, 20% and 24%, respectively and leaded to a reduction of blood cholesterol by 15%, 28%, 33% and 43% for 2%, 4%, 6% and 8% of garlic paste. This author proposed that egg yolk and blood cholesterol reduction when hens were given garlic paste might be attributed to the reduction of synthetic enzyme activity. However, Attia et al. [57] demonstrated that the organic source of Cu decreased plasma cholesterol by 12.8% compared to 9.2% inorganic source and confirmed the hypothesis of Kim et al. [61] who reported that higher levels of Cu depressed hepatic glutathione formation thus the cholesterol one.

Table 4. Effects of various diets on lipids profile.

	Diets		Statistics	
	Control (C)	CFSGLSCS	SEM $^\delta$	p-Value
Triglyceride, mg/g yolk	202.2 ± 14.94	213.74 ± 19.4	5.22	0.13
Triglyceride, mg/egg	2859.14 ± 234.9	3143.43 ± 234.9	100.38	0.59
Total cholesterol, mg/g yolk	17.01 ^{a} ± 1.1	16.09 ^{b} ± 0.73	0.28	0.0317
Total cholesterol, mg/egg	240.98 ± 22.4	236.25 ± 19.00	6.33	0.60
Total lipids (g/egg)	4.59 ^{b} ± 0.45	5.23 ^{a} ± 0.46	0.138	0.0038
Serum cholesterol (mg/dL)	158.42 ^{a} ± 32.1	122.88 ^{b} ± 24.2	10.55	0.0242

Note: C = control; CFSGLSCS = diet contained: 2.9 kg of fenugreek seed, 2.9 kg of linseed, 76 g of CuSO$_4$ and 970 g of garlic mixed with 92 kg of basal diet; $^\delta$ SEM = Standard Error of the mean; ^{a,b}: Mean in the same row having different superscripts are significantly different ($p < 0.05$).

4. Conclusions

The results of the present studies clearly showed that fenugreek seeds (3%), garlic (1%), linseeds (3%) and copper sulfate (0.078%) combination is a primary factor causing significant reduction of egg yolk cholesterol concentration (from 17.01 mg/g to 16.09 mg/g yolk) and blood cholesterol (from 158.42 g/egg to 122.88 g/egg) without imposing any adverse effect on performances parameters. However, response to the dietary incorporation of linseed in terms of the fatty acids profile needs to be evaluated.

Author Contributions: Conceptualization, B.L.M., A.S. and H.A.; Data curation, A.D., M.L. and R.R.; Formal analysis, B.O., B.L.M. and Z.J.; Methodology, B.L.M., Z.J. and R.R.; Supervision, A.S. and H.A.; Validation, A.D. and M.L.; Writing—original draft, B.O., B.L.M. and A.S.; Writing—review & editing, A.D., M.L. and R.R.

Funding: This research received no external funding.

Conflicts of Interest: The authors declare no conflict of interest.

References

1. Santini, A.; Tenore, G.C.; Novellino, E. Nutraceuticals: A paradigm of proactive medicine. *Eur. J. Pharm. Sci.* **2017**, *96*, 53–61. [CrossRef] [PubMed]
2. Daliu, P.; Santini, A.; Novellino, E. A decade of nutraceutical patents: Where are we now in 2018? *Expert Opin. Ther. Pat.* **2018**, *28*, 875–882. [CrossRef] [PubMed]

3. Durazzo, A.; D'Addezio, L.; Camilli, E.; Piccinelli, R.; Turrini, A.; Marletta, L.; Marconi, S.; Lucarini, M.; Lisciani, S.; Gabrielli, P.; et al. From plant compounds to botanicals and back: A current snapshot. *Molecules* **2018**, *23*, 1844. [CrossRef] [PubMed]
4. Durazzo, A.; Lucarini, M. Extractable and non-extractable antioxidants. *Molecules* **2019**, *24*, 1933. [CrossRef] [PubMed]
5. Durazzo, A.; Lucarini, M.; Souto, E.B.; Cicala, C.; Caiazzo, E.; Izzo, A.A.; Novellino, E.; Santini, A. Polyphenols: A concise overview on the chemistry, occurrence and human health. *Phyt. Res.* **2019**, 1–23. [CrossRef] [PubMed]
6. Meluzzi, A.; Sirri, F.; Manfreda, G.; Tallarico, N.; Franchini, A. Effects of dietary vitamin E on the quality of table eggs enriched with n-3 long-chain fatty acids. *Poult. Sci.* **2000**, *79*, 539–545. [CrossRef] [PubMed]
7. Anton, M.; Nau, F.; Nys, Y. Bioactive egg components and their potential uses. *Wourld's Poult. Sci. J.* **2006**, *62*, 429–438. [CrossRef]
8. Naviglio, D.; Gallo, M.; Le Grottaglie, L.; Scala, C.; Ferrara, L.; Santini, A. Determination of cholesterol in Italian chicken eggs. *Food Chem.* **2012**, *132*, 701–708. [CrossRef]
9. Abdouli, H.; Belhouane, S.; Hcini, E. Effect of fenugreek seeds on hens' egg yolk color and sensory quality. *J. New Sci.* **2014**, *5*, 20–24.
10. Abdouli, H.; Omri, B.; Tayachi, L. Effect of whole fenugreek seed before and after its maceration in water on hens' laying performance and egg cholesterol profile. *J. New Sci.* **2014**, *8*, 28–34.
11. Weggemans, R.M.; Zock, P.L.; Katan, M.B. Dietary cholesterol from eggs increases the ratio of total cholesterol to high-density lipoprotein cholesterol in humans: A meta-analysis. *Am. J. Clin. Nutr.* **2001**, *73*, 885–891. [CrossRef] [PubMed]
12. Omri, B.; Mourou, I.; Abdouli, H.; Tayachi, L. Effect of fenugreek seed supplementation on hens' egg fatty acids profile and atherogenic and thrombogenic health lipid indices. *J. New Sci.* **2015**, *2*, 405–410.
13. Lamas, A.; Anton, X.; Miranda, J.M.; Roca-Saavedra, P.; Cardelle-Cobas, A.; Rodriguez, J.A.; Franco, C.M.; Cepeda, A. Technological development of functional egg products by an addition of n-3 polyunsaturated-fatty-acid-enriched oil. *CyTA-J. Food* **2016**, *14*, 289–295. [CrossRef]
14. Aida, H.; Hamandiz, M.; Gagic, A.; Mihaljevic, M.; Krinic, J. Egg yolk lipid modifications by fat supplemented diets of laying hens. *Acta Vet.* **2005**, *55*, 41–51. [CrossRef]
15. Rahardja, D.P.; Hakim, M.R.; Pakiding, W.; Lestari, V.S. Hypocholesterolemic effect of garlic powder in laying hen: Low cholesterol egg. *J. Ind. Trop. Anim. Agric.* **2010**, *35*, 16–21. [CrossRef]
16. Safaa, H.M. Effect of dietary garlic or fenugreek on cholesterol metabolism in laying hens. *Egypt Poult. Sci.* **2007**, *27*, 1207–1221.
17. Bakalli, R.I.; Pesti, G.M.; Ragland, W.L.; Konjofca, V. Dietary copper in excess of nutritional requirement reduces plasma and breast muscle cholesterol of chickens. *Poult. Sci.* **1995**, *74*, 360–365. [CrossRef]
18. Pesti, G.M.; Bakalli, R.I. Studies on the effect of feeding cupric sulfate pentahydrate to laying hens on egg cholesterol content. *Poult. Sci.* **1998**, *77*, 1540–1545. [CrossRef]
19. Caston, L.J.; Squires, E.J.; Lesson, S. Hen performance, egg quality and the sensory evaluation of eggs from SCWL hens fed dietary flax. *Can. J. Anim. Sci.* **1994**, *74*, 347–353. [CrossRef]
20. Nasra, B.A.; Yahya, Z.E.; Abd El-Ghany, F.A. Effect of dietary supplementation with phytoestrogens sources before sexual maturity on productive performance of Mandarah hens. *Egypt Poult. Sci.* **2010**, *30*, 829–846.
21. Bean, L.D.; Leeson, S. Long-term effects of feeding flaxseed on performance and egg fatty acid composition of brown and white hens. *Poult. Sci.* **2003**, *82*, 388–394. [CrossRef]
22. Quershi, A.A.; Din, Z.Z.; Buirmeileh, N.; Burger, W.C.; Ahmad, Y.; Elson, C. Suppression of avian hepatic lipid metabolism by solvent extracts of garlic: Impact on serum lipids. *J. Nutr.* **1983**, *113*, 1746–1755. [CrossRef]
23. Sharma, R.K.; Singh, R.A.; Pal, R.N.; Aggarwal, C.K. Cholesterol content of chicken eggs as affected by feeding garlic, sarpagandha, and nicotinic acid. Haryana Agriculture University. *J. Res.* **1979**, *9*, 263–265.
24. Botsoglou, N.A.; Yannakopoulos, A.L.; Fletouris, D.J.; Tserveni-Goussi, A.C.; Psomas, I. Yolk fatty acid composition and cholesterol content in response to level and form of dietary flaxseed. *J. Agric. Food Chem.* **1998**, *46*, 4652–4656. [CrossRef]
25. Caston, L.; Leeson, S. Dietary flaxseed and egg composition. *Poult. Sci.* **1990**, *69*, 1617–1620. [CrossRef]
26. Sim, J.S. Flaxseed as a high energy/protein/omega-3 fatty acid ingredient for poultry. In Proceedings of the 53rd Flax Institute of the United States, Bismarck, ND, USA, 25–26 January 1990; Carter, J.R., Ed.; NDSU: Fargo, ND, USA, 1990; pp. 65–71.

27. Jiang, Z.; Ahn, D.U.; Ladner, L.; Sim, J.S. Influence of feeding full fat flax and sunflower seeds on internal and sensory qualities of eggs. *Poult. Sci.* **1992**, *71*, 378–382. [CrossRef]
28. Sari, M.; Aksit, M.; Özdogan, M.; Basmacıoglu, H. Effects of addition of flaxseed to diets of laying hens on some production characteristics, levels of yolk and serum cholesterol, and fatty acid composition of yolk. *Arch. Für Geflügelkunde* **2002**, *2*, 75–79.
29. Mabrouki, S.; Omri, B.; Abdouli, H. Chemical, functional and nutritional characteristics of raw, autoclaved and germinated fenugreek seeds. *J. New Sci.* **2015**, *16*, 541–551.
30. Omri, B.; Chalghoumi, R.; Abdouli, H. Effect of unprocessed, autoclaved and pre-germinated fenugreek seeds on hens 'laying performance, egg quality characteristics and chemical composition'. *Rev. Colomb. Cienc. Pecu.* **2017**, *30*, 147–158. [CrossRef]
31. Yeh, Y.Y.; Liu, L. Cholesterol-lowering effect of garlic extracts and organosulfur compounds: Human and animal studies. *J. Nutr.* **2001**, *131*, 989S–993S. [CrossRef]
32. Motamedi, S.M.; Taklimi, S.M.M. Investigating the effect of fenugreek seed powder and garlic powder in the diet on immune response of commercial laying hens' egg. *Indian J. Sci. Res.* **2014**, *3*, 277–283.
33. Adebiyi, F.G.; Ologhobo, A.D.; Adejumo, I.O. Raw *Allium sativum* as performance enhancer and hypocholesterolemic agent in laying hens. *Asian J. Anim. Vet. Adv.* **2018**, *13*, 210–217.
34. Pekel, A.Y.; Alp, M. Effects of different dietary copper sources on laying hen performance and egg yolk cholesterol. *J. Appl. Poult. Res.* **2011**, *20*, 506–513. [CrossRef]
35. Jegede, A.V.; Oso, A.O.; Fafiolu, A.O.; Sobayo, R.A.; Idowu, O.M.O.; Oduguwa, O.O. Effect of dietary copper on performance, serum and egg yolk cholesterol and copper residues in yolk of laying chickens. *Slovak J. Anim. Sci.* **2015**, *48*, 29–36.
36. Omri, B.; Chalghoumi, R.; Abdouli, H. Study of the Effects of Dietary supplementation of linseeds, fenugreek seeds and tomato-pepper mix on laying hen's performances, egg yolk lipids and antioxidants profiles and lipid oxidation status. *J. Anim. Sci. Livest. Prod.* **2017**, *1*, 2.
37. Omri, B.; Chalghoumi, R.; Izzo, L.; Ritieni, A.; Lucarini, M.; Durazzo, A.; Abdouli, A.; Santini, A. Effect of dietary incorporation of linseed alone or together with tomato-red pepper mix on laying hens' egg yolk fatty acids profile and health lipid indexes. *Nutrients* **2019**, *11*, 813. [CrossRef]
38. Yassein, S.A.; El-Mallah, G.M.; Sawsan, M.A.; El-Ghamry, A.A.; Abdel-Fattah, M.M.; El-Harriry, D.M. Response of laying hens to dietary flaxseed levels on performance, egg quality criteria, fatty acid composition of egg and some blood parameters. *Int. J. Res. Stud. Biosci.* **2015**, *3*, 27–34.
39. Nascimento, G.A.J. Prediction Equations of the Energetic Values of Poultry Feedstuffs for Utilizing the Meta-Analysis Principle. Ph.D. Thesis, University Lavras, Minas Gerais, Brazil, 2007.
40. Van Soest, P.J.; Robertson, J.B.; Lewis, B.A. Methods of dietary fiber, neutral detergent fiber and non-starch carbohydrates in relation to animal nutrition. *J. Dairy Sci.* **1991**, *74*, 3583–3597. [CrossRef]
41. AOAC. *Association of Official Analytical Chemists. Official Methods of Analysis*, 10th ed. Association of Official Analytical Chemists: Washington, DC, USA, 1984.
42. Pasin, G.; Smith, G.M.; O'Mahony, M. Rapid determination of total cholesterol in egg yolk using commercial diagnostic cholesterol reagent. *Food. Chem.* **1998**, *61*, 255–259. [CrossRef]
43. SAS. *Statistical Analysis System*, version 6; SAS Institute Inc.: Raleigh, NC, USA, 1989.
44. Moustafa, K.K. Effect of using commercial and natural growth promoters on the performance of commercial laying hens. *Egypt. J. Poult. Sci.* **2006**, *26*, 941–965.
45. Ademeola, S.G.; Sikiru, A.B.; Akinwumi, O.; Olamiyi, O.F.; Egbewande, O.O. Performance, yolk lipid, egg organoleptic properties and haematological parameters of laying hens fed cholestryamine and garlic oil. *Glob. Vet.* **2011**, *6*, 542–546.
46. Olobatoke, R.Y.; Mulugeta, S.D. Effect of dietary garlic powder on layer performance, fecal bacterial load, and egg quality. *Poult. Sci.* **2011**, *90*, 665–670. [CrossRef]
47. Sibel, C.; Mesut, K.; Zeynep, E.; Mikail, B.; Altug, K.; Vesile, D.; Ali, K.O. Effect of galiric powder on egg yolk and serum cholesterol and performances of laying hens. *Bull. Vet. Inst. Pulawy* **2009**, *53*, 515–519.
48. Chowdhury, S.R.; Chowdhury, S.D.; Smith, T.K. Effects of dietary garlic on cholesterol metabolism in laying hens. *Poult Sci.* **2002**, *81*, 1856–1862. [CrossRef]
49. Ahmad, S.; Ahsan, H.; Yousaf, M.; Kamran, Z.; Ata, R.; Sohail, M.U.; Shahid, R. Effect of feeding whole linseed as a source of polyunsaturated fatty acids on performance and egg characteristics of laying hens kept at high ambient temperature. *Braz. J. Poult. Sci.* **2013**, *15*, 21–26. [CrossRef]

50. Criste-Rodica, D.; Tudora-Dumitra, P.; Ciurescu, C.; Ropota, M.; Rachieru, D. Effects of moderate (5%) levels of linseed in layer diets. *Arch. Zootech.* **2009**, *12*, 11–21.
51. Idowu, O.M.O.; Laniyan, T.F.; Kuye, O.A.; Oladele-Ojo, V.O.; Eruvbetine, D. Effect of Copper Salts on performance, cholesterol, residues in liver, eggs and excreta of laying hens. *Arch. Zootech.* **2006**, *55*, 327–338.
52. Kaya, A.; Kaya, H.; Macit, M.; Çelbi, Ş.; Esenbuğa, N.; Yŏrŭk, M.A.; Karaoğlu, M. Effects of Dietary Inclusion of Plant Extract Mixture and Copper into Layer Diets on Egg Yield and Quality, Yolk Cholesterol and Fatty Acid Composition. *Kafkas Univ. Vet. Fak. Derg.* **2013**, *19*, 673–679. [CrossRef]
53. Rahimi, S.h.; Rafiei, A.; Lotfollahian, H.; Afsharnaderi, A. Influence of combined usage of garlic powder and copper on egg yolk cholesterol concentration in laying hens. *J. Vet. Res.* **2008**, *63*, 1–6.
54. Aderemi, F.; Olufemi, A.; Oluseyi, A. Evaluating pepper (Capsicum annuum) and garlic (*Allium sativum*) on performance egg trait and serum parameters of old layers. *J. Biol. Agric. Healthc.* **2013**, *3*, 90–95.
55. Al-Nasser, A.Y.; Al-Saffar, A.E.; Abdullah, F.K.; Al-Bahouh, M.E.; Gehan, R.; Magdy, M.M. Effect of adding flaxseed in the diet of laying hens on both production of omega-3 enriched eggs and on production performance. *Int. J. Poult. Sci.* **2011**, *10*, 825–831. [CrossRef]
56. Krawczyk, J.; Bzducha, E.S.; Chomentowska, Z.K.; Semik, E. Efficiency of feeding linseed to heritage breeds hens. *Ann. Anim. Sci.* **2011**, *11*, 135–142.
57. Attia, Y.A.; Abdalah, A.A.; Zeweil, H.S.; Bovera, F.; Tag El-Din, A.A.; Araft, M.A. Effect of inorganic or organic copper additions on reproductive performance, lipid metabolism and morphology of organs of dual-purpose breeding hens. *Arch. Geflugelk.* **2011**, *75*, 169–178.
58. Basu, S.K. Seed Production Technology for Fenugreek (*Trigonella foenumgraecum* L.) in the Canadian Prairies. Master's Thesis, Department of Biological Sciences University of Lethbridge, Lethbridge, AB, Canada, 2006; p. 202.
59. Acharya, S.N.; Srichamroen, A.; Basu, S.K.; Ooraikul, B.; Basu, T. Improvement in the nutraceutical properties of fenugreek (*Trigonella foenum-graecum* L.). *Songklanakarin J. Sci. Technol.* **2006**, *28*, 1–9.
60. Acharya, S.N.; Thomas, J.E.; Basu, S.K. Fenugreek (*Trigonella foenum-graecum* L.) an alternative crop for semiarid regions of North America. *Crop. Sci.* **2008**, *48*, 841–853. [CrossRef]
61. Kim, J.W.; Chao, P.Y.; Allen, A. Inhibition of elevated hepatic glutathione abolishes copper deficiency cholesterolemia. *FASEB J.* **1992**, *6*, 2467–2471. [CrossRef]
62. Itokawa, Y.; Inoue, K.; Sasagawa, S.; Fujiwara, M. Effect of S-methylcysteine sulfoxide, S-allylcysteine sulfoxide and related sulfur-containing amino acids on lipid metabolism of experimental hypercholesterolemic rats. *J. Nutr.* **1973**, *103*, 88–92. [CrossRef]
63. Ali, M.; Al-Qattan, K.K.; Al-Enezi, F.; Khanafer, R.M.; Mustafa, T. Effect of allicin from garlic powder on serum lipids and blood pressure in rats fed with a high cholesterol diet. *Prostaglandins Leukot. Essent. Fatty Acids* **2000**, *62*, 253–259. [CrossRef]
64. Sauvaire, Y.; Ribes, G.; Baccou, J.C.; Loubatieères-Mariani, M.M. Implication of steroid saponins and sapogenins in the hypocholesterolemic effect of fenugreek. *Lipids* **1991**, *26*, 191–197. [CrossRef]

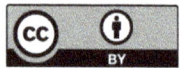

© 2019 by the authors. Licensee MDPI, Basel, Switzerland. This article is an open access article distributed under the terms and conditions of the Creative Commons Attribution (CC BY) license (http://creativecommons.org/licenses/by/4.0/).

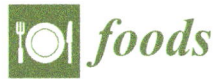

Review

Antioxidant and Anti-Inflammatory Properties of Cherry Extract: Nanosystems-Based Strategies to Improve Endothelial Function and Intestinal Absorption

Denise Beconcini [1,2,3,*], Francesca Felice [2], Angela Fabiano [3], Bruno Sarmento [4,5,6], Ylenia Zambito [3,7] and Rossella Di Stefano [2,7,*]

1. Department of Life Sciences, University of Siena, via Aldo Moro 2, 53100 Siena, Italy
2. Cardiovascular Research Laboratory, Department of Surgery, Medical, Molecular, and Critical Area Pathology, University of Pisa, via Paradisa 2, 56100 Pisa, Italy; francesca.felice@for.unipi.it
3. Department of Pharmacy, University of Pisa, via Bonanno 33, 56100 Pisa, Italy; angela.fabiano@unipi.it (A.F.); ylenia.zambito@unipi.it (Y.Z.)
4. i3S-Instituto de Investigação e Inovação em Saúde, University of Porto, Rua Alfredo Allen 208, 4200-153 Porto, Portugal; bruno.sarmento@ineb.up.pt
5. INEB—Instituto de Engenharia Biomédica, Universidade do Porto, Rua Alfredo Allen, 208, 4200-135 Porto, Portugal
6. CESPU, Instituto de Investigação e Formação Avançada em Ciências e Tecnologias da Saúde, Rua Central de Gandra, 1317, 4585-116 Gandra, Portugal
7. Interdepartmental Research Center Nutraceuticals and Food for Health, University of Pisa, via Borghetto 80, 56100 Pisa, Italy
* Correspondence: denisebeconcini@gmail.com (D.B.); rossella.distefano@unipi.it (R.D.S.)

Received: 31 December 2019; Accepted: 14 February 2020; Published: 17 February 2020

Abstract: Cherry fruit has a high content in flavonoids. These are important diet components protecting against oxidative stress, inflammation, and endothelial dysfunction, which are all involved in the pathogenesis of atherosclerosis, which is the major cause of cardiovascular diseases (CVD). Since the seasonal availability of fresh fruit is limited, research has been focused on cherry extract (CE), which also possesses a high nutraceutical potential. Many clinical studies have demonstrated the nutraceutical efficacy of fresh cherries, but only a few studies on CE antioxidant and anti-inflammatory activities have been carried out. Here, the results concerning the antioxidant and anti-inflammatory activities of CE are reviewed. These were obtained by an in vitro model based on Human Umbilical Vein Endothelial Cells (HUVEC). To clarify the CE mechanism of action, cells were stressed to induce inflammation and endothelial dysfunction. Considering that antioxidants' polyphenol compounds are easily degraded in the gastrointestinal tract, recent strategies to reduce the degradation and improve the bioavailability of CE are also presented and discussed. In particular, we report on results obtained with nanoparticles (NP) based on chitosan derivatives (Ch-der), which improved the mucoadhesive properties of the chitosan polymers, as well as their positive charge, to favor high cellular interaction and polyphenols intestinal absorption, compared with a non-mucoadhesive negative surface charged poly(lactic-co-glycolic) acid NP. The advantages and safety of different nanosystems loaded with natural CE or other nutraceuticals are also discussed.

Keywords: cherry; nutraceuticals; polyphenols; antioxidant; anti-inflammatory; intestinal absorption; nanoparticles; nanosystems; HUVEC

1. Introduction

Cardiovascular diseases (CVD) have always been recognized as the leading cause of death and invalidity in the Occidental world. Atherosclerosis (ATS), a fibroproliferative inflammatory disease due to endothelial dysfunction, is considered the major cause of CVD. Cardiovascular risk factors such as smoking, hypertension, dyslipidemia, diabetes, obesity, and a sedentary lifestyle lead to oxidative stress, which is the most important known factor involved in endothelial dysfunction (Figure 1).

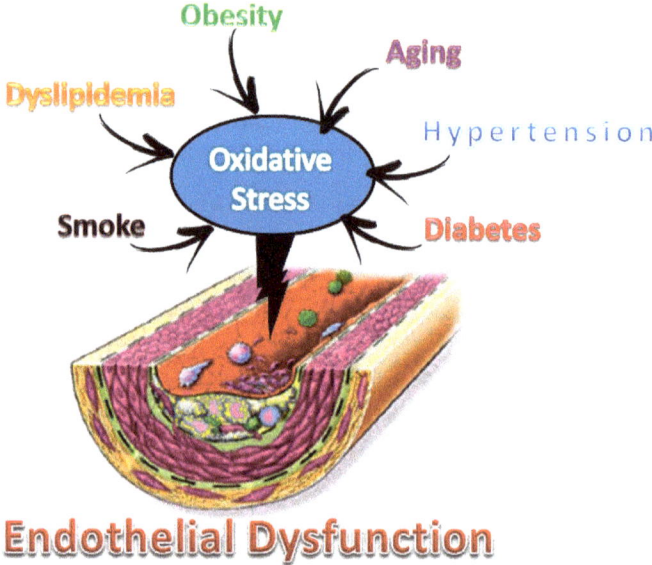

Figure 1. Main cardiovascular risk factors and their involvement in endothelial dysfunction.

Recent studies have demonstrated that a Mediterranean-type diet has a preventive effect on ATS and CVD [1–3]. In particular, the consumption of nutraceuticals contained in plant derivatives has showed a very important role in preventing ATS plaque formation. Among agri-food products, soft fruit such as strawberries, grapes, apples, cherries, etc. are widely consumed due to their good taste based on the balance between sugar and acid content in the fruit. Among soft fruit, sweet cherries (*Prunus avium* L.) have been studied for their high content in biologically active substances, such as phenolic acids. It is known that p-coumaric, p-hydroxybenzoic, chlorogenic, ferulic, and gallic acid, which are found in a lot of different sweet cherry cultivars, have antioxidant properties. Indeed, antioxidants have strong scavenging activity for superoxide and 2,2-diphenyl-1-picrylhydrazil (DPPH) radicals. Moreover, sweet cherries have an anti-inflammatory effect principally due to a decrease in plasma C-reactive protein (CPR) and nitric oxide (NO) levels [4].

However, a low bioavailability is the major problem of using antioxidants from cherry extract in therapy. A poor intestinal absorption along with oxidation in the gastrointestinal tract (GI) and marked metabolism in liver make it unlikely that high concentrations of these antioxidants are found in the organism for long after ingestion and reach the blood, which is the action site. From here, the notion came of preparing nanoparticles loaded with these natural extracts. This nanosystem prolongs the polyphenols residence in the GI lumen, reducing the intestinal clearance mechanisms and increasing the interaction with the intestinal epithelium, which is the absorption surface. Moreover, the nanoparticles can penetrate the tissues through the capillaries and are internalized in cells [5].

Despite the enormous success and consequent use of many synthetic polymers to prepare nanoparticles, using this polymer type in the nutraceutical field is not advisable, as substances of natural origin are required for this purpose. For this reason, we will only review nanosystems that are based on polymers of natural origin (chitosan and its derivatives), made of endogenous monomers (poly(lactic-co-glycolic acid)), or consist of natural phospholipids (liposomes).

2. Cardiovascular Diseases

CVD are disorders that include coronary heart disease, cerebrovascular disease, and peripheral vessel disease. According to the World Health Organization (WHO) report [6], CVD have been responsible for 17.9 million deaths per year, 85% of which are due to heart attack and stroke. The WHO stated that most CVD can be prevented by adopting a healthy lifestyle, e.g., reducing the use of alcohol and tobacco as well as improving diet and physical activities. Consequently, detection and management using counseling and medicines, as appropriate, is a promising strategy to reduce CVD risk factors.

The dominant pathogenesis of CVD is represented by ATS, which is an inflammatory disease that is increasing worldwide as a result of the adoption of the Western lifestyle, and it is likely to reach epidemic proportions in the coming decades [7]. The major direct cause of CVD appears to be the atherosclerotic plaques [8]. Nowadays, it is well-known that ATS is a chronic metabolic and inflammatory process affecting the intima of medium-sized and large arteries. This process is characterized by the formation of plaques made of a cholesterol-rich core (atheroma) surrounded by a fibrous cap (Figure 2). ATS risk factors such as smoking, hypertension, dyslipidemia, diabetes, a sedentary lifestyle, and obesity lead to the activation (dysfunction) of the endothelium [9]. The activated endothelium exhibits an increased permeability, generates reactive oxygen species (ROS), and expresses inflammatory adhesion proteins and chemokines, contributing to the formation of the atherosclerotic plaque, which can be classified into types I and II (early lesions) or types II to VI (advanced lesions) on the basis of the lesion progression [9]. In addition, neoangiogenesis contributes to the progression of atherosclerotic plaque and complications [10].

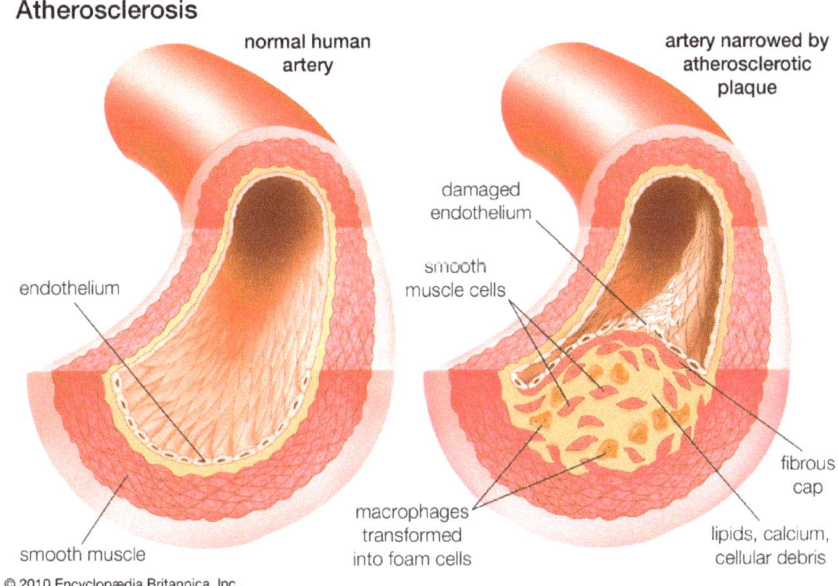

Figure 2. Atherosclerotic plaque formation in a damaged endothelium.

3. Inflammation

Cytokines are often classified in pro-inflammatory (tumor necrosis factor-α (TNF-α), interleukin-1 (IL-1), interleukin-12 (IL-12), interleukin-18 (IL-18), interferon γ (IFNγ)) or anti-inflammatory (interleukin-4 (IL-4), interleukin-10 (IL-10), interleukin-13 (IL-13), transforming growth factor-β (TGF-β)) molecules, according to their activities during the inflammation process (Figure 3). Cytokines, secondary mediators of inflammation, are produced by monocytes, neutrophils and natural killer T (NKT) cells in response to microbial infection, toxic reagents, trauma, antibodies, or immune complexes. After inflammation has been triggered, there is a release of cytokines, the production of which is maintained and amplified by several other factors [11].

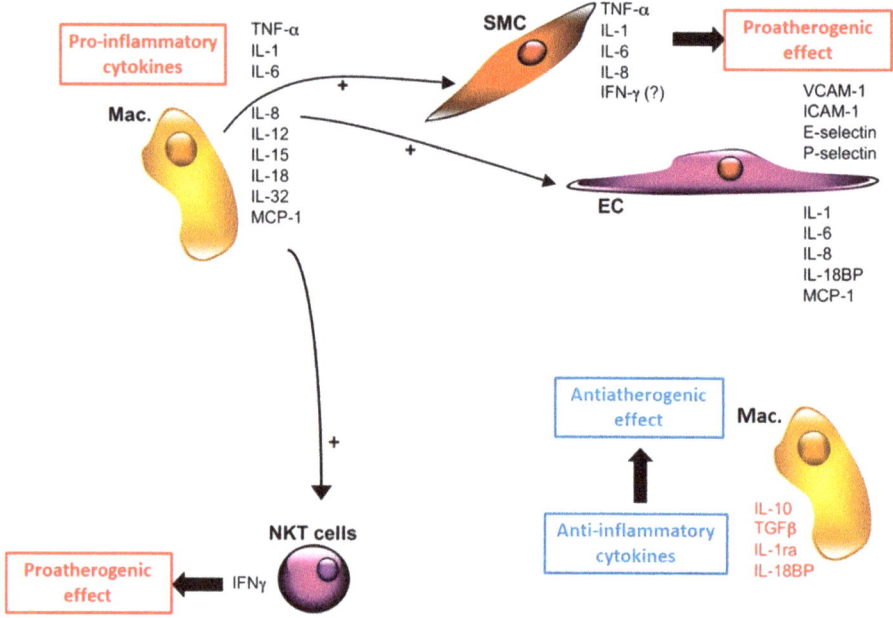

Figure 3. Cytokines involved in atherogenesis (adapted from [11]); Mac. = macrophage, SMC = smooth muscle cells.

Caspases are cysteine proteases that have an important role in the execution of apoptosis. A subfamily of caspases known as inflammatory caspases is involved in innate immunity. Caspase-1 is the prototypic member of this subfamily: its activation requires the assembly of the inflammasome, which is a unique intracellular complex that cleaves and activates IL-1 and IL-18 and contributes to the production of all the other cytokines [11]. Recently, the activation of Nucleotide-binding domain and Leucine-rich repeat Receptor containing a Pyrin domain 3 (NLRP3) inflammasome activation, the oxidative stress causing immune cell dysregulation, and chronic infections have showed a pivotal role in ATS and in inflammaging, which is a condition involved in CVD [12,13].

4. Role of Oxidative Stress

Oxidative stress results from an imbalance between free radicals and antioxidants in the body that could promote endothelial dysfunction and lead to cardiovascular dysfunctions [14].

There are tight relations between ROS generation and vascular functions in the normal physiological state and various pathologies, ATS being among them [15]. A high concentration of ROS can damage endothelium cellular structures and components, resulting in cellular death [16].

Cells expressed in the atherosclerotic plaque can generate ROS in response to activation by cytokines (TNF-α, IL-1), growth factors (platelet-derived growth factor (PDGF)), vasoactive peptides (angiotensin II), and platelet-derived products (thrombin, serotonin). Although different enzymes are present in the atherosclerotic plaque, NADPH oxidase-like activity appears to be the most important enzymatic source of ROS in the vascular wall [11].

Model for the Study of Endothelial Dysfunction

Endothelial cells (EC) lining the blood vessels are very sensitive to injury caused by oxidative stress [17]. The injury leads to compensatory responses that alter the normal homeostatic properties of the EC, increases the adhesiveness of the endothelium to leukocytes and platelets, as well as its permeability [18], and induces a procoagulant state and the release of vasoactive molecules, cytokines, and growth factors. If the inflammatory response is not effectively neutralized or the offending agents are not removed, the process can continue indefinitely [18].

Human Umbilical Vein Endothelial Cells (HUVEC) have been considered a good standard model for EC in normal and diseased conditions [19–24]. HUVEC were cultured for the first time in 1973 and isolated by the perfusion of healthy donors' umbilical veins with trypsin or collagenase [20]. HUVEC offer several advantages not only because they are relatively easy to recover and isolate from the umbilical vein, but also because they can be made to proliferate, and they can be maintained by a standard protocol. Moreover, HUVEC have been shown to be responsive to physiological and/or pathological stimuli such as high glucose, lipopolysaccharide (LPS), and shear stress [21–23].

Many in vitro studies performed on EC demonstrated the beneficial effects of natural products and their derivatives in protection from aging and oxidative stress [25–27].

5. Nutraceutical Intervention

The term "nutraceutical" derives from the fusion of the words "nutrition" and "pharmaceutical" [28]. According to DeFelice, nutraceutical can be defined as "a food (or a part of food) that provides medical or health benefits, including the prevention and/or treatment of disease".

Since the term nutraceutical has no regulatory meaning in marketing, different definitions have been proposed to help distinguish between functional food, nutraceuticals, and dietary supplements [29,30]. In 1994, Zeisel [31] provided two additional useful definitions of nutraceutical and functional food. A nutraceutical can be defined as "a diet supplement that delivers a concentrated form of a biologically active component of food in a non-food matrix to enhance health". Functional food is not a dietary supplement, but it includes "any food or food ingredient that may provide a health benefit beyond the traditional nutrients it contains" [32].

For these reasons, the interest in nutraceuticals and functional food has gained ground for its safety and potential nutritional and therapeutic effects. From here, it can be stated that because any functional food/nutraceutical is a source of macro and micronutrients, depending on the dose, it has the potentiality to be used as a drug [33].

In particular, nutraceuticals have showed a physiological benefit or provided protection against chronic inflammatory disorders, such as CVD [34].

Therefore, lowering inflammation is the most promising strategy for the prevention of atherosclerosis and its complications. Many clinical studies, e.g., the Lyon Diet Hearth Study [1], have demonstrated the protective effects in the primary and secondary prevention of CVD [2,3]. The consumption of plant derivatives, with a high intake of fruit and vegetables, such as plant sterols/stanols, red year rice, green tea catechins, curcumin, berberine, garlic etc., reducing physiological threats, including CVD and ATS risk factors [35], and improving the immune responses and defense system [36–38], could be used in monotherapy or combination therapy to significantly reduce CVD-related complications [39].

The constant increase of the nutraceutical market led the nutraceutical industry to develop innovative research in the delivery systems of molecules that have poor solubility or adsorption. These molecules without an appropriate oral formulation have limited efficacy [40].

6. Polyphenols and Sweet Cherry (*Prunus avium* L.)

Polyphenols are biologically active substances that are contained in plants derivatives or produced as secondary metabolites, which can be chemically distinguished into three main classes: phenolic acids, flavonoids, and non-flavonoids (stilbenes—resveratrol and lignans) (Figure 4). Polyphenols found in fruit, vegetables, nuts, and their derivatives have antioxidant and anti-inflammatory activities. Among phenolic acids, hydroxycynnamic, e.g., p-coumaric acid, and hydrobenzoic acids, e.g., gallic acid, have important antioxidant properties. Most polyphenols are represented by flavonoids, such as anthocyanins (cyanidin) and anthoxantins (flavonols—quercetin, flavanols—catechin etc.), which have both antioxidant and anti-inflammatory properties [41–43]. Flavonoids are found in chocolate, tea, and wine. Since oxidative stress is a determining factor in many chronic and degenerative pathologies, e.g., ATS, numerous efforts have been made to study antioxidant compounds that could prevent these diseases and hamper their progression. Indeed, numerous types of polyphenols (e.g., p-coumaric acid, gallic acid, and ferulic acid) have been found to have radical scavenging and antioxidant activity [44]. The literature also shows by in vitro and/or in vivo models that polyphenols could reduce the inflammation, inhibit the edema, and stop the progression of tumors, as a virtue of their proapoptotic and anti-angiogenic actions. In addition, they could modulate the immune system, prevent the bones disturbances associated with the osteoporosis, increase the capillary resistance by acting on the constituents of blood vessels, protect the cardiovascular system, etc. [45].

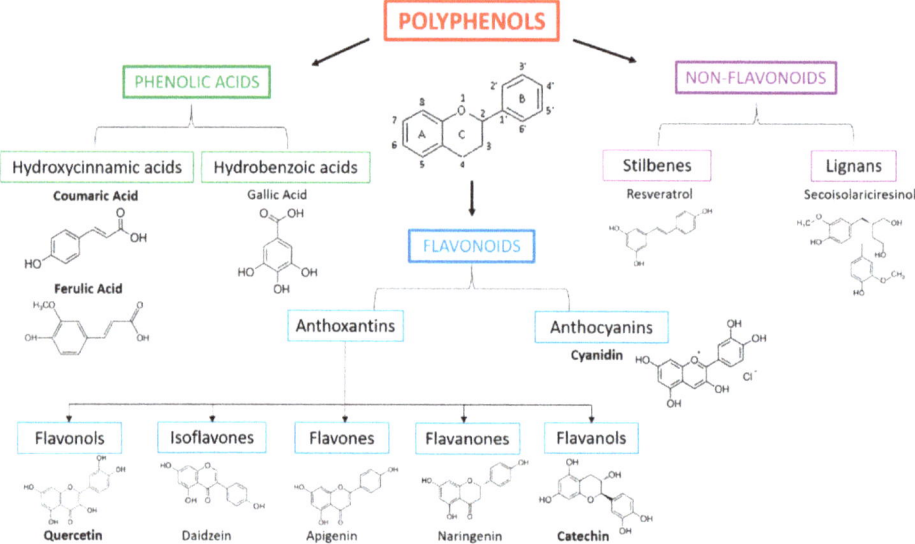

Figure 4. Schematic classification of polyphenols and examples of chemical structures. The main molecules present in sweet cherries are represented in bold.

Among plant products, cherry fruit has been studied for its nutritional properties and beneficial effects [46,47]. Cherries are within the Rosaceae family and belong to the genes *Prunus* and subspecies *Cerasus*, according to the Linneus classification. Sweet cherry (*Prunus avium*) and tart or sour cherry (*Prunus cerasus*) have global trading importance and are now growing widely around the world. Depending on pre- and post-harvest factors, sweet cherry contains high levels of nutrients and bioactive compounds, which present various health benefits [48–50]. Średnicka-Tober et al. [51] showed the in vitro antioxidant potential of different cultivars of commercial sweet cherries, having a high variability in phenolics profile, and the ability to prevent disease. Other studies [52,53] confirmed the high phenol content variability and demonstrated that local sweet cherry varieties represent an interesting source of bioactive molecules and promote sustainability and biodiversity. Several clinical studies have showed that cherry fruit or juice consumption plays an important role in inflammatory diseases [54–56] by preventing or reducing inflammation related to muscle damage from intense strength exercise and also by accelerating recovery from strenuous physical activity. Ben Lagha et al. [57] reported that the tart cherry fractions and their bioactive constituents have antiplaque action due to their ability to inhibit the adherence properties of oral pathogens and increase the epithelial barrier function. Moreover, a recent study has confirmed the importance of cherry fruit in ATS risk factors prevention due to the effect of its polyphenols to reduce inflammation and endothelial dysfunction [58]. Nowadays, the interest is also moving toward the possibility of using coffee cherry extracts for brain health improvement, although further studies are required [59].

The most representative molecules in cherries are polyphenols, such as phenolic acids and flavonoids (see Figure 4), which also represent the most abundant antioxidants in the diet [60]. In particular, cherry extracts (CE) have a high content in phenols that reflects their nutraceutical potential, which could prevent chronic diseases [52]. Anthocyanins, the water-soluble subclass of flavonoids, are the ones responsible for the red color of cherry fruit and for the major part of CE vasoprotective properties [61], e.g., anti-inflammatory, anti-atherogenic, and vasodilatory action in vitro [62]. The antioxidant ability and the protective effect against oxidative stress of CE phenols have been investigated and demonstrated mainly by in vivo studies [48]. Regarding their anti-inflammatory activity, some studies have demonstrated that anthocyanins, such as cyanidin-3-o-glucoside and quercetin, inhibit LPS-induced inflammation and the release of endothelial-derived vasoactive factors after vascular endothelial damage [43,63,64]. A possible CE phenols mechanism of action in the cells has been recently reported by Console et al. [65]. In particular, they demonstrated the activation of recombinant human mitochondrial carnitine/acylcarnitine transporter, which was reconstituted in liposomes, by polyphenolic extract from *Prunus avium* L, thus confirming their antioxidant properties and showing their involvement in the mitochondrial fatty acid oxidation pathway.

In our own experience, the sweet CE polyphenols from *Prunus avium* L. showed a potential antioxidant effect by protecting HUVEC against oxidative stress, in addition to an ability to reduce ROS [66]. CE also demonstrated the ability to reduce inflammatory cytokines production, which resulted to be as efficient as that of the strong anti-inflammatory drug dexamethasone [67].

However, the use of antioxidants extracted from fruit is restricted because of their poor oral bioavailability. Indeed, they have a poor intestinal absorption, because of the oxidation in the intestinal tract and metabolic degradation in liver. Hence, there is a low probability of finding effective concentrations of these substances in the blood that is their site of action for a long time after ingestion. From this, the importance is clear of a formulation that could maintain the structural integrity of polyphenols, increase their water solubility and bioavailability, and transport them toward the physiological target [45].

7. Nanotechnology in Nutraceutical

To avoid the problem of polyphenols' low oral bioavailability, nanotechnology has been applied in nutraceutical and nanomedicine [68], which resulted in new drug delivery systems. The delivery of nutraceuticals provides protective mechanisms that are able to (1) maintain the active molecular form until the time of consumption and (2) deliver the active form to the physiological target within the organism [69].

From a technological point of view, nanocarriers are promising candidate as nutraceuticals delivery because they have a minimum influence on the appearance of final food products such as beverages [70].

Many types of nanosystems are increasingly studied to increase the stability of bioactives during storage and consumption, such as polymeric nanoparticles (NP), solid lipid NP, and liposomes. These nanosystems could deliver molecules with low bioavailability such as polyphenols [71]. In particular, nanoparticles are able to encapsulate phenolic compounds via hydrogen bonds and hydrophobic interactions, consequently increasing their aqueous solubility and preventing the oxidation in the GI tract [72]. NP having subcellular size improve the bioavailability of nutraceutical compounds. In particular, NP are able to prolong the polyphenols residence time in the GI tract, decreasing the intestinal clearance mechanisms and the interaction with the biological target [73]. Furthermore, NP can also penetrate into tissue through fine capillaries, cross the epithelial lining fenestration (e.g., in the liver), and are generally taken up efficiently by cells [74], thus allowing the efficient delivery of active compounds to target sites in the body.

Nanoparticles are solid colloidal particles with diameters in the range of 1–1000 nm. They are distinguished into nanospheres and nanocapsules. In particular, nanospheres have the drug dispersed inside the polymeric matrix or adsorbed on their surface. The polymeric matrix can be natural or synthetic: generally, natural polymers are preferred because of their biocompatibility, biodegradability, and relative non-toxicity; moreover, polymeric NP have various different structures and bio-imitative characteristics [75]. The ability of mucoadhesive polymeric nanoparticles to be internalized by cells and promote the absorption of phenolic compounds has been demonstrated [76,77]. In particular, more mucoadhesive NP were more able to enhance the bioavailability of the encapsulated drug than less mucoadhesive ones [78]. Among mucoadhesive polymeric matrices, natural chitosan and its derivatives are considered polymers of prime interest. Another polymer that has been approved by the United States Food and Drug Administration and European Medicine Agency and is considered one of the best biomaterials available for drug delivery [79] is synthetic poly(lactic-co-glycolic acid) (PLGA).

Therefore, bioavailability, targeting, and controlled release are the main advantages of using natural product-based nanomedicine [80]. The increased solubility and bioavailability, and improved sustained release by nanoencapsulation may elevate the phytochemicals' bioactivities [81]. However, the problem related to the nanosystems potential toxicity needs to be investigated. The minimal systemic toxicity of a nanosystem, based on biodegradable and biocompatible PLGA, could be of some advantage and represent an alternative to chitosan derivatives [82].

From here, the idea emerged of developing nanosystems based on mucoadhesive chitosan derivatives, which showed the ability to promote polyphenols intestinal absorption and antioxidant activity for the entrapment and the delivery of CE polyphenols. In addition, a comparison was made between such nanosystems and those based on non-mucoadhesive PLGA, which have different physical–chemical properties, in order to evaluate and select the best delivery system for CE polyphenols [82].

In addition to polymeric nanocarriers, an interesting strategy for drug delivery is represented by lipid-based nanocarriers, including vesicles, which were introduced as drug delivery vehicles for the first time in the 1970s. Vesicles are denominated either as liposomes, if the amphiphilic molecules are represented by phospholipids, or niosomes if they are based on non-ionic surfactants [83,84]. Liposomes have a spherical bilayer structure with sizes ranging from 20 nm to several µm. They are made of natural or synthetic phospholipids and cholesterol, and they can be loaded with either hydrophilic or hydrophobic molecules. Liposomes have shown many advantages, such as cell-like membrane structure [85,86], high biocompatibility, low immunogenicity, protection of the drugs or active groups, prolongation of drug half-life, reducing drug toxicity, and increasing efficiency. Moreover, structural and surface modifications can be made by using targeting ligands to generate a novel generation of liposomes and promote receptor-mediated endocytosis [87], thus expanding the application of liposomes in biomedicine [88]. Liposomes can be classified on the basis of their structural parameters, preparation methods [89], composition, and therapeutic applications. Their ability to encapsulate natural substances, e.g., plant-derived essential oils, grape seed extracts (GSE), curcumin, and enhance their antioxidant and anti-inflammatory activity has been demonstrated [90–92].

The liposome coating with chitosan led to a system for the controlled and sustained release of GSE polyphenols in water-based food [92]. Then, liposomes represent innovative vectors for the prolonged and sustained release of nutraceuticals and other active molecules, and their structure can be easily modified for multiple specific therapeutic applications.

A more recent trend in nanotechnology is represented by the use of complex systems. However, there are only a few data regarding the application of these systems as vehicles for nutraceuticals. Ma et al. [93] demonstrated the ability of nitric oxide-releasing chitosan nanoparticles (GSNO-Ch NP) to maintain the quality of sweet cherries during cold storage, thus improving their antioxidant properties. In effect, the authors showed that the combined treatment with S-nitrosoglutathione (GSNO) and Ch NP can preserve the soluble solid content and enhance the activity of antioxidants enzymes, in addition to reducing nitric oxide production, during its storage, better than GSNO or Ch alone.

7.1. Nanoparticles Based on Chitosan Derivatives

Chitosan (Figure 5) is a cationic polysaccharide composed of D-glucosamine and N-acetyl-D-glucosamine units, which are linked by β-(1,4)-glycosidic bonds. It is obtained by the incomplete deacetylation of chitin, which is a homopolymer of β-(1,4)-linked N-acetil-D-glucosamine present in the shell of crustaceans and molluscs, the cell walls of fungi, and the cuticle of insects. Chitosan is biocompatible, biodegradable, mucoadhesive, and non-toxic, and it has antimicrobial, antiviral, and immunoadjuvant activities.

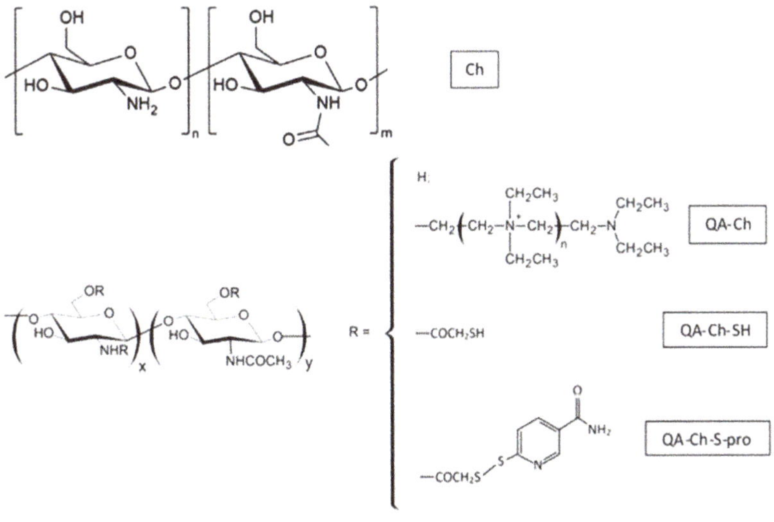

Figure 5. Chemical structures of chitosan (Ch) derivatives: quaternary ammonium chitosan (QA-Ch), its thiolated derivative (QA-Ch-SH) and S-protected quaternary ammonium chitosan (QA-Ch-S-pro).

Chitosan obtained by a heterogeneous reaction is not soluble in water, although it is soluble in acid conditions. Water-soluble chitosan is instead obtained with homogeneous reaction. The acetylation of highly deacetylated chitin can also produce soluble chitosan. As a result, chitosan is available on the market in various forms that are different in molecular weight (MW) and deacetylation degree. Moreover, chitosan can be chemically modified because of the presence of –NH$_2$ and –OH groups on the repetition units, leading to different derivatives. Chitosan has been found to enhance drug penetration across the cell monolayer, such as the intestinal epithelia [94]. Due to its absorption-enhancing effect, chitosan can be used for the development of new therapeutic drug delivery systems [95] administered by the oral route. Thus, the mucoadhesive properties of chitosan could be applied in nanomedicine with the purpose of improving the effectiveness of nutraceuticals and drug delivery systems in age-related and diet-related diseases, e.g., ATS [96].

However, the use of chitosan is restricted because of its limited mucoadhesive strength and low water solubility at neutral and basic pH. For these reasons, various chemical modifications of chitosan have been studied in order to improve its solubility and consequently its applications [97]. In its protonated form, chitosan facilitates the paracellular transport of hydrophilic drugs combining the bioadhesion to a transient widening of the tight junction in the membrane. However, it is incapable of enhancing the absorption in the more basic environment of the small intestine. Therefore, positive charges have been introduced on the chitosan polymer chains [98,99] to obtain chitosan derivatives with increased solubility properties, especially at neutral and basic pH values.

A promising class of chitosan derivatives called N,O-[N,N-diethylaminomethyl(diethyldimethy leneammonium)$_n$ methyl chitosan, or quaternary ammonium chitosan (QA-Ch) (Figure 5), was prepared by reacting chitosan with 2-diethylaminoethyl chloride under different conditions [4].

QA-Ch has a high fraction of free, unsubstituted, primary amino groups that are potentially available for the covalent attachment of thiol-bearing compounds via the formation of 3-marcaptopropionamide moieties. This has led to water-soluble thiolated chitosan-quaternary ammonium conjugates (QA-Ch-SH), which are also called thiomers (Figure 5). Thiol groups tend to keep the polymer adherent to the epithelium by reacting with the thiol groups of the epithelium mucus to form disulfide bonds, thus favoring the permeability-enhancing action of the positive ions. The synergism of quaternary ammonium and thiol groups has been evidenced [100]. Indeed, it has been demonstrated that the thiomer was more effective than the non-thiolated parent polymer in promoting absorption. The quaternary ammonium ions of the thiomer are responsible for the permeabilization of epithelium and the polymer mucoadhesion, while the thiols increase the latter. This synergistic effect is the basis of the polymer bioactivity [100].

To confirm the NP penetration mechanism, sections of the intestinal wall were observed under a fluorescence microscope following incubation with NP [101]. Microphotographs showed discrete fluorescent spots across the gut section, which were representative of integral NP penetration from the mucosal to serosal side of the intestine. This demonstrated that the NP did not disintegrate in their transit across the intestinal wall [101].

Despite the innumerable qualities, the thiomers have shown instability problems in solution; in particular, the thiol groups can be subject to oxidation at pH values ≥ 5. The early oxidation of thiols can limit the interaction with glycoproteins in the mucus, drastically reducing the effectiveness of these polymers. To overcome this problem, it was necessary to design and develop a second generation of oxidation-stable thiomer, called S-protected chitosan (QA-Ch-S-pro) (Figure 5). The protection of the sulfhydryl ends with mercaptonicotinamide groups allows increasing the mucoadhesive and cohesive properties of the thiomers, independently of the pH of the environment. Moreover, the amplified adhesive properties of the polymer make it possible to prolong the contact time with the mucosal membranes, the residence time of any vehiculated drugs, or small molecules, thus increasing the concentration gradient of these at the absorption site. Consequently, the more facilitated transport allows increasing the bioavailability of the drugs, with consequent reduction of the dose and the frequency of administration. Thus, chitosan-S-protected polymers can be considered a promising category of mucoadhesive polymers for the future development of new, effective, and safe non-invasive delivery systems for polyphenols.

The antioxidant, anti-inflammatory, antidiabetic, and anticancer properties of chitosan and its derivatives [96], especially when combined with such natural antioxidants as polyphenols, are promising for the prevention, delay, mitigation, and treatment of age-related dysfunctions and diseases, such as CVD. Moreover, NP are able to enhance the absorption of phenolic compounds because they are able to disrupt the tight junctions of biological membranes and can be directly uptaken by epithelial cells via endocytosis (Figure 6) [102].

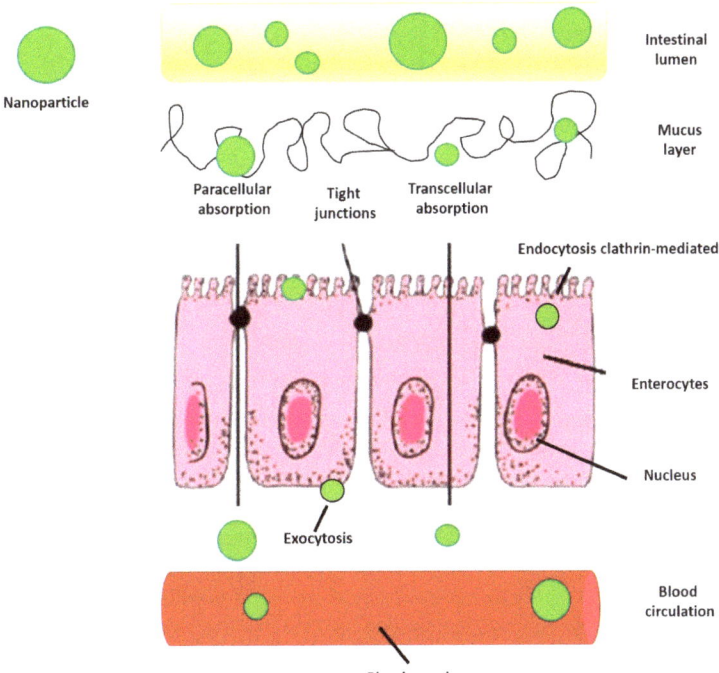

Figure 6. Cellular uptake of nanoparticles (NP) carrying polyphenols by intestinal epithelial cells.

To prepare Ch-der NP, different techniques have been used [103], but the choice of a particular method should consider the nature of the drug to be entrapped, the delivery system, the administration route, and the absorption site. One of the established methods for the preparation of mucoadhesive Ch-der NP, which is intended for oral absorption, is the ionotropic gelation with de-polymerized hyaluronic acid (HA) [104], which is very simple because it does not require the use of organic solvents. The NP are obtained by the addition of a solution of HA containing or not the drug to a dilute solution of chitosan, under stirring. Nanoparticle size strictly depends on the concentration of both chitosan and HA. The efficacy of Ch-der NP prepared with this method to encapsulate red grape polyphenols, thereby promoting their oral absorption and producing beneficial effects on endothelial cells, has been demonstrated [76,77]. Moreover, a recent study on Caco-2 cells demonstrated that Ch der NP were easily internalized by adsorptive endocytosis [97].

Chitosan and its derivatives were used also to prepare nanoparticles complex systems. Ba et al. [105] prepared zein-carboxymethyl chitosan-tea polyphenols (zein-CMCS-TP) for the delivery of β-carotene. These ternary complexes had more stability against heat and acid conditions and antioxidant activity than single protein and protein-polysaccharide binary systems. Zein NP coated with alginate/chitosan were used also to encapsulate resveratrol [106]. These complexes reduce the photodegradation of resveratrol, could improve its stability, and could represent a useful potential delivery system for application in functional food and pharmaceutical products.

7.2. Poly(Lactic-co-glycolic Acid) Nanoparticles

The polyester PLGA is a synthetic copolymer of poly lactic acid (PLA) and poly glycolic acid (PGA) (Figure 7). PLGA is biocompatible and biodegradable, and it is used not only as a delivery vehicle for drugs, proteins, and other macromolecules, but also for the development of NP containing nutraceuticals [107]. It is soluble in a wide range of common solvents including chlorinated solvents, tetrahydrofuran, acetone, or ethyl acetate. In water, PLGA is degraded by the hydrolysis of its ester linkages (Figure 7). PLGA NP can be used to encapsulate either hydrophilic or hydrophobic small molecules by using different formulation methods.

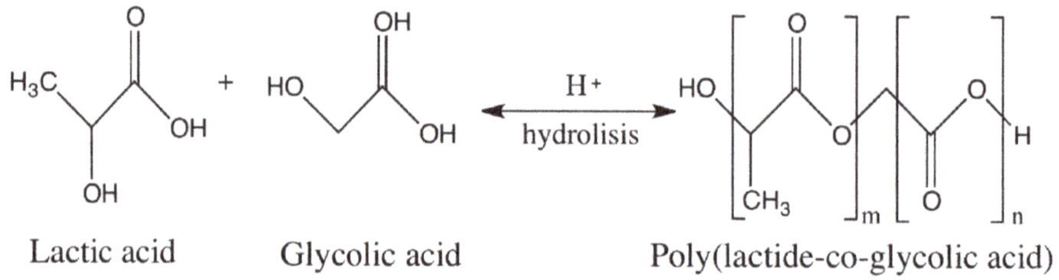

Figure 7. Degradation of poly(lactic-co-glycolic acid) (PLGA) based on the hydrolysis of the copolymer.

The most common technique for the preparation of PLGA NP that is able to encapsulate small hydrophilic molecules is the double emulsion technique (w/o/w), which is a modification of the emulsification-solvent evaporation technique [108]. PLGA NP are internalized by cells partly through pinocytosis and also through clathrin-mediated endocytosis and enter the cytoplasm within 10 min of incubation [107]. The controlled release, biocompatibility, and biodegradability properties of PLGA NP have produced an overall decrease in cytotoxicity; therefore, they have been used as delivery systems for polyphenols rich-materials from fruit and other nutraceuticals [108–111]. The negative surface charges of PLGA could also be modified by PEGylation of the polymer [112] or coating NP with chitosan [113]. In the first case, NP with a neutral surface were obtained; in the second case, the NP surface was positively charged. In both cases, the NP cellular uptake was improved. Another advantage of using PLGA nanoparticles or nanospheres is in the possibility of reducing local inflammation through a long-term treatment, thanks to the slow biodegradation of NP and the consequent release of the drug [114]. In particular, PLGA NP have been successfully used for the preparation of polyphenol nanoformulations in cancer therapy [115].

In addition to simple PLGA NP, more complex and recent strategies have been applied for the delivery of nutraceuticals different from cherry. PEG-lipid-PLGA hybrid NP were prepared by Yu et al. [116] to enhance the liposolubility and the oral delivery of berberine, which is a natural compound that presents potential anti-cancer and anti-inflammatory activity. Complex nanoparticles systems could be also prepared by the combination of PLGA with Ch. Abd-Rabou et al. [117] used polyethylene glycol/chitosan-blended PLGA (PLGA-Ch-PEG) to prepare *Moringa oleifera* leaves extract-loaded nanocomposites, which could be used as a natural source of anti-cancer compounds. Another study reported the possibility of co-encapsulating Nigella sativa oil (NSO) and plasmid DNA (pDNA) in chitosan-PLGA NP, in order to improve the gene therapy for Alzheimer neurodegenerative disease [118].

7.3. Liposomes

Liposomes are bilayer vesicles with an aqueous core entirely covered by a phospholipid membrane. They are attractive encapsulation systems for water-soluble phenolic compounds [119] (Figure 8).

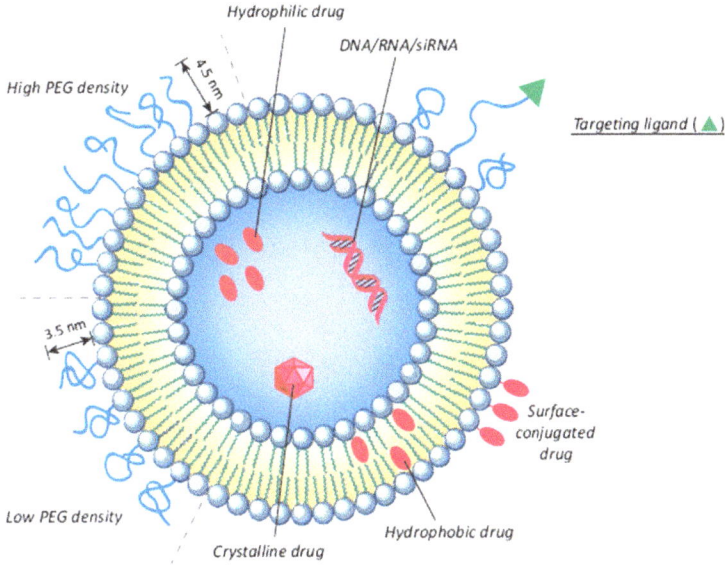

Figure 8. Structural and design considerations for liposomal drug delivery (adapted from [87]).

The thin layer evaporation technique is one of the simplest and most used methods [120] to prepare liposomes by hydrating lipid films [85,121,122], which involves the encapsulation of active principles in the organic phase (with lipophilic actives) or in the aqueous phase (with hydrophilic ones) during the initial steps of liposomal preparation. However, using this technique, the encapsulation efficiency is generally higher with lipophilic molecules than with hydrophilic ones. Another limitation of using conventional liposomes is represented by a rapid elimination from the bloodstream, which could reduce the therapeutic efficacy [123].

In the food area, these vesicles could be used for the encapsulation of functional bioactives. Among the bioactive substances, the essential oils have been thoroughly studied, since many of them have strong antioxidant and antimicrobial properties [124]. However, the difficulties with their dispersion in aqueous formulations and their high oxidation sensitivity require their encapsulation in water-dispersible systems and protection from degradation. A recent work [125] demonstrated the ability of multilamellar liposomes prepared by the dry film hydration technique to incorporate essential oil from Brazilian cherry (*Eugenia uniflora* L.) leaves, which is a plant that is known for its anti-inflammatory properties.

Liposomal aqueous dispersions have low stability; therefore, anhydrous liposomal preparations have been studied. Anhydrous preparations have the advantage of being stable and can be hydrated to regenerate the liposomal dispersion at the time of use. For this reason, transforming the aqueous liposomal dispersion into powder means creating a release system that is more fit for industrial production. This was the goal of Akgün et al. [126], who showed a promising industrially applicable delivery system for sour cherry phenols that were efficiently loaded in a liposomal powder incorporated into a stirred-type yoghurt system. Since the spray-drying process did not degrade phenolic compounds encapsulated in liposomes, this technique could represent another strategy for reducing polyphenols degradation and enhancing their beneficial activity.

8. Intestinal Absorption

The oral route is the preferred one for drug administration because it is the physiological mechanism of nutrients and other exogenous molecules [127]. A drug administered by the oral route is mainly absorbed in the small intestine. The small intestinal epithelium is mainly composed of enterocytes, which have well-ordered projections, called microvilli, on their apical side. Microvilli increase the absorptive area, making up a total intestinal surface area of 300–400 m^2. The intestine also comprises mucus-secreting goblet cells, which are the second most abundant cell type.

Mucus has an essential role in the GI tract. In fact, it has transport activity as well as lubricant and protective properties. It is the first physical barrier encountered by biopharmaceuticals after their oral administration [128]. Mucus is a complex hydrogel composed of proteins, carbohydrates, lipids, salts, antibodies, bacteria, and cellular debris. The main protein components of mucus are mucins, which are responsible for the gel properties of mucus [129]. An example of the dynamic barrier properties of mucus is represented by its ability to act as a selective barrier to the diffusion of acids, due to interactions that change depending on the environmental pH and pKa of the acid.

Since the primary site of absorption after oral administration is represented by the small intestine, rather than the colon [127], it is important to establish the best epithelial cells-based model that is able to simulate the intestinal barrier, in order to evaluate the nutrients intake. After being transported across the epithelial lining, molecules reach the lamina propria, which contains a network of capillaries responsible for their drainage into blood circulation and thus to their action site. All epithelial cells are interconnected by tight junctions, which have an important role in retaining the polarization of the cells and maintaining the integrity of the epithelium [130].

Nanoparticles have the potential to enhance the absorption of phenolic phytochemicals because they are able to disrupt tight junctions and/or they could be directly uptaken by epithelial cells via endocytosis [102] (see Figure 6).

The in vitro model most widely accepted to study the human oral drug absorption is the colon epithelial cancer cells (Caco-2) monolayer. Caco-2 clones from adenocarcinoma have morphologic and functional characteristics similar to enterocytes: e.g., they show tight junctions, apical and basolateral sides, and a brush border with microvilli on the apical surface. However, these Caco-2 monolayers have several limitations. One of these is represented by tight junctions being tighter than those present in the small intestine. In addition, they are more similar to colon epithelium cells, as they have a reduced permeability to drugs through the paracellular route. Hence, many research groups have proposed to use the co-culture of Caco-2/methotrexate mucus-secreting subclones HT29-MTX, as a model that is able to mime the human intestinal epithelium better than the simple Caco-2 monolayer. The mucus-producing HT29-MTX cell line is used as a model to study the mucus role in the transport of drugs through the intestinal tract. Mucus-secreting goblet cells are usually obtained from adenocarcinoma cell line HT29. HT29 cells are treated with methotrexate to get mature goblet cells, which are so-called HT29-MTX.

Triple Cell Co-Culture (Caco-2/HT29-MTX/Raji B) as a Model of Study

A more recent in vitro model based on a triple cell co-culture of Caco-2/HT29-MTX/Raji B, as represented in Figure 9, has been developed in order to reproduce the intestinal epithelium [127,130]. Caco-2 cells cultured with Raji B lymphocytes acquire the M cell phenotype. Caco-2 cells losing the brush border organization, the microvilli, and the typical digestive function from enterocytes play an important role in the immune system, and they have the ability to take up bacteria, viruses, nanoparticles, and microparticles by endocytosis. Previous studies [127,130] proved that the three cell types, when cultured together, present the features of the human intestinal barrier.

In our studies [66,67,82], we tested Ch-der and PLGA NP on both HUVEC and Caco-2 cells in order to evaluate NP cytotoxicity, their ability to protect polyphenols from degradation in the GI, and the mucoadhesive properties that are able to promote intestinal absorption. Our results demonstrated that Ch-der NP, based on mucoadhesive QA-Ch and QA-Ch-S-pro derivatives, were able to encapsulate CE polyphenols and protect them from GI degradation [66]. In particular, QA-Ch and QA-Ch-S-pro NP enhanced the anti-inflammatory and antioxidant activity, respectively, of the lowest CE polyphenolic concentration tested (2 µg/mL). This was ineffective when non-encapsulated [66,67]. PLGA NP were able to encapsulate higher polyphenolic concentrations, maintain their beneficial activities, and promote intestinal permeation [82]. Both Ch-der NP had the ability to reduce ROS production, but only QA-Ch-S-pro NP significantly protected HUVEC from oxidative stress [66], which was probably because of the highest affinity between CE and NP. It is probable that the presence of protected thiol groups on the surface, acting as reducing groups [131], enhances the polyphenols' antioxidant effect. Moreover, QA-Ch-S-pro NP were able to promote CE polyphenols intestinal permeability through the in vitro triple co-culture model based on epithelial cells (Caco-2/HT29-MTX/Raji B) better than non-mucoadhesive PLGA NP [82]. For its part, QA-Ch NP showed the ability of reducing inflammatory cytokines production, nitric oxide, and NLRP3 production in stressed HUVEC, to the same extent as the anti-inflammatory synthetic drug dexamethasone [67]. Although all the NP types were efficiently internalized by HUVEC after 2 h of incubation, the mucoadhesive properties and the positive surface charge of Ch-der NP showed higher cellular interaction than the non-mucoadhesive and negatively charged PLGA NP [67].

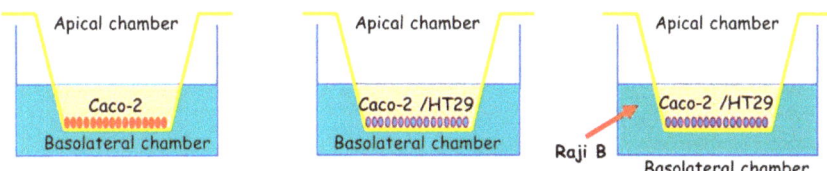

Figure 9. Scheme of Caco-2/HT29 (HT29-MTX)/Raji B triple cell co-culture model preparation (adapted from [127]).

The results obtained have shown that all the types of NP tested are promising from the nutraceutical standpoint. Chitosan NP, thanks to their chemical–physical properties, could be used as efficient transport systems for polyphenols; nevertheless, if higher polyphenolic concentrations are needed, the use of PLGA NP, as nanosystems with low cytotoxicity, could be more convenient [82].

Triple cell co-cultures of Caco-2/HT29-MTX/Raji B were also used as a model to assess the liposomes' permeation ability. Otero et al. [132] demonstrated that non-encapsulated bacteriophages were able to cross the intestinal barrier with respect to the encapsulated ones, which was probably because liposomes containing bacteriophages had a prolonged residence time in the stomach, thus adhering to the intestinal wall and protecting phages until they release. In another study, Belubbi et al. [133] encapsulated nelfinavir mesylate (NFV) in liposomes and studied their permeability using the triple cell co-culture method. They found that the liposomes had a high NFV encapsulation efficiency, but no liposomes permeation was observed. However, the authors demonstrated that these liposomes were able to protect the drug in the gastric environment.

Although no liposomes containing polyphenolic compounds have already been investigated using triple cell co-cultures of a Caco-2/HT29 MTX/Raji B model, these results suggest that liposomes can protect the encapsulated drugs from degradation in the GI tract and that the triple cell co-culture model can yield sound information about polyphenols' transcytosis.

9. Conclusions

Many clinical studies have reported that the consumption of cherries and their derivatives has a beneficial effect on human health. In addition, in vitro studies have demonstrated that natural polyphenols-rich sweet cherry extracts are able to protect endothelial cells from oxidative stress. Regarding inflammatory stress protection, CE was found to be as efficient as the most used anti-inflammatory synthetic drug dexamethasone.

The encapsulation of CE in nanoparticles based on chitosan derivatives improves the intestinal absorption of cherry polyphenols and enhances their antioxidant and anti-inflammatory activity. The mucoadhesive properties of the NP favor cellular internalization and promote the CE biological effects.

For all these reasons, the use of nanosystems based on chitosan derivatives represents a good and innovative strategy for the delivery of polyphenols from cherry extracts. PLGA-based nanosystems are a valid alternative in case higher polyphenol concentrations are needed. The differences in nutraceutical properties between the different types of nanoparticles loaded with cherry extracts have been attributed to the chemical differences between NP surfaces. Indeed, the surface properties of the nanoparticles influence their ability to be internalized by the cells and to cross the mucus that lines the intestine.

Other types of carriers, such as liposomes, should be taken into account for the development of future delivery systems for polyphenols or essential oils. A more recent approach is the use of complex systems based on nanoparticles to enhance the stability of phytochemicals and thus preserve the therapeutic properties of the encapsulated bioactive compounds.

In conclusion, considering that the fresh cherry fruit is a seasonal fruit, the use of nanosystems protects CE from degradation in the GI, thus allowing cherry consumption and its benefits to not be limited by seasonality.

Author Contributions: Conceptualization, D.B., F.F., Y.Z., and R.D.S.; methodology, D.B., F.F., and A.F.; investigation, D.B. and A.F.; resources, R.D.S., B.S., and Y.Z.; writing—original draft preparation, D.B.; writing—review and editing, Y.Z., A.F., and R.D.S.; supervision, R.D.S. and Y.Z.; project administration, R.D.S. All authors have read and agreed to the published version of the manuscript.

Funding: This research received no external funding.

Acknowledgments: Thanks to the Tuscany Region for support. Thanks to Claudio Cantini, Roberto Berni, and the National Research Council of Italy—Trees and Timber Institute (CNR-IVALSA) for providing *Prunus avium* L. cherry fresh fruits and extracts to study.

Conflicts of Interest: The authors declare no conflict of interest.

References

1. Kris-Etherton, P.; Eckel, R.H.; Howard, B.V.; St. Jeor, S.; Bazzarre, T.L. Benefits of a Mediterranean-Style, National Cholesterol Education Program/American Heart Association Step I Dietary Pattern on Cardiovascular Disease. *Circulation* **2001**, *103*, 1823–1825. [CrossRef] [PubMed]
2. Estruch, R.; Ros, E.; Salas-Salvadó, J.; Covas, M.I.; Corella, D.; Arós, F.; Gómez-Gracia, E.; Ruiz-Gutiérrez, V.; Fiol, M.; Lapetra, J.; et al. Primary prevention of cardiovascular disease with a Mediterranean diet. *N. Engl. J. Med.* **2013**, *368*, 1279–1290. [CrossRef] [PubMed]
3. Torres, N.; Guevara-Cruz, M.; Velázquez-Villegas, L.A.; Tovar, A.R. Nutrition and Atherosclerosis. *Arch. Med. Res.* **2015**, *46*, 408–426. [CrossRef]
4. Kelley, D.S.; Rasooly, R.; Jacob, R.A.; Kader, A.A.; Mackey, B.E. Consumption of Bing sweet cherries lowers circulating concentrations of inflammation markers in healthy men and women. *J. Nutr.* **2006**, *136*, 981–986. [CrossRef] [PubMed]
5. Zambito, Y.; Fogli, S.; Zaino, C.; Stefanelli, F.; Breschi, M.C.; Di Colo, G. Synthesis, characterization and evaluation of thiolated quaternary ammonium-chitosan conjugates for enhanced intestinal drug permeation. *Eur. J. Pharm. Sci.* **2009**, *33*, 343–350. [CrossRef] [PubMed]
6. World Health Organization. Cardiovascular Diseases (CVDs). Available online: https://www.who.int/en/news-room/fact-sheets/detail/cardiovascular-diseases-(cvds) (accessed on 17 May 2017).
7. Taleb, S. Inflammation in atherosclerosis. *Arch. Cardiovasc. Dis.* **2016**, *109*, 708–715. [CrossRef]
8. Frostegård, J. Immunity, atherosclerosis and cardiovascular disease. *BMC Med.* **2013**, *11*, 117. [CrossRef]
9. Ross, R. Atherosclerosis—An inflammatory disease. *N. Engl. J. Med.* **1999**, *340*, 115–126. [CrossRef]
10. Camaré, C.; Pucelle, M.; Nègre-Salvayre, A.; Salvayre, R. Angiogenesis in the atherosclerotic plaque. *Redox Biol.* **2017**, *12*, 18–34. [CrossRef]
11. Tedgui, A.; Mallat, Z. Cytokines in atherosclerosis: Pathogenic and regulatory pathways. *Physiol. Rev.* **2006**, *86*, 515–581. [CrossRef]
12. Ferrucci, L.; Fabbri, E. Inflammageing: Chronic inflammation in ageing, cardiovascular disease, and frailty. *Nat. Rev. Cardiol.* **2018**, *15*, 505–522. [CrossRef] [PubMed]
13. Hoseini, Z.; Sepahvand, F.; Rashidi, B.; Sahebkar, A.; Masoudifar, A.; Mirzaei, H. NLRP3 inflammasome: Its regulation and involvement in atherosclerosis. *J. Cell. Physiol.* **2018**, *233*, 2116–2132. [CrossRef] [PubMed]

14. Higashi, Y.; Maruhashi, T.; Noma, K.; Kihara, Y. Oxidative stress and endothelial dysfunction: Clinical evidence and therapeutic implications. *Trends Cardiovasc. Med.* **2014**, *24*, 165–169. [CrossRef] [PubMed]
15. Goncharov, N.; Avdonin, P.; Nadeev, A.; Zharkikh, I.; Jenkins, R. Reactive Oxygen Species in Pathogenesis of Atherosclerosis. *Curr. Pharm. Des.* **2014**, *21*, 1134–1146. [CrossRef] [PubMed]
16. Sinha, K.; Das, J.; Pal, P.B.; Sil, P.C. Oxidative stress: The mitochondria-dependent and mitochondria-independent pathways of apoptosis. *Arch. Toxicol.* **2013**, *87*, 1157–1180. [CrossRef]
17. Dejana, E.; Spagnuolo, R.; Bazzoni, G. Interendothelial junctions and their role in the control of angiogenesis, vascular permeability and leukocyte transmigration. *Thromb. Haemost.* **2001**, *86*, 308–315.
18. Yingshun, X.; Melendez, A.J. Secreted proinflammatory mediators in atherosclerosis: New insights and potential novel therapeutics applications. *IJIB* **2007**, *1*, 65–71.
19. Understanding the Vasculature with the Help of HUVECs. Available online: https://www.promocell.com/in-the-lab/understanding-vasculature-help-huvecs/2017 (accessed on 21 July 2017).
20. Jaffe, E.A.; Nachman, R.L.; Becker, C.G.; Minick, C.R. Culture of human endothelial cells derived from umbilical veins. Identification by morphologic and immunologic criteria. *J. Clin. Investig.* **1973**, *52*, 2745–2756. [CrossRef]
21. Patel, H.; Chen, J.; Das, K.C.; Kavdia, M. Hyperglycemia induces differential change in oxidative stress at gene expression and functional levels in HUVEC and HMVEC. *Cardiovasc. Diabetol.* **2013**, *12*, 142. [CrossRef]
22. Walshe, T.E.; Dela Paz, N.G.; D'Amore, P.A. The role of shear-induced transforming growth factor-β signaling in the endothelium. *Arterioscler. Thromb. Vasc. Biol.* **2013**, *33*, 2608–2617. [CrossRef]
23. Jang, J.; Jung, Y.; Kim, Y.; Jho, E.H.; Yoon, Y. LPS-induced inflammatory response is suppressed by Wnt inhibitors, Dickkopf-1 and LGK974. *Sci. Rep.* **2017**, *7*, 41612. [CrossRef] [PubMed]
24. Cao, Y.; Gong, Y.; Liu, L.; Zhou, Y.; Fang, X.; Zhang, C.; Li, Y.; Li, J. The use of human umbilical vein endothelial cells (HUVECs) as an in vitro model to assess the toxicity of nanoparticles to endothelium: A review. *J. Appl. Toxicol.* **2017**, *37*, 1359–1369. [CrossRef] [PubMed]
25. Hafizah, A.H.; Zaiton, Z.; Zulkhairi, A.; Ilham, A.M.; Anita, M.N.; Zaleha, A.M. Piper sarmentosum as an antioxidant on oxidative stress in human umbilical vein endothelial cells induced by hydrogen peroxide. *J. Zhejiang Univ. Sci. B* **2010**, *11*, 357–365. [CrossRef] [PubMed]
26. Lin, X.L.; Liu, Y.; Liu, M.; Hu, H.; Pan, Y.; Fan, X.J.; Zou, W.W. Inhibition of hydrogen peroxide-induced human umbilical vein endothelial cells aging by allicin depends on Sirtuin1 activation. *Med. Sci. Monit.* **2017**, *23*, 563. [CrossRef]
27. Felice, F.; Maragò, E.; Sebastiani, L.; Di Stefano, R. Apple juices from ancient Italian cultivars: A study on mature endothelial cells model. *Fruits* **2015**, *70*, 361–369. [CrossRef]
28. Brower, V. Nutraceuticals: Poised for a healthy slice of the healthcare market? *Nat. Biotechnol.* **1998**, *16*, 728–732. [CrossRef]
29. Kalra, E.K. Nutraceutical—Definition and introduction. *AAPS J.* **2003**, *5*, 27–28. [CrossRef]
30. Aronson, J.K. Defining 'nutraceuticals': Neither nutritious nor pharmaceutical. *Br. J. Clin. Pharmacol.* **2017**, *83*, 8–19. [CrossRef]
31. Zeisel, S.H. Regulation of "Nutraceuticals". *Science* **1999**, *285*, 1853–1855. [CrossRef]
32. Ross, S. Functional foods: The Food and Drug Administration perspective. *Am. J. Clin. Nutr.* **2000**, *71*, 1735s–1738s. [CrossRef]
33. Santini, A.; Tenore, G.C.; Novellino, E. Nutraceuticals: A paradigm of proactive medicine. *Eur. J. Pharm. Sci.* **2017**, *96*, 53–61. [CrossRef]
34. Rajasekaran, A.; Sivagnanam, G.; Xavier, R. Nutraceuticals as therapeutic agents: A Review. *Res. J. Pharm. Technol.* **2008**, *1*, 328–340.
35. Zhao, C.N.; Meng, X.; Li, Y.; Li, S.; Liu, Q.; Tang, G.Y.; Li, H. Fruits for Prevention and Treatment of Cardiovascular Diseases. *Nutrients* **2017**, *9*, 598. [CrossRef] [PubMed]
36. Suleria, H.A.R.; Butt, M.S.; Anjum, F.M.; Saeed, F.; Khalid, N. Onion: Nature protection against physiological threats. *Crit. Rev. Food Sci. Nutr.* **2015**, *55*, 50–66. [CrossRef] [PubMed]
37. Butt, M.S.; Imran, A.; Sharif, M.K.; Ahmad, R.S.; Xiao, H.; Imran, M.; Rsool, H.A. Black tea polyphenols: A mechanistic treatise. *Crit. Rev. Food Sci. Nutr.* **2014**, *54*, 1002–1011. [CrossRef] [PubMed]
38. Sultan, M.T.; Buttxs, M.S.; Qayyum, M.M.N.; Suleria, H.A.R. Immunity: Plants as effective mediators. *Crit. Rev. Food Sci. Nutr.* **2014**, *54*, 1298–1308. [CrossRef]

39. Chiu, H.-F.; Shen, Y.-C.; Venkatakrishnan, K.; Wang, C.-K. Popular functional foods and nutraceuticals with lipid lowering activity and in relation to cardiovascular disease, dyslipidemia, and related complications: An overview. *J. Food Bioact.* **2018**, *2*, 16–27. [CrossRef]
40. Gleeson, J.P.; Ryan, S.M.; Brayden, D.J. Oral delivery strategies for nutraceuticals: Delivery vehicles and absorption enhancers. *Trends Food Sci. Technol.* **2016**, *53*, 90–101. [CrossRef]
41. Wang, H.; Nair, M.G.; Strasburg, G.M.; Chang, Y.C.; Booren, A.M.; Gray, J.I.; DeWitt, D.L. Antioxidant and antiinflammatory activities of anthocyanins and their aglycon, cyanidin, from tart cherries. *J. Nat. Prod.* **1999**, *62*, 294–296. [CrossRef]
42. Grzesik, M.; Naparło, K.; Bartosz, G.; Sadowska-Bartosz, I. Antioxidant properties of catechins: Comparison with other antioxidants. *Food Chem.* **2018**, *241*, 480–492. [CrossRef]
43. Wang, J.; Mazza, G. Inhibitory effects of anthocyanins and other phenolic compounds on nitric oxide production in LPS/IFN-γ-activated RAW 264.7 macrophages. *J. Agric. Food Chem.* **2002**, *50*, 850–857. [CrossRef] [PubMed]
44. Martínez, V.; Mitjans, M.; Vinardell, M.P. Cytoprotective Effects of Polyphenols against Oxidative Damage. *Polyphen. Hum. Health Dis.* **2014**, *1*, 275–288.
45. Munin, A.; Edwards-Lévy, F. Encapsulation of natural polyphenolic compounds: A review. *Pharmaceutics* **2011**, *3*, 793–829. [CrossRef] [PubMed]
46. Kelley, D.S.; Adkins, Y.; Laugero, K.D. A review of the health benefits of cherries. *Nutrients* **2018**, *10*, 368. [CrossRef]
47. McCune, L.M.; Kubota, C.; Stendell-Hollis, N.R.; Thomson, C.A. Cherries and Health: A Review. *Crit. Rev. Food Sci. Nutr.* **2010**, *51*, 1–12. [CrossRef]
48. Ferretti, G.; Bacchetti, T.; Belleggia, A.; Neri, D. Cherry antioxidants: From farm to table. *Molecules* **2010**, *15*, 6993–7005. [CrossRef]
49. Gonzales, G.B.; Smagghe, G.; Grootaert, C.; Zotti, M.; Raes, K.; Van Camp, J. Flavonoid interactions during digestion, absorption, distribution and metabolism: A sequential structure–activity/property relationship-based approach in the study of bioavailability and bioactivity. *Drug Metab. Rev.* **2015**, *47*, 175–190. [CrossRef]
50. Chockchaisawasdee, S.; Golding, J.B.; Vuong, Q.V.; Papoutsis, K.; Stathopoulos, C.E. Sweet cherry: Composition, postharvest preservation, processing and trends for its future use. *Trends Food Sci. Technol.* **2016**, *55*, 72–83. [CrossRef]
51. Średnicka-Tober, D.; Ponde, A.; Hallmann, E.; Głowacka, A.; Rozpara, E. The Profile and Content of Polyphenols and Carotenoids in Local and Commercial Sweet Cherry Fruits (*Prunus avium* L.) and Their Antioxidant Activity In Vitro. *Antioxidants* **2019**, *8*, 534. [CrossRef]
52. Berni, R.; Cantini, C.; Romi, M.; Hausman, J.F.; Guerriero, G.; Cai, G. Agrobiotechnology Goes Wild: Ancient Local Varieties as Sources of Bioactives. *Int. J. Mol. Sci.* **2018**, *19*, 2248. [CrossRef]
53. Berni, R.; Romi, M.; Cantini, C.; Hausman, J.F.; Guerriero, G.; Cai, G. Functional Molecules in Locally-Adapted Crops: The Case Study of Tomatoes, Onions, and Sweet Cherry Fruits from Tuscany in Italy. *Front. Plant Sci.* **2018**, *9*, 1983. [CrossRef] [PubMed]
54. Coelho, L.; De Lima, R.; De Oliveira Assumpção, C.; Prestes, J.; Denadai, B.S. Consumption of cherries as a strategy to attenuate exercise-induced muscle damage and inflammation in humans. *Nutr. Hosp.* **2015**, *32*, 1885–1893.
55. Kelley, D.S.; Adkins, Y.; Reddy, A.; Woodhouse, L.R.; Mackey, B.E.; Erickson, K.L. Sweet Bing Cherries Lower Circulating Concentrations of Markers for Chronic Inflammatory Diseases in Healthy Humans. *J. Nutr.* **2013**, *143*, 340–344. [CrossRef] [PubMed]
56. Keane, K.M.; George, T.W.; Constantinou, C.L.; Brown, M.A.; Clifford, T.; Howatson, G. Effects of Montmorency tart cherry (*Prunus Cerasus*, L.) consumption on vascular function in men with early hypertension. *Am. J. Clin. Nutr.* **2016**, *103*, 1531–1539. [CrossRef]
57. Ben Lagha, A.; LeBel, G.; Grenier, D. Tart cherry (*Prunus cerasus* L.) fractions inhibit biofilm formation and adherence properties of oral pathogens and enhance oral epithelial barrier function. *Phytother. Res.* **2019**. [CrossRef]
58. Lietava, J.; Beerova, N.; Klymenko, S.V.; Panghyova, E.; Varga, I.; Pechanova, O. Effects of Cornelian Cherry on Atherosclerosis and Its Risk Factors. *Oxid. Med. Cell. Longev.* **2019**, *6*, 1–8. [CrossRef]

59. Robinson, J.L.; Hunter, J.M.; Reyes-Izquierdo, T.; Argumedo, R.; Brizuela-Bastien, J.; Keller, R.; Pietrzkowski, Z. Cognitive short- and long-term effects of coffee cherry extract in older adults with mild cognitive decline. *Neuropsychol. Dev. Cognit. B Aging Neuropsychol. Cognit.* **2019**. [CrossRef]
60. Scalbert, A.; Manach, C.; Morand, C.; Rémésy, C.; Jiménez, L. Dietary polyphenols and the prevention of diseases. *Food Sci. Nutr.* **2005**, *45*, 287–306. [CrossRef]
61. Kashi, D.S.; Shabir, A.; Da Boit, M.; Bailey, S.J.; Higgins, M.F. The Effcacy of administering fruit-derived polyphenols to improve health biomarkers, exercise performance and related physiological responses. *Nutrients* **2019**, *11*, 2389. [CrossRef]
62. Edwards, M.; Czank, C.; Woodward, G.M.; Cassidy, A.; Kay, C.D. Phenolic metabolites of anthocyanins modulate mechanisms of endothelial function. *J. Agric. Food Chem.* **2015**, *63*, 2423–2431. [CrossRef]
63. Fratantonio, D.; Cimino, F.; Molonia, M.S.; Ferrari, D.; Saija, A.; Virgili, F.; Speciale, A. Cyanidin-3-O-glucoside ameliorates palmitate-induced insulin resistance by modulating IRS-1 phosphorylation and release of endothelial derived vasoactive factors. *Biochim. Biophys. Acta Mol. Cell Biol. Lipids* **2017**, *1862*, 351–357. [CrossRef] [PubMed]
64. Xue, F.; Nie, X.; Shi, J.; Liu, Q.; Wang, Z.; Li, X.; Zhou, J.; Su, J.; Xue, M.; Chen, W.D.; et al. Quercetin inhibits LPS-induced inflammation and ox-LDL-induced lipid deposition. *Front. Pharmacol.* **2017**, *8*, 1–8. [CrossRef] [PubMed]
65. Console, L.; Giangregorio, N.; Cellamare, S.; Bolognino, I.; Palasciano, M.; Indiveri, C.; Incampo, G.; Campana, S.; Tonazzi, A. Human mitochondrial carnitine acylcarnitine carrier: Molecular target of dietary bioactive polyphenols from sweet cherry (*Prunus avium* L.). *Chem. Biol. Interact.* **2019**, *307*, 179–185. [CrossRef] [PubMed]
66. Beconcini, D.; Fabiano, A.; Zambito, Y.; Berni, R.; Santoni, T.; Piras, A.M.; Di Stefano, R. Chitosan-Based Nanoparticles Containing Cherry Extract from *Prunus avium* L. to Improve the Resistance of Endothelial Cells to Oxidative Stress. *Nutrients* **2018**, *10*, 1598. [CrossRef] [PubMed]
67. Beconcini, D.; Felice, F.; Zambito, Y.; Fabiano, A.; Piras, A.M.; Macedo, M.H.; Sarmento, B.; Di Stefano, R. Anti-Inflammatory Effect of Cherry Extract Loaded in Polymeric Nanoparticles: Relevance of Particle Internalization in Endothelial Cells. *Pharmaceutics* **2019**, *11*, 500. [CrossRef] [PubMed]
68. Saha, M. Nanomedicine: Promising Tiny Machine for the Healthcare in Future-A Review. *Oman Med. J.* **2009**, *24*, 242–247. [CrossRef]
69. Fang, Z.; Bhandari, B. Encapsulation of polyphenols—A review. *Trends Food Sci. Technol.* **2010**, *21*, 510–523. [CrossRef]
70. McClements, D.J.; Jafari, S.M. General Aspects of Nanoemulsions and Their Formulation. In *Nanoemulsions: Formulation, Applications, and Characterization*; Academic Press: Cambridge, MS, USA, 2018; pp. 3–20. ISBN 9780128118399.
71. Aditya, N.P.; Espinosa, Y.G.; Norton, I.T. Encapsulation systems for the delivery of hydrophilic nutraceuticals: Food application. *Biotechnol. Adv.* **2017**, *35*, 450–457. [CrossRef]
72. Punia, S.; Sandhu, K.S.; Kaur, M.; Siroha, A.K. Nanotechnology: A Successful Approach to Improve Nutraceutical Bioavailability. In *Nanobiotechnology in Bioformulations*; Springer: Cham, Switzerland, 2019; pp. 119–133.
73. Kawashima, Y. Nanoparticulate systems for improved drug delivery. *Adv. Drug Deliv. Rev.* **2001**, *47*, 1–2. [CrossRef]
74. Desai, M.P.; Labhasetwar, V.; Walter, E.; Levy, R.J.; Amidon, G.L. The mechanism of uptake of biodegradable microparticles in Caco-2 cells is size dependent. *Pharm. Res.* **1997**, *14*, 1568–1573. [CrossRef]
75. El-Say, K.M.; El-Sawy, H.S. Polymeric nanoparticles: Promising platform for drug delivery. *Int. J. Pharm.* **2017**, *528*, 675–691. [CrossRef] [PubMed]
76. Felice, F.; Zambito, Y.; Di Colo, G.; D'Onofrio, C.; Fausto, C.; Balbarini, A.; Di Stefano, R. Red grape skin and seeds polyphenols: Evidence of their protective effects on endothelial progenitor cells and improvement of their intestinal absorption. *Eur. J. Pharm. Biopharm.* **2012**, *80*, 176–184. [CrossRef] [PubMed]
77. Felice, F.; Zambito, Y.; Belardinelli, E.; D'Onofrio, C.; Fabiano, A.; Balbarini, A.; Di Stefano, R. Delivery of natural polyphenols by polymeric nanoparticles improves the resistance of endothelial progenitor cells to oxidative stress. *Eur. J. Pharm. Sci.* **2013**, *50*, 393–399. [CrossRef] [PubMed]

78. Fabiano, A.; Piras, A.M.; Uccello-Barretta, G.; Balzano, F.; Cesari, A.; Testai, L.; Citi, V.; Zambito, Y. Impact of mucoadhesive polymeric nanoparticulate systems on oral bioavailability of a macromolecular model drug. *Eur. J. Pharm. Biopharm.* **2018**, *130*, 281–289. [CrossRef]
79. Makadia, H.K.; Siegel, S.J. Poly Lactic-co-Glycolic Acid (PLGA) as biodegradable controlled drug delivery carrier. *Polymers* **2011**, *3*, 1377–1397. [CrossRef]
80. Watkins, R.; Wu, L.; Zhang, C.; Davis, R.M.; Xu, B. Natural product-based nanomedicine: Recent advances and issues. *Int. J. Nanomed.* **2015**, *10*, 6055–6074.
81. Wang, S.; Su, R.; Nie, S.; Sun, M.; Zhang, J.; Wu, D.; Moustaid-Moussa, N. Application of nanotechnology in improving bioavailability and bioactivity of diet-derived phytochemicals. *J. Nutr. Biochem.* **2014**, *25*, 363–376. [CrossRef]
82. Beconcini, D.; Fabiano, A.; Di Stefano, R.; Macedo, M.H.; Felice, F.; Zambito, Y.; Sarmento, B. Cherry Extract from *Prunus avium* L. to Improve the Resistance of Endothelial Cells to Oxidative Stress: Mucoadhesive Chitosan vs. Poly(lactic-co-glycolic acid) Nanoparticles. *Int. J. Mol. Sci.* **2019**, *20*, 1759. [CrossRef]
83. Bilia, A.R.; Piazzini, V.; Risaliti, L.; Vanti, G.; Casamonti, M.; Wang, M.; Bergonzi, M.C. Nanocarriers: A successful tool to increase solubility, stability and optimise bioefficacy of natural constituents. *Curr. Med. Chem.* **2019**, *26*, 4631–4656. [CrossRef]
84. Sinico, C.; Caddeo, C.; Valenti, D.; Fadda, A.M.; Bilia, A.R.; Vincieri, F.F. Liposomes as carriers for verbascoside: Stability and skin permeation studies. *J. Liposome Res.* **2008**, *18*, 83–90. [CrossRef]
85. Bangham, A.D.; Standish, M.M.; Watkins, J.C. Diffusion of univalent ions across the lamellae of swollen phospholipids. *J. Mol. Biol.* **1965**, *13*, 238–252. [CrossRef]
86. Van Hoogevest, P.; Wendel, A. The use of natural and synthetic phospholipids as pharmaceutical excipients. *Eur. J. Lipid Sci. Technol.* **2014**, *116*, 1088–1107. [CrossRef] [PubMed]
87. Çağdaş, M.; Sezer, A.D.; Bucak, S. Liposomes as potential drug carrier systems for drug delivery. In *Application of Nanotechnology in Drug Delivery*; IntechOpen: London, UK, 2014.
88. Li, M.; Du, C.; Guo, N.; Teng, Y.; Meng, X.; Sun, H.; Li, S.; Yu, P.; Galons, H. Composition design and medical application of liposomes. *Eur. J. Med. Chem.* **2019**, *164*, 640–653. [CrossRef] [PubMed]
89. Akbarzadeh, A.; Rezaei-Sadabady, R.; Davaran, S.; Joo, S.W.; Zarghami, N.; Hanifehpour, Y.; Samiei, M.; Kouhi, M.; Nejati-Koshki, K. Liposome: Classification, preparation, and applications. *Nanoscale Res. Lett.* **2013**, *8*, 102. [CrossRef] [PubMed]
90. Risaliti, L. Nanocarriers for the Oral and Topical Delivery of Natural Compounds. Ph.D. Thesis, University of Florence, Florence, Italy, 2019.
91. Gibis, M.; Ruedt, C.; Weiss, J. In vitro release of grape-seed polyphenols encapsulated from uncoated and chitosan-coated liposomes. *Food Res. Int.* **2016**, *88*, 105–113. [CrossRef] [PubMed]
92. Feng, T.; Wei, Y.; Lee, R.J.; Zhao, L. Liposomal curcumin and its application in cancer. *Int. J. Nanomed.* **2017**, *12*, 6027–6044. [CrossRef] [PubMed]
93. Ma, Y.; Fu, L.; Hussain, Z.; Huang, D.; Zhu, S. Enhancement of storability and antioxidant systems of sweet cherry fruit by nitric oxide-releasing chitosan nanoparticles (GSNO-CS NPs). *Food Chem.* **2019**, *285*, 10. [CrossRef]
94. Artursson, P.; Lindmark, T.; Davis, S.S.; Illum, L. Effect of chitosan on the permeability of monolayers of intestinal epithelial cells (Caco-2). *Pharm. Res.* **1994**, *11*, 1358–1361. [CrossRef]
95. Peniche, H.; Peniche, C. Chitosan nanoparticles: A contribution to nanomedicine. *Polym. Int.* **2011**, *60*, 883–889. [CrossRef]
96. Kerch, G. The potential of chitosan and its derivatives in prevention and treatment of Age-related diseases. *Mar. Drugs* **2015**, *13*, 2158–2182. [CrossRef]
97. Ways, T.M.M.; Lau, W.M.; Khutoryanskiy, V.V. Chitosan and its derivatives for application in mucoadhesive drug delivery systems. *Polymers* **2018**, *10*, 267. [CrossRef] [PubMed]
98. Kotzé, A.F.; Lueßen, H.L.; De Leeuw, B.J.; De Boer, B.G.; Coos Verhoef, J. Comparison of the effect of different chitosan salts and N-trimethyl chitosan chloride on the permeability of intestinal epithelial cells (Caco-2). *J. Controll. Release* **1998**, *51*, 35–46. [CrossRef]
99. Kotzé, A.F.; De Leeuw, B.J.; Lueßen, H.L.; De Boer, A.G.; Verhoef, J.C.; Junginger, H.E. Chitosans for enhanced delivery of therapeutic peptides across intestinal epithelia: In vitro evaluation in Caco-2 cell monolayers. *Int. J. Pharm.* **1997**, *159*, 243–253. [CrossRef]

100. Ylenia, Z.; di Colo, G. Thiolated quaternary ammonium–chitosan conjugates for enhanced precorneal retention, transcorneal permeation and intraocular absorption of dexamethasone. *Eur. J. Pharm. Biopharm.* **2010**, *75*, 194–199.
101. Fabiano, A.; Mattii, L.; Braca, A.; Felice, F.; Di Stefano, R.; Zambito, Y. Nanoparticles based on quaternary ammonium-chitosan conjugate: A vehicle for oral administration of antioxidants contained in red grapes. *J. Drug Deliv. Sci. Technol.* **2016**, *32*, 291–297. [CrossRef]
102. Li, Z.; Jiang, H.; Xu, C.; Gu, L. A review: Using nanoparticles to enhance absorption and bioavailability of phenolic phytochemicals. *Food Hydrocoll.* **2015**, *43*, 153–164. [CrossRef]
103. Hembram, K.C.; Prabha, S.; Chandra, R.; Ahmed, B.; Nimesh, S. Advances in preparation and characterization of chitosan nanoparticles for therapeutics. *Artif. Cells Nanomed. Biotechnol.* **2016**, *44*, 305–314. [CrossRef]
104. Zambito, Y.; Felice, F.; Fabiano, A.; Di Stefano, R.; Di Colo, G. Mucoadhesive nanoparticles made of thiolated quaternary chitosan crosslinked with hyaluronan. *Carbohydr. Polym.* **2013**, *92*, 33–39. [CrossRef]
105. Ba, C.; Fu, Y.; Niu, F.; Wang, M.; Jin, B.; Li, Z.; Chen, G.; Zhang, H.; Li, X. Effects of environmental stresses on physiochemical stability of β-carotene in zein-carboxymethyl chitosan-tea polyphenols ternary delivery system. *Food Chem.* **2020**, *311*, 125878. [CrossRef]
106. Khan, M.A.; Yue, C.; Fang, Z.; Hu, S.; Cheng, H.; Bakry, A.M.; Liang, L. Alginate/chitosan-coated zein nanoparticles for the delivery of resveratrol. *J. Food Eng.* **2019**, *258*, 4553. [CrossRef]
107. Danhier, F.; Ansorena, E.; Silva, J.M.; Coco, R.; Le Breton, A.; Préat, V. PLGA-based nanoparticles: An overview of biomedical applications. *J. Controll. Release* **2012**, *161*, 505–522. [CrossRef] [PubMed]
108. Sousa, F.; Cruz, A.; Fonte, P.; Pinto, I.M.; Neves-Petersen, M.T.; Sarmento, B. A new paradigm for antiangiogenic therapy through controlled release of bevacizumab from PLGA nanoparticles. *Sci. Rep.* **2017**, *7*, 3736. [CrossRef] [PubMed]
109. Pereira, M.C.; Oliveira, D.A.; Hill, L.E.; Zambiazi, R.C.; Borges, C.D.; Vizzotto, M.; Mertens-Talcott, S.; Talcott, S.; Gomes, C.L. Effect of nanoencapsulation using PLGA on antioxidant and antimicrobial activities of guabiroba fruit phenolic extract. *Food Chem.* **2018**, *240*, 396–404. [CrossRef] [PubMed]
110. Kumar, P.; Singh, A.K.; Raj, V.; Rai, A.; Keshari, A.K.; Kumar, D.; Maity, B.; Prakash, A.; Maiti, S.; Saha, S. Poly(lactic-co-glycolic acid)-loaded nanoparticles of betulinic acid for improved treatment of hepatic cancer: Characterization, in vitro and in vivo evaluations. *Int. J. Nanomed.* **2018**, *13*, 975. [CrossRef]
111. Silva, L.M.; Hill, L.E.; Figueiredo, E.; Gomes, C.L. Delivery of phytochemicals of tropical fruit by-products using poly (DL-lactide-co-glycolide) (PLGA) nanoparticles: Synthesis, characterization, and antimicrobial activity. *Food Chem.* **2014**, *165*, 362–370. [CrossRef]
112. Danhier, F. To exploit the tumor microenvironment: Since the EPR effect fails in the clinic, what is the future of nanomedicine? *J. Controll. Release* **2016**, *244*, 108–121. [CrossRef]
113. Tahara, K.; Sakai, T.; Yamamoto, H.; Takeuchi, H.; Hirashima, N.; Kawashima, Y. Improved cellular uptake of chitosan-modified PLGA nanospheres by A549 cells. *Int. J. Pharm.* **2009**, *382*, 198–204. [CrossRef]
114. Gref, R.; Minamitake, Y.; Peracchia, M.T.; Trubetskoy, V.; Torchilin, V.; Langer, R. Biodegradable long-circulating polymeric nanospheres. *Science* **1994**, *263*, 1600–1603. [CrossRef]
115. Davatgaran-Taghipour, Y.; Masoomzadeh, S.; Farzaei, M.H.; Bahramsoltani, R.; Karimi-Soureh, Z.; Rahimi, R.; Abdollahi, M. Polyphenol nanoformulations for cancer therapy: Experimental evidence and clinical perspective. *Int. J. Nanomed.* **2017**, *12*, 2689–2702. [CrossRef]
116. Yu, F.; Ao, M.; Zheng, X.; Li, N.; Xia, J.; Li, Y.; Li, D.; Hou, Z.; Qi, Z.; Chen, X.D. PEG-lipid-PLGA hybrid nanoparticles loaded with berberine-phospholipid complex to facilitate the oral delivery efficiency. *Drug Deliv.* **2017**, *24*, 825–833. [CrossRef]
117. Abd-Rabou, A.A.; Abdalla, A.M.; Ali, N.A.; Zoheir, K.M.A. Moringa oleifera root induces cancer apoptosis more effectively than leave nanocomposites and its free counterpart. *APJCP* **2017**, *18*, 2141–2149.
118. Doolaanea, A.A.; Mansor, N.I.; Mohd Nor, N.H.; Mohamed, F. Co-encapsulation of Nigella sativa oil and plasmid DNA for enhanced gene therapy of Alzheimers disease. *J. Microencapsul.* **2016**, *33*, 114–126. [CrossRef] [PubMed]
119. Rashidinejad, A.; Birch, E.J.; Sun-Waterhouse, D.; Everett, D.W. Delivery of green tea catechin and epigallocatechin gallate in liposomes incorporated into low-fat hard cheese. *Food Chem.* **2014**, *156*, 176–183. [CrossRef] [PubMed]
120. Kapoor, B.; Gupta, R.; Gulati, M.; Singh, S.K.; Khursheed, R.; Gupta, M. The Why, Where, Who, How, and What of the vesicular delivery systems. *Adv. Colloid Interface Sci.* **2019**, *271*, 101985. [CrossRef] [PubMed]

121. Bangham, A.D.; Hill, M.W.; Miller, N.G.A. Preparation and use of liposomes as models of biological membranes. In *Methods in Membrane Biology*; Springer: Boston, MA, USA, 1974; pp. 1–68.
122. Deamer, D.; Bangham, A.D. Large volume liposomes by an ether vaporization method. *Biochim. Biophys. Acta Biomembr.* **1976**, *443*, 629–634. [CrossRef]
123. Gabizon, A.; Chisin, R.; Amselem, S.; Druckmann, S.; Cohen, R.; Goren, D.; Fromer, I.; Peretz, T.; Sulkes, A.; Barenholz, Y. Pharmacokinetic and imaging studies in patients receiving a formulation of liposome-associated adriamycin. *Br. J. Cancer* **1991**, *64*, 1125–1132. [CrossRef]
124. Bilia, A.R.; Piazzini, V.; Guccione, C.; Risaliti, L.; Asprea, M.; Capecchi, G.; Bergonzi, M.C. Improving on nature: The role of nanomedicine in the development of clinical natural drugs. *Planta Med.* **2017**, *83*, 366–381. [CrossRef]
125. Yoshida, P.A.; Yokota, D.; Foglio, M.A.; Rodrigues, R.A.F.; Pinho, S.C. Liposomes incorporating essential oil of Brazilian cherry (*Eugenia uniflora* L.): Characterization of aqueous dispersions and lyophilized formulations. *J. Microencapsul.* **2010**, *27*, 416–425. [CrossRef]
126. Akgün, D.; Gültekin-Özgüven, M.; Yücetepe, A.; Altin, G.; Gibis, M.; Weiss, J.; Özçelik, B. Stirred-type yoghurt incorporated with sour cherry extract in chitosan-coated liposomes. *Food Hydrocoll.* **2020**, *101*, 105532. [CrossRef]
127. Lozoya-Agullo, I.; Araújo, F.; González-Álvarez, I.; Merino-Sanjuán, M.; González-Álvarez, M.; Bermejo, M.; Sarmento, B. Usefulness of Caco-2/HT29-MTX and Caco-2/HT29-MTX/Raji B coculture models to predict intestinal and colonic permeability compared to Caco-2 monoculture. *Mol. Pharm.* **2017**, *14*, 1264–1270. [CrossRef]
128. Araújo, F.; das Neves, J.; Martins, J.P.; Granja, P.L.; Santos, H.A.; Sarmento, B. Functionalized materials for multistage platforms in the oral delivery of biopharmaceuticals. *Prog. Mater. Sci.* **2017**, *89*, 306–344. [CrossRef]
129. Angela, M. The effect of gastro-intestinal mucus on drug absorption. *Adv. Drug Deliv. Rev.* **1993**, *11*, 201–220.
130. Araújo, F.; Sarmento, B. Towards the characterization of an in vitro triple co-culture intestine cell model for permeability studies. *Int. J. Pharm.* **2013**, *458*, 128–134. [CrossRef] [PubMed]
131. Kafedjiiski, K.; Hoffer, M.; Werle, M.; Bernkop-Schnürch, A. Improved synthesis and in vitro characterization of chitosan–thioethylamidine conjugate. *Biomat* **2006**, *27*, 127–135. [CrossRef]
132. Otero, J.; García-Rodríguez, A.; Cano-Sarabia, M.; Maspoch, D.; Marcos, R.; Cortés, P.; Llagostera, M. Biodistribution of liposome-encapsulated bacteriophages and their transcytosis during oral phage therapy. *Front. Microbiol.* **2019**, *10*, 689. [CrossRef]
133. Belubbi, T.; Shevade, S.; Dhawan, V.; Sridhar, V.; Majumdar, A.; Nunes, R.; Araújo, F.; Sarmento, B.; Nagarsenker, K.; Steiniger, F.; et al. Lipid Architectonics for Superior Oral Bioavailability of Nelfinavir Mesylate: Comparative in vitro and in vivo Assessment. *AAPS PharmSciTech* **2018**, *19*, 3584–3598. [CrossRef]

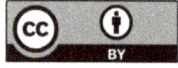

© 2020 by the authors. Licensee MDPI, Basel, Switzerland. This article is an open access article distributed under the terms and conditions of the Creative Commons Attribution (CC BY) license (http://creativecommons.org/licenses/by/4.0/).

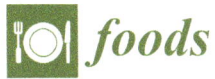

Review

Phytochemicals and Traditional Use of Two Southernmost Chilean Berry Fruits: Murta (*Ugni molinae* Turcz) and Calafate (*Berberis buxifolia* Lam.)

Carolina Fredes [1], Alejandra Parada [1], Jaime Salinas [2] and Paz Robert [3,*]

1. Departamento Ciencias de la Salud, Carrera de Nutrición y Dietética, Facultad de Medicina, Pontificia Universidad Católica de Chile, Santiago 7820436, Chile; cpfredes@uc.cl (C.F.); acparada@uc.cl (A.P.)
2. Instituto Forestal, Sede Coyhaique, Coyhaique 5951840, Chile; jsalinas@infor.cl
3. Departamento Ciencia de los Alimentos y Tecnología Química, Facultad de Ciencias Químicas y Farmacéuticas, Universidad de Chile, Santiago 8380592, Chile
* Correspondence: proberts@uchile.cl; Tel.: +56-229-781-666

Received: 30 November 2019; Accepted: 30 December 2019; Published: 6 January 2020

Abstract: Murta and calafate have been traditionally used by indigenous and rural peoples of Chile. Research on murta and calafate has gained interest due to their attractive sensory properties as well as a global trend in finding new fruits with potential health benefits. The objective of this review was to summarize the potential use of murta and calafate as sources of nutraceuticals regarding both the traditional and the up-to-date scientific knowledge. A search of historical documents recorded in the Digital National Library as well as scientific articles in the Web of Science database were performed using combinations of keywords with the botanical nomenclature. Peer-reviewed scientific articles did meet the inclusion criteria ($n = 38$) were classified in phytochemicals (21 papers) and biological activity (17 papers). Murta and calafate are high oxygen radical absorbance capacity (ORAC)-value fruits and promising sources of natural antioxidants, antimicrobial, and vasodilator compounds with nutraceutical potential. The bioactivity of anthocyanin metabolites in murta and calafate must continue to be studied in order to achieve adequate information on the biological activity and health-promoting effects derived for the consumption of murta and calafate fruit.

Keywords: anti-inflammatory; antimicrobial; antioxidant; anthocyanins; medicinal foods; nutraceuticals

1. Introduction

Historically, indigenous peoples of Chile have had a deep relationship with nature; flora native to their territories has been used for various purposes, such as food, fuel, religious ceremonies, decoration, dyeing, and medicine [1]. In this context, the Mapuche ("people of the earth" in the Mapuzugun language) hold a vast, rich body of knowledge about flora that has been learned and transmitted within the culture throughout space and time [2,3]. Moreover, southernmost communities, such as the Aónikenk ("people of the south" in the Aónikoaish language) and the Yámana ("human being" in the Yahgan language), collected several edible plant roots, wild fruits, and seeds to survive in extremally harsh conditions [4]. In these particular areas, two small berry-type fruits known as murta, murtilla, or uñi (*Ugni molinae* Turcz, *Myrtaceae*) and calafate (*Berberis buxifolia* Lam., *Berberidaceae*) grow in the wild of the Patagonia. Murta is an evergreen bush that naturally grows in Chile from south of Talca (35° SL) to the Palena River (44° SL) (Figure 1), forming part of the deciduous forests of *Nothofagus* as well as the southern evergreen forests [5]. In these habitats, murta grows alongside other edible Chilean fruit plants such as peumo (*Cryptocarya alba*), boldo (*Peumus boldus*), keule (*Gomortega queule*), avellano or gevuin

(*Gevuina avellana*), diverse michay species (*Berberis darwinii*, *B. serrata*, *B. dentata*), litre (*Lithraea caustica*), pitra (*Myrceugenia planipes*), and luma (*Amomyrtus luma*) [1]. Calafate is an evergreen spiny bush which naturally grows in Chile from Curicó (35° SL) to the Cape Horn Archipelago (56° SL) [6]. Nevertheless, it is most abundant from Valdivia (40° SL) to the Strait of Magellan (54° SL) (Figure 1).

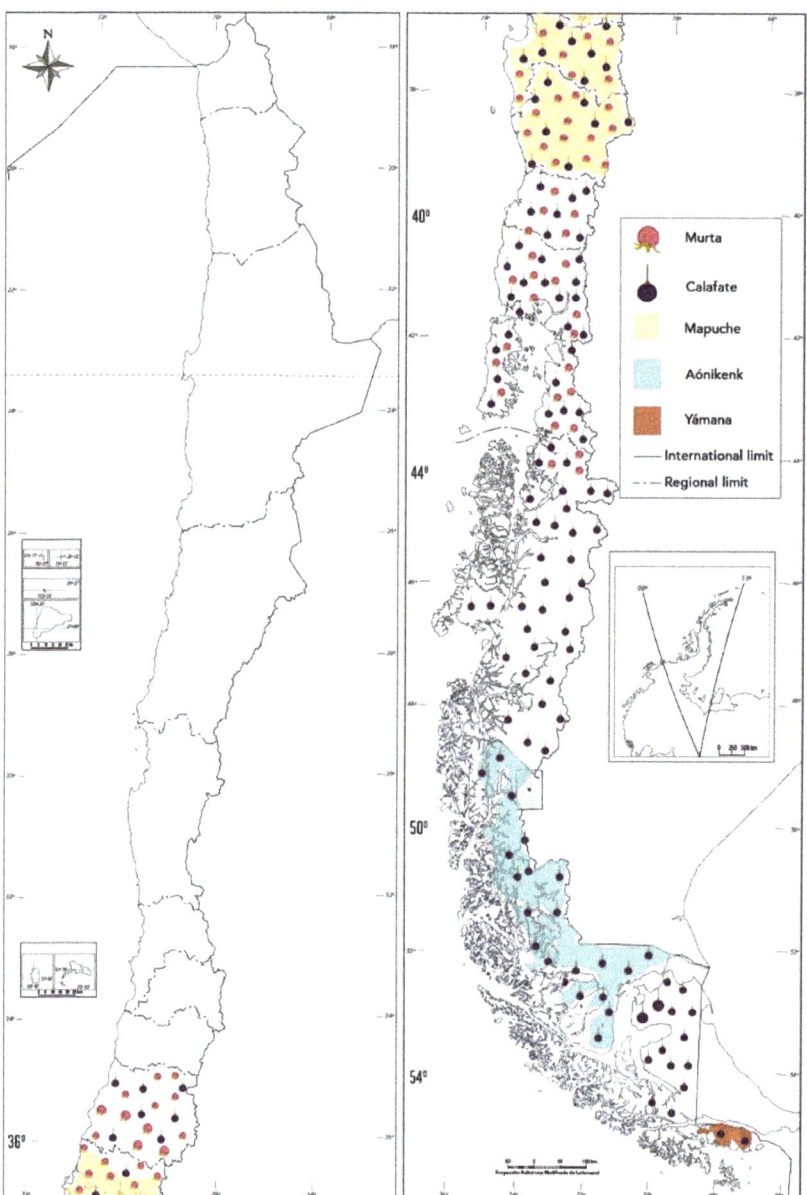

Figure 1. Distribution of murta (**red**) and calafate (**blue**) in a Chilean map, and the territory of Mapuche (**winter white**), Aónikenk (**soft blue**) and Yámana (**brown**).

During the last decade, interest in studying these berry-type fruits has increased, due to their attractive sensory properties as well as a global trend in finding new fruits with potential health benefits.

Berry-type fruits are well known for their high polyphenol, and especially anthocyanin content [7]. Specifically, wild berry-type fruits stand out over their cultivated counterparts in terms of polyphenol content [8]. Furthermore, the extreme weather conditions that predominate during southern Chilean summers (a high-temperature oscillation) may favor the plant biosynthesis of anthocyanins [9]. Both murta and calafate fruits can be sources of anthocyanins with nutraceutical potential. Lee [10] defined Nutraceuticals as foods or part of foods that provide both health benefits to reduce the risk of chronic diseases and basic nutrition. Therefore, this review summarizes the potential use of murta and calafate as sources of nutraceuticals regarding both the traditional and the up-to-date scientific knowledge. This review would like to contribute to the development of both new research and indigenous peoples, in line with the 2030 agenda for sustainable development goals of the United Nations with its promise to "leave no one behind".

2. Traditional Knowledge around Murta and Calafate

The search strategy of historical documents was focused in revising manuscripts written by recognized naturalists of the Chilean flora such as Juan Ignacio Molina (1740–1829) [11], Claude Gay (1800–1873) [12,13], Charles Darwin (1809–1882) [4], and Ernesto Wilhelm de Mosbach (1882–1963) [1] available in Digital National Library database (www.memoriachilena.cl). At the same time, ethnobotany and ethnopharmacology books were also suitable publications that were extensively reviewed.

2.1. Murta and Calafate in the Mapuche and Rural Culture

The Mapuche are the most prominent indigenous peoples in Chile, due to both their social and demographic weight and cultural identity. Mapuche have historically settled between the Itata (36° SL) and Toltén (38° SL) Rivers (Figure 1) in Chile [2]. In this sense, Figure 1 contrasts the wild distribution of murta and calafate and the historically territory occupied by the Mapuche people.

The first records regarding the traditional uses of murta fruit (Figure 2a) by the Mapuche indicate the preparation of a sweet stomach wine that was an appetite stimulant, and "whose aroma was appreciated as the most delicate Muscat" [11]. In this sense, the aromatic properties of murta fruits were early recognized; Gay [13] indicated that country people eat murta fruits with a great pleasure and prepared pleasant and aromatic confections. Nowadays people from the countryside consume murta as dried fruits and in the preparation of jams [14].

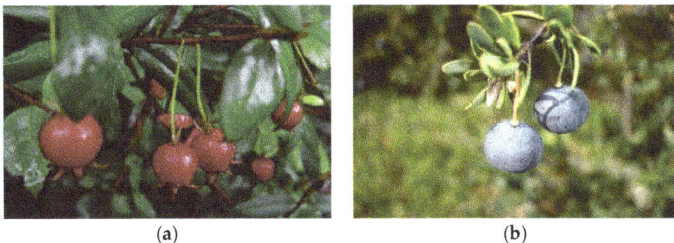

Figure 2. Murta (**a**) and calafate (**b**) fruits.

Mapuche used the word *maki* to name black fruits [1]. In this sense, calafate (Figure 2b) were appreciated as fruit rich in pigments where the root and bark of calafate were also used to obtain purple and yellow dyes [14].

The Mapuche tradition of using plants for medicinal purposes was recorded in the archives of the several settlers and naturalists who, in turn, enriched them with the contribution of medicinal plants from Europe and other regions [15]. Since 2008, the traditional use of medicinal plants has been recognized by the Chilean Health Ministry [16]. The traditional use of murta includes making a leaf infusion to treat urinary and throat infections, while the fruit is known for its astringent power [14,17].

In the case of calafate, traditional uses include using its roots to control fevers, as an anti-inflammatory, and to ease stomach pains, indigestion, and colitis [14,17].

2.2. Calafate in the Extreme South Communities of Chile

Historical records on the use of native flora as food and medicine by extreme south communities are more limited than the information available about the indigenous peoples of the central and southern zone of Chile. Among the communities of the extreme south Chile, the Aónikenk were an exclusively cultural entity defined by a particular tradition, language, and lifestyle [18], who occupied the territory located between the Santa Cruz River (50° SL) and the Strait of Magellan (54° SL) (Figure 1). The Aónikenk had a significant collecting tradition in which not only women participated but also involved men, children, and occasionally elderly people [18]. Calafate as well as other native fruits like zarzaparrilla (*Ribes magellanicum*), chaura (*Pernettya mucronata*), murtilla (*Empetrum rubrum*), and strawberry (*Rubus geoides*) were consumed mainly as fresh fruits during the harvest season (November to March) [4]. Furthermore, Aónikenk women occasionally painted their faces with calafate juice, believing it would whiten the skin tone [18].

The Yámana were the southernmost ethnic group in the world who lived in the territory of the Cape Horn Archipelago (56° SL) in the south of Tierra del Fuego Island and the Beagle Channel (Figure 1) [18]. Yámana were maritime hunter-gatherers who spent much of their lives in their anan (tree bark canoe). Men collected firewood, fruits, and vegetables [19]. A Yámana legend says that whoever tastes the bittersweet flavor of calafate will return to the extreme south territory [20].

3. Scientific Knowledge around Murta and Calafate

The search strategy of scientific literature is detailed in the flow diagram of Figure 3.

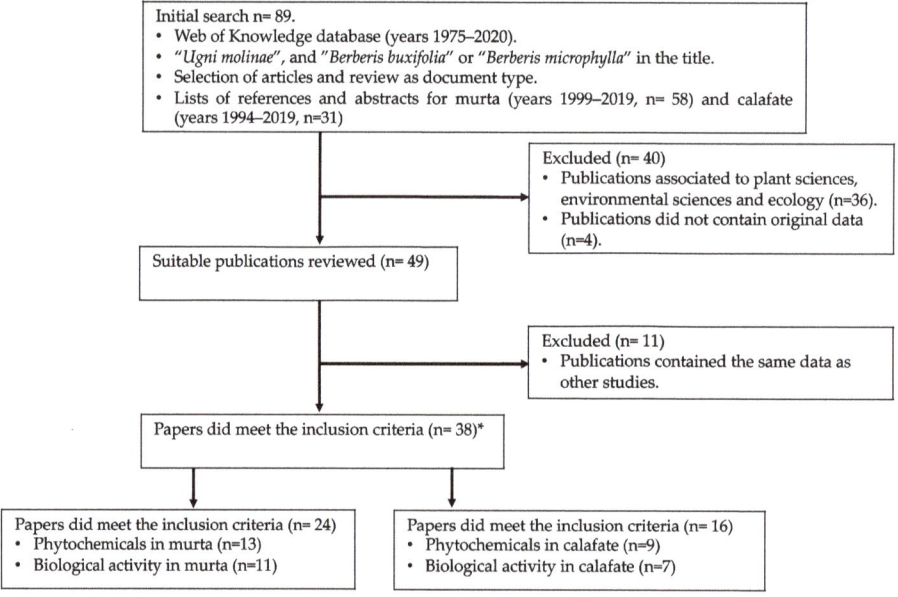

Figure 3. Summary of the search and selection protocols used to identify scientific articles included in the review.

Relevant publications were identified through an initial search in Web of Science database using the current botanical nomenclature in the title. The time interval for obtaining the records was between 1975 and 2020. Since 1994, the search results identified a higher number of documents on murta (58 records) than on calafate (31 records). Each abstract was revised and publications associated to plant sciences, environmental sciences and ecology that did not report any information about nutritional and phytochemical composition of murta and calafate (36 records) were excluded. At the same time, publications that did not contain original data (four records) were also excluded. Suitable publications were extensively reviewed and scientific articles contained the same data as other studies (11 papers) were excluded. Papers did meet the inclusion criteria were classified in phytochemicals (21 papers) and biological activity (17 papers) in terms to analyze the the up-to-date scientific evidence of murta and calafate as sources of nutraceuticals.

3.1. Nutritional Content of Murta and Calafate Fruits

Murta fruit has a soluble solid content (SS) around 19 °Brix, a titratable acid around 8 meq Na OH/100 g, and a pH around 4.3 [21]. The sensory properties of murta fruit include the sweetness of a strawberry, the pungency of a guava, and the texture of a dried blueberry [22]. Furthermore, volatile compounds identified in murta fruit aroma have been described as fruity, sweet, and floral; ethyl hexanoate and 4-methoxy-2,5-dimethyl-furan-3-one are the most potent compounds found in murta [23]. The proximate analysis of murta fruit shows a content in moisture of 76.9%, protein of 1.2 g/100 g, fat of 0.9 g/100 g, crude fibre of 2.5 g/100 g, ash of 0.5 g/100 g and carbohydrates (by difference) of 18.5 g/100g expressed on fresh weight (FW) [24]. Furthermore, murta has a content in ascorbic acid of 210 mg/100 g [25].

Calafate fruit has a SS content between 25–31 °Brix and a titratable acid around 2 g malic acid/100 g (15 meq NaOH/100 g) [26]. Calafate fruit has a higher SS content than murta, and the highest SS content in comparison to other berries such as maqui (19 °Brix), pomegranate (15 °Brix), blueberry (14 °Brix), blackberry (13 °Brix), red raspberry (11 °Brix), and strawberry (9 °Brix) [27]. The proximate composition, sugars, and ascorbic acid of calafate fruit shows a content in moisture of 75%, protein of 2.6 g/100 g, ether extract of 0.18 g/100 g, crude fibre of 7.0 g/100 g, ash of 0.9 g/100 g, glucose of 3.0 g/100 g, fructose of 0.8 g/100 g and ascorbic acid of 74.0 mg/100 g expressed on FW [28].

3.2. Phytochemicals in Murta and Calafate Fruits

Phytochemicals (i.e., phenolic compounds, terpenoids, alkaloids, and nitrogen-containing compounds) can be defined as non-nutrient chemicals found in plants that demonstrate biological activity against chronic diseases [29,30]. Furthermore, several phytochemicals such as phenolic compounds and terpenoids have been used throughout human history as condiments and pigments [31]

3.2.1. Anthocyanins in Murta and Calafate Fruit

Anthocyanins are the common coloring compounds found in a large number of plants and are responsible for the purple, red, blue, and orange colors of berry-type fruits [32]. Chemically, anthocyanins are phenolic compounds belonging to the flavonoid class, with two benzene rings joined by a linear three-carbon chain, possessing the C6–C3–C6 basic skeleton [33]. Anthocyanins are formed by the modification of anthocyanidins by glycosyl and aromatic or aliphatic acyl moieties [34]. The basic structure of an anthocyanidin is a flavonoid ion (2-phenylbenzopyrilium) that can vary based on the different positions of hydroxyl groups (OH) or methoxyls (OCH$_3$) (Figure 4a). Six anthocyanidins (cyanidin, delphinidin, pelargonidin, peonidin, malvidin, and petunidin) are the most common in plants [33,35] and are present in berry-type fruits [32,36].

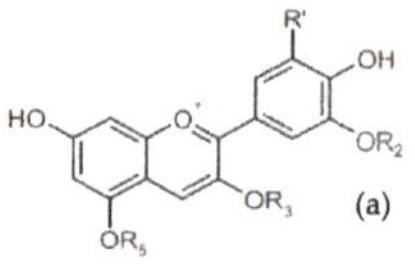

Figure 4. Anthocyanidin basic chemical structure (**a**), anthocyanins in murta (**b**) and calafate (**c**), and their different glycosylation patters.

(b) Murta anthocyanins adapted from Junqueira-Gonzalves et al. [39] and Ruiz et al. [42].

Compound	R'	R₂	R₃	R₅	Name
1	OH	OH	Glu	H	delphinidin-3-O-glucoside
2	OCH₃	OH	Glu	H	petunidin-3-O-glucoside
3	OCH₃	OH	Gal	H	petunidin-3-O-galactoside
4	OH	OH	Gal	H	delphinidin-3-O-galactoside
5	OCH₃	H	Glu	H	peonidin-3-O-glucoside
6	OH	H	Glu	H	cyanidin-3-O-glucoside
7	OH	H	Ara	H	cyanidin-3-O-arabinoside
8	OCH₃	OCH₃	Ara	H	malvidin-3-O-arabinoside
9	OH	OH	Ara	H	delphinidin-3-O-arabinoside
10	OCH₃	OCH₃	Glu	H	malvidin-3-O-glucoside

(c) Calafate anthocyanins adapted from Ruiz et al. [42]

Compound	R'	R₂	R₃	R₅	Name
1	OH	OH	Hex	Hex	delphinidin-3,5-dihexoside
2	OH	OH	Rut	Glu	delphinidin-3-rutinoside-5-glucoside
3	OH	H	Hex	Hex	cyanidin-3,5-dihexoside
4	OCH₃	OH	Hex	Hex	petunidin-3,5-dihexoside
5	OCH₃	OH	Rut	Glu	petunidin-3-rutinoside-5-glucoside
6	OCH₃	H	Hex	Hex	peonidin-3,5-dihexoside
7	OCH₃	OCH₃	G	Hex	malvidin-3,5-dihexoside
8	OH	OH	Glu	H	delphinidin-3-O-glucoside
9	OH	OH	Rut	H	delphinidin-3-O-rutinoside
10	OCH₃	OCH₃	Rut	Glu	malvidin-3-rutinoside-5-glucoside
11	OH	H	Glu	H	cyanidin-3-O-glucoside
12	OH	H	Rut	H	cyanidin-3-O-rutinoside
13	OCH₃	OH	Glu	H	petunidin-3-O-glucoside
14	OCH₃	OH	Rut	H	petunidin-3-O-rutinoside
15	OCH₃	H	Glu	H	peonidin-3-O-glucoside
16	OCH₃	H	Rut	H	peonidin-3-O-rutinoside
17	OCH₃	OCH₃	Glu	H	malvidin-3-O-glucoside
18	OCH₃	OCH₃	Rut	H	malvidin-3-O-rutinoside

The use of LC-MS as an analytical chemistry technique has allowed for the identification and/or tentative identification of the anthocyanin profile of murta and calafate. In a first report, two anthocyanins (cyanidin-3-O-glucoside and peonidin-3-O-glucoside) were identified in murta whereas 18 anthocyanins (3-O-monoglycosylated and 3,5-O-diglycosylated delphinidins, cyanidins, petunidins, peonidins, and malvidins) were most abundant in calafate [28,37,38]. As can be expected by the wide variability of colors observed in murta ecotypes, subsequent studies [39] have described a greater number of anthocyanins where 3-O-glucosides of delphinidin, petunidin, and malvidin have been also identified in murta fruit. Based on these findings, murta (Figure 4a) and calafate (Figure 4b) could be used as promising sources of a wide variety of anthocyanins.

3.2.2. Phenolic Acids and Other Flavonoids in Murta and Calafate Fruit

The identification of other phenolic compounds in murta and calafate indicate the presence of phenolic acids (gallic acid, benzoic acid, p-coumaric acid, and hydrocaffeic acid), flavan-3-ols (epicatechin) and flavonols (quercetin, rutin, luteolin, kaempferol, and myricetin) in murta fruits [39,40]. On the other hand, 20 hydroxycinnamic acids and flavonols such as hyperoside, isoquercitrin, quercetin, rutin, myricetin, and isorhamnetin are more abundant in calafate fruits [39,41,42]. Furthermore, among flavonoid subclasses, murta shows higher flavonol and flava-3-ols content (0.29 and 0.27 μmoL/g FW respectively) than calafate (0.16 and 0.24 μmoL/g FW respectively) whereas calafate has a higher anthocyanin content (17.8 μmoL/g FW) than murta (0.21 μmoL/g FW) associated with the deep-blue color of the calafate fruit [28].

The existing research on murta and calafate show that phenolic compounds are the main phytochemicals studied in these berry-type fruits.

3.3. Phytochemical Changes in Murta and Calafate

The main factors that affect the polyphenol content in plants are genotype, environment, stage at fruit harvest, and storage and processing [15]. When wild plants are studied, domestication emerges as a key factor affecting polyphenol content due to changes in the allocation of nutrients within the plant (domestication syndrome) that occur during the continuous process of selection [43].

3.3.1. Genotype vs. Environment

Phytochemical changes in murta have been studied in its leaves and stems and its fruits. The total amount of flavonols (rutin, kaempferol, and quercetin) in wild murta plant (leaves) is significantly higher (~20%) than in cultivated murta plants, showing the domestication effect [44]. Results on the flavonol content in murta fruit have been inconsistent. In one study, no significant differences between wild and cultivated murta fruits were found [44,45]. Conversely, in another study by Augusto [40], the total phenolic compounds in the fruits of wild and selected murta (14-4) genotype were 19.4 and 40.3 mg GAE/g in dry weight, respectively. Consistent with the results of phenolic compound content, the antioxidant capacity (AC) of the wild murta genotype was lower than the selected murta (14-4) genotype for both DPPH (76.5 and 134.4 mu moL TEAC/g) and ABTS (157.0 and 294.0 mu moL TEAC/g) tests [40]. These results show that phenolic content and AC in murta fruits did not decrease as a result of the domestication process.

In addition to differences in polyphenol content among different murta genotypes, the effect of the environment may cause the same variety to present differences depending on the harvest year. In this context, Alfaro et al. [46] indicate that genotype and growing season have a significant effect on the polyphenol content and AC of murta fruits; the lowest polyphenol content (283 ± 72 mg GAE/100 g DW) was obtained for the 14-4 genotype in 2008, and the highest value (2152 ± 290 mg GAE/100 g DW) was observed for the variety South Pearl-INIA in 2007. Furthermore, a canonical discriminant analysis of seasonal differences showed that the South Pearl-INIA variety had the greatest variation in polyphenol content in relation to the other genotypes studied [46]. The same authors indicate that rainfall and frosts were the most relevant climate factors that may explain the seasonal variation of total polyphenol content of murta fruits [46].

In the case of calafate, the effect of genotype and environment on phytochemical changes is scarce. Mariangel et al. [47] indicated that the phenolic composition of calafate fruit can vary according to the geographical area of fruit collection. However, it is difficult to determine if these differences are attributed to the different genotypes evaluated and/or to the effect of the environment. On the other hand, Arena et al. [48] demonstrated that calafate fruits from field conditions with different light intensities (i.e., 100%, 57%, 24% of natural irradiance) show significant differences in anthocyanin content. Fruits grown under high light intensity (299.7 mg/100 g FW) had an anthocyanin content 2.9 times higher than fruits grown under medium light intensity (103.8 mg/100 g FW) [48]. The authors associated a higher anthocyanin content with a higher photosynthetic rate and a concomitant increase in SS and sugar content measured under the same conditions [48].

3.3.2. Stage at Fruit Harvest

Berry-type fruits harvested at different maturity stages present different chemical characteristics as well as phenolic compound profiles; in immature fruits proanthocyanidins are predominant while in mature fruits anthocyanins predominate [49–51]. From an ecological point of view, plants with immature fruits—without viable seeds—have high phenolic and proanthocyanidin contents that act as deterrent compounds to prevent their consumption by insects and herbivores [52]. In contrast, ripe fruits have attractive colors (anthocyanins and other pigments) and a sweet taste to stimulate their consumption by herbivores and the consequent dispersion of seeds [52].

Phytochemical changes during fruit development and ripening have been studied in calafate fruits as well as other berry-type fruits [49–51,53]. Early studies attempted to understand the main changes in phenolic compounds and AC during the process of fruit maturation and ripening in order to establish the best maturity index for calafate fruit according to phenolic compound content [26,54]. According to this study, for calafate fruits collected in March, the maximum anthocyanin content (761 mg/100 g FW) coincided with the highest accumulation of SS (25 °Brix) 126 days after flowering [54].

3.3.3. Storage and Fruit Processing

In fruits, anthocyanins are mainly found in the epicarp (peel) [55] where they are stored in the cell vacuole and remain stable in intact fruits [56]. During fruit processing, the plant cell loses its compartmentalization and anthocyanins are exposed to the action of enzymes (polyphenol oxidase), other fruit components, and environmental conditions that favor their degradation [57]. Several factors such as temperature, pH, light, oxygen, ascorbic acid, metal ions, sugars, and enzymes may affect the stability of anthocyanins during processing and storage [58]. The mechanism of anthocyanin degradation has been studied in some plant species such as roselle (*Hibiscus sabdariffa*); a metal-catalyzed oxidation followed by condensation (brown polymer) and a deglycosylation followed by scission (phloroglucinaldehyde and phenolic acids) were identified as two pathways of anthocyanin degradation [59].

Fleshy fruits have high moisture content, thereby they are classified as highly perishable commodities [60]. The dehydration of murta and calafate fruits emerges as an attractive conservation alternative given also the high seasonality of their production, allowing for the commercialization of value-added dehydrated fruit products throughout the year. Different drying processes for murta, such as freeze-drying [61,62], convective drying, combined infrared-convective drying [63], vacuum drying [62,64,65], atmospheric drying [62,64], infrared-radiation [62], and sun-drying [62] have been evaluated in order to preserve the polyphenols, the AC, and/or the microstructure of fresh murta fruit. Lopez et al. [62] reported that freeze-drying showed the highest retention of total flavonoids as well as anthocyanins and the least damage of murta microstructure. No studies on the drying of calafate fruit have been published.

The understanding of the phytochemical changes in murta and calafate facilitates the design and development of formulations and the evaluation of the efficacy of new nutraceutical products.

3.4. Validation of Traditional Use and New Insights in the Research of Murta and Calafate

Different methods of biological activity have been used to validate the traditional uses of murta and calafate as well as to examine some potential uses of calafate shoots and fruits (Table 1).

Some studies identified phytochemicals such as triterpenoids, phenolic compounds, and isoquinoline alkaloids. However, in many cases it is difficult to correlate a specific compound to a specific biological effect. In addition, some studies lacked detailed information about the genotype and time of harvest of raw materials. This information is particularly important because, as was discussed previously, genotype, environment, and time of harvest have been shown to affect the phytochemistry of murta and calafate.

Table 1. Traditional medicinal use, biological activity, and phytochemicals reported for murta and calafate.

Plant Organ	Traditional Use	Biological Activity	Phytochemicals	Reference
Murta leaf	Urinary and throat infection	Antioxidant	NR	[66]
		Antioxidant	Phenolic acids, hydrolyzable tannins, epicatechin, myricetin, quercetin	[67]
		Analgesic	Flavonoids and triterpenoids	[68]
		Anti-inflammatory	Triterpenoids	[69]
		Anti-inflammatory	Triterpenoids and phenolic compounds	[70,71]
		Antimicrobial	Catechin, rutin, isoquercitrin, ellagic acid, quercitrin, narcissin, isorhamnetin-3-O-glucoside	[72–75]
Murta fruit	Astringent	Antimicrobial	Isoquinoline alkaloids	[39]
		Vasodilator	Gallic acid, catechin, quercetin-3-β-D-glucoside, myricetin, quercetin, and kaempferol	[76,77]
Calafate root	Control fever, anti-inflammatory, stomach pain, indigestion, colitis	Antimicrobial	Isoquinoline alkaloids	[78,79]
		Hypoglycaemic	NR	[80]
Calafate shoot	NR	Antimicrobial	Isoquinoline alkaloids	[78,79,81]
Calafate fruit	NR	Antioxidant	NR	[82]
		Anti-inflammatory	Phenolic compounds	[83]

NR: Not reported.

3.4.1. Antioxidant Capacity

Based on a traditional use of murta leaf that suggests antioxidant, anti-inflammatory, and antimicrobial activity, an early study of murta leaf AC (ORAC method) in vivo was evaluated in the plasma of healthy volunteers before and after the ingestion of a murta leaf infusion (1%) twice a day for three days [66]. The results indicated a significant increase (from 2.258 to 3.108 µM TE/L) in the AC of the volunteers' plasma. Later, murta leaf AC was attributed to the presence of polyphenols such as phenolic acids, hydrolyzable tannins, flavanols (epicatechin), and flavonols (myricetin, quercetin) [67]. In another study, Albrecht et al. [82] examined the beneficial effect of calafate fruit on oxidative stress induced by chloramphenicol. Calafate-fruit aqueous extracts were shown to reduce oxidative stress caused by chloramphenicol in human blood cells by significantly diminishing reactive oxygen species (ROS). In parallel with the decrease of ROS, the fruit extract protected the viability of leukocytes [82].

3.4.2. Anti-Inflammatory Activity

To study the biological activity of murta-leaf triterpenoids, the topical anti-inflammatory activity of alphitolic, asiatic, and corosolic acids isolated from murta leaf were evaluated in vivo in a mouse ear model; inflammation was induced with either arachidonic acid or 12-O-tetradecanoylphorbol-13 acetate [69]. Only corosolic acid was active in the arachidonic acid-induced inflammation assay, with similar potency to nimesulide, while the three triterpene acids together inhibited 12-O-tetradecanoylphorbol-13 acetate-induced inflammation with potencies comparable to that of indomethacin [69]. Furthermore, Goity et al. [70] and Arancibia-Radich et al. [71] indicated that the differences in the anti-inflammatory activity of murta leaf is associated to the different quantitative composition of phenolic compounds and triterpenoids.

The anti-inflammatory potential of calafate fruit has been studied by Reyes-Farias et al. [83] where aqueous extracts were able to modulate the proinflammatory state generated by the interaction between adipocytes and macrophages in vitro.

3.4.3. Antimicrobial Activity

The antimicrobial activity of murta leaf extract against clinically important microorganisms with antibiotic resistance (*Staphylococcus aureus*, *Enterobacter aerogenes*, *Pseudomonas aeruginosa*, and *Candida albicans*) in vitro has been shown by Avello et al. [72] and Shen et al. [73]. Furthermore, Shene et al. [74] described the antimicrobial activity of murta leaf in human gut bacteria and Di Castillo et al. [75] showed the antimicrobial activity of murta leaf against *Escherichia coli* and *Listeria monocytogenes*.

Junqueira-Gonzalves et al. [39] studied the antibacterial activity (*E. coli* (ATCC 25922) and *Salmonella typhi* (ATCC 14028)) of ethanolic and acidic methanolic extracts. A methanolic murta fruit extract (100 µL) was equivalent to the activity of all of the antibiotics (tetracycline, clotrimazole, gentamicin, amikacin, ceftriaxone, cefuroxim, cefotaxim, ampicillin, ciprofloxacin, and ampicillin/sulbactam) tested in the case of *S. typhi*. However, in the case of *E. coli*, 100 µL of the extract was equivalent to the activity of tetracycline, amikacin, cefuroxim, cefotaxim, ampicillin, and ciprofloxacin.

The antimicrobial activity of calafate roots and shoots (stem and leaves) against Gram-positive bacteria (*Staphylococcus aureus*, *Bacillus cereus*, *Staphylococcus epidermidis*, and *Bacillus subtilis*) has been associated with the presence of isoquinoline alkaloids [78,81]. Calafate root had the highest alkaloid yield and berberine was the main alkaloid identified [79].

3.4.4. Analgesic Activity

Delporte et al. [68] studied the analgesic activity of dichloromethane, ethyl acetate, and methanol extracts from murta leaves on acute pain in mice. Murta-leaf extracts produced antinociception in chemical and thermal pain models through a mechanism partially linked to either lipooxygenase and/or cyclooxygenase via the arachidonic acid cascade and/or opioid receptors. Flavonoids and triterpenoids were associated with the antinociceptive activity [68].

3.4.5. New Insights in the Research of Murta and Calafate

In order to explore in the potential beneficial effect of murta and calafate fruit on the management of cardiovascular disease, Jofre et al. [76] and Calfío and Huidobro-Toro [77] studied the antioxidant and vasodilator activity of murta and calafate fruit in rat models. Dose-dependent vasodilator activity in the presence of endothelium was shown in aortic rings. Its hypotensive mechanism is partially mediated by nitric oxide synthase/guanylate cyclase and large-conductance calcium-dependent potassium channels [76]. Similarly, vascular responses of main glycosylated anthocyanins found in calafate fruit were endothelium-dependent and mediated by NO production [77]. Nevertheless, the authors propose that the anthocyanin-induced vasodilation is not due to an antioxidant mechanism [77]. Furthermore, Furrianca et al. [80] showed that a calafate-root ethanolic extract had hypoglycemic effects, stimulating glucose uptake in non-resistant and insulin-resistant liver (HepG2) cells by activating AMPK protein.

3.5. Potential Health Benefits Associated with Murta and Calafate Fruit Consumption

The high consumption of anthocyanin-rich foods has been associated with several health benefits in humans [84–87]. Internationally, these potential anti-inflammatory, antioxidant, hypoglycaemic, and cardioprotective health benefits found in berry-type fruits are used as a strategy to promote consumption. Antioxidant capacity measured in vitro is commonly determined in studies of phenolic profiling [9,88] however the in vitro method of measuring total antioxidant capacity is questionable due to it having almost zero relevance for human (animal) physiology. Nevertheless, the ORAC value as a way to determine AC in vitro is considered a quality parameter in the international market of berry-type agri-foods [88]. Speisky et al. [89] reported 27 fruit species grown in Chile, where the total phenolic content of murta (863 mg GAE/100g FW) and calafate (1201 mg GAE/100g FW) were higher than well-known polyphenol-rich fruits such as blackberry (671 mg GAE/100g FW) and blueberry (529 mg

GAE/100g FW). Murta and calafate were grouped among the highest ORAC (10,000–25,000 μmoL TE/100 g FW) fruits where calafate had the highest ORAC (25,662 μmoL TE/100 g FW) value; 2.8-fold higher than blackberry and 2.9-fold higher than blueberry [89].

As was mentioned previously, polyphenols are susceptible to degradation by heat, oxygen, and changes in pH, among others that may occur not only during product storage, but also into the gastrointestinal (GI) tract [57]. For example, it is well known that anthocyanins are unstable at high pH, and the shift from the acidic pH (pH 2) of the stomach to the almost neutral pH of the duodenum (pH 6) may be responsible for their specific hydrolysis and/or degradation [90–92]. Bioaccessibility, defined as the amount of compounds that are released from the food matrix after digestion [90] is measured to determine the impact of the food matrix on the protection and/or release of bioactive compounds as well as the stability of bioactive compounds during GI digestion. Ah-Hen et al. [93] compared the bioaccessibility of murta fruit and juice during an in vitro GI digestion process showing that juice as food matrix released bioactive compounds earlier in the gastric stage, while murta fruit released bioactive compounds in the small intestine. However, both murta fruit and juice achieved a high bioaccessibility index of polyphenols (70%) after being digested by the small intestine [93].

According to anthocyanin metabolism, its degradation is a result of chemical instability and the impact of bacterial catabolism, resulting in a number of circulating phenolic metabolites [94]. Along this line, Bustamante et al. [95] performed a pharmacokinetic study of phenolic compounds in gerbil plasma after the consumption of calafate, where the amount of 16 phenolic acids increased 4–8 h post-intake. Although all catabolites were found in concentration peaks between 0.1 and 1 mu M, no parental anthocyanins were detected [95]. Currently, it is postulated that anthocyanin bioactivity in vivo results from lesser studied, though more bioavailable, phenolic metabolites [96,97] and some authors have demonstrated that these phenolic metabolites are more active on inflammatory biomarkers than their precursor structures (parent anthocyanins) [97,98]. In this sense, the bioactivity of anthocyanin metabolites in murta and calafate must continue to be studied in order to achieve adequate information on the biological activity and health-promoting effects derived for the consumption of murta and calafate fruit.

4. Conclusions and Future Perspectives

This review, for the first time, approximates the traditional knowledge of murta and calafate with the scientific research on both species. Scientific knowledge of murta and calafate is much more limited compared to other South American fruits such as maqui (*Aristotelia chilensis* (Mol.) Stuntz) and acai (*Euterpe oleracea* Mart.) for which there are 96 and 232 records (article, proceedings paper, book chapter, and review) available in the Web of Science database, respectively. Advances in the study of the nutritional composition of fruits, the identification of phytochemicals, the validation of traditional use, and the biological activity of certain phytochemicals indicate that murta and calafate are promising sources of natural antioxidants, antimicrobial, and vasodilator compounds with nutraceutical potential. Like international studies on nutraceuticals in other berry-type fruits such as blueberries [95–97] future studies are needed to establish the mechanisms of action of both murta and calafate anthocyanins (and their metabolites) in antioxidant and anti-inflammatory activity. These studies are needed in order to further the study of the potential health benefits associated with the consumption of these berry-type fruits. From the nutritional point of view, murta appears to be a good source of ascorbic acid, similar to other fruits in the Myrtaceae family such as camu camu (*Myrciaria dubia* (Kunth) McVaugh, 397 mg/100 g FW) and white guava (*Psidium guajava* L., 142 mg/100 g FW), which are internationally recognized as good sources of vitamin C [99].

Plant domestication is a necessary strategy to guarantee the sustainable use of Chilean botanical resources and to standardize the quality of the raw materials derived from murta and calafate. Murta domestication programs are around 20 years old, while calafate has only very recently been domesticated. At the same time, sustainable harvesting of wild murta and calafate performed by several indigenous and rural communities can be an alternative for supplying raw materials for future research. This review will be a useful reference for new research on murta and calafate, respecting and recognizing the traditional knowledge in the hands of indigenous and rural peoples from south and extreme south of Chile.

Author Contributions: C.F. performed the historical and scientific search of literature; C.F. and P.R. structured the review and analyzed the main papers; A.P. provided the review on nutritional composition; J.S. provided the review on botany and distribution. All authors have read and agreed to the published version of the manuscript.

Funding: This research received no external funding.

Acknowledgments: We are sincerely grateful to the Biblioteca Nacional of Chile for granting us access to and permission to use images of Abate José Ignacio Molina, Claudio Gay, and Charles Darwin, and to Carlos Aldunate, Director of the Museo Chileno de Arte Precolombino for the permission to use the picture of Father Ernesto Wilhem de Mösbach.

Conflicts of Interest: The authors declare no conflict of interest.

References

1. Wilhem De Mösbach, E. *Botánica Indígena*; Editorial Andrés Bello: Santiago, Chile, 1992; pp. 26–33.
2. Estomba, D.; Ladio, A.; Lozada, M. Medicinal wild plant knowledge and gathering patterns in a Mapuche community from North-western Patagonia. *J. Ethnopharmacol.* **2006**, *103*, 109–119. [CrossRef]
3. Lozada, M.; Ladio, A.; Weigandt, M. Cultural transmission of ethnobotanical knowledge in a rural community of northwestern Patagonia, Argentina. *Econ. Bot.* **2006**, *60*, 374–385. [CrossRef]
4. Darwin, C. *Viaje de un Naturalista Alrededor del Mundo*; Joaquín Gil: Buenos Aires, Argentina, 1945; p. 618.
5. Seguel, I.; Torralbo, L. Murtilla: El berry nativo del Sur de Chile. *Rev. Tierra Adentro* **2004**, *57*, 20–25.
6. Hoffmann, A. *Flora Silvestre de Chile. Zona Araucana. Árboles, Arbustos y Enredaderas Leñosas*; Fundación Claudio Gay: Santiago, Chile, 1982; p. 258.
7. Seeram, N.P. Berry fruits: Compositional elements, biochemical activities, and the impact of their intake on human health, performance, and disease. *J. Agric. Food Chem.* **2008**, *56*, 627–629. [CrossRef] [PubMed]
8. Halvorsen, B.L.; Holte, K.; Myhrstad, M.C.W.; Barikmo, I.; Hvattum, E.; Remberg, S.F.; Wold, A.-B.; Haffner, K.; Baugerod, H.; Andersen, L.F.; et al. A systematic screening of total antioxidants in dietary plants. *J. Nutr.* **2002**, *132*, 461–471. [CrossRef] [PubMed]
9. Fredes, C.; Yousef, G.G.; Robert, P.; Grace, M.H.; Lila, M.A.; Gómez, M.; Gebauer, M.; Montenegro, G. Anthocyanin profiling of wild maqui berries (*Aristotelia chilensis* [Mol.] Stuntz) from different geographical regions in Chile. *J. Sci. Food Agric.* **2014**, *94*, 2639–2648. [CrossRef] [PubMed]
10. Lee, S. Strategic design of delivery systems for nutraceuticals. In *Nanotechnology Applications in Food: Flavor, Stability, Nutrition, and Safety*; Oprea, O.E., Grumezescu, A.M., Eds.; Academic Press, Elsevier Inc.: London, UK, 2017; pp. 65–86.
11. Molina, J.I. *Compendio de la Historia Geográfica, Natural y Civil del Reyno de Chile*; Don Antonio de Sancha: Madrid, España, 1788; p. 418.
12. Gay, C. *Historia Física y Política de Chile. Botánica. Tomo Primero*; Museo de Historia Natural de Santiago: Santiago, Chile, 1845; p. 535.
13. Gay, C. *Historia Física y Política de Chile. Botánica. Tomo Segundo*; Museo de Historia Natural de Santiago: Santiago, Chile, 1846; p. 372.
14. Montenegro, G. *Chile Nuestra Flora Útil*; Universidad Católica de Chile: Santiago, Chile, 2002; p. 267.
15. Fredes, C.; Montenegro, G. Chilean plants as a source of polyphenols. In *Natural Antioxidants and Biocides from Wild Medicinal Plants*; Céspedes, C., Sampietro, D., Seigler, D., Rai, M., Eds.; CAB International: Wallingford, UK, 2013; pp. 116–136.
16. Minsal-Ministerio de Salud. Medicamentos Herbarios Tradicionales. 2009. Available online: https://www.minsal.cl/wp-content/uploads/2018/02/Libro-MHT-2010.pdf (accessed on 10 April 2018).
17. Muñoz, O.; Montes, M.; Wilkomirsky, T. *Plantas Medicinales de Uso en Chile. Química y Farmacología*; Editorial Universitaria: Santiago, Chile, 2001; p. 330.
18. Martinic, M. *Los Aónikenk: Historia y Cultura*; Universidad de Magallanes: Punta Arenas, Chile, 1995; p. 387.
19. Barros, A. *Aborígenes Australes de América*; Editorial Lord Cochrane: Santiago, Chile, 1975; pp. 15–25.
20. Cárdenas, R. *Poemas Migratorios*; Armando Menedin: Santiago, Chile, 1974; pp. 29–30.

21. Torres, A.; Seguel, I.; Contreras, G.; Castro, M. Physico-chemical characterization of murta (murtilla) fruits *Ugni molinae* Turcz. *Agric. Técnica* **1999**, *59*, 260–270.
22. Schreckinger, M.E.; Lotton, J.; Lila, M.A.; De Mejia, E.G. Berries from South America: A comprehensive review on chemistry, health potential, and commercialization. *J. Med. Food* **2010**, *13*, 233–246. [CrossRef]
23. Scheuermann, E.; Seguel, I.; Montenegro, A.; Bustos, R.; Hormazabal, E.; Quiroz, A. Evolution of aroma compounds of murtilla fruits (*Ugni molinae* Turcz) during storage. *J. Sci. Food Agric.* **2008**, *88*, 485–492. [CrossRef]
24. Ah-Hen, K.S.; Vega-Gálvez, A.; Moraga, N.O.; Lemus-Mondaca, R. Modelling of rheological behaviour of pulps and purées from fresh and frozen-thawed murta (*Ugni molinae* Turcz) berries. *Int. J. Food Eng.* **2012**, *8*. [CrossRef]
25. Arancibia-Avila, P.; Namiesnik, J.; Toledo, F.; Werner, E.; Martinez-Ayala, A.M.; Rocha-Guzmán, N.E.; Gallegos-Infante, J.A.; Gorinstein, S. The influence of different time durations of thermal processing on berries quality. *Food Control* **2012**, *26*, 587–593. [CrossRef]
26. Arena, M.E.; Zuleta, A.; Dyner, L.; Constenla, D.; Ceci, L.; Curvetto, N. *Berberis buxifolia* fruit growth and ripening: Evolution in carbohydrate and organic acid contents. *Sci. Hortic.* **2013**, *158*, 52–58. [CrossRef]
27. Fredes, C.; Montenegro, G.; Zoffoli, J.; Santander, F.; Robert, P. Comparison of total phenolic, total anthocyanin and antioxidant activity of polyphenol-rich fruits grown in Chile. *Cienc. Investig. Agrar.* **2014**, *41*, 49–60. [CrossRef]
28. Ruiz, A.; Hermosin-Gutierrez, I.; Mardones, C.; Vergara, C.; Herlitz, E.; Vega, M.; Dorau, C.; Winterhalter, P.; Von Baer, D. Polyphenols and antioxidant activity of calafate (*Berberis microphylla*) fruits and other native berries from southern Chile. *J. Agric. Food Chem.* **2010**, *58*, 6081–6089. [CrossRef] [PubMed]
29. Liu, R.H. Potential synergy of phytochemicals in cancer prevention: Mechanism of action. *J. Nutr.* **2004**, *134*, 3479S–3485S. [CrossRef]
30. Reilly, K. On-farm and fresh produce management. In *Handbook of Plant Food Phytochemicals: Sources Stability and Extraction*; Tiwari, B.K., Brunton, N., Brennan, C., Eds.; Wiley-Blackwell Publishing Co.: Hoboken, NJ, USA, 2013; pp. 201–235.
31. Springob, K.; Kutchan, T.M. Introduction to the different classes of natural products. In *Plant-Derived Natural Products*; Osbourn, A.E., Lanzotti, V., Eds.; Springer: New York, NY, USA, 2009; pp. 1–50.
32. Robert, P.; Fredes, C. The encapsulation of anthocyanins from berry-type fruits: Trends in foods. *Molecules* **2015**, *20*, 5875–5888. [CrossRef]
33. Manach, C.; Scalbert, A.; Morand, C.; Rémésy, C.; Jiménez, L. Polyphenols: Food sources and bioavailability. *Am. J. Clin. Nutr.* **2004**, *79*, 727–747. [CrossRef]
34. Castañeda-Ovando, A.; Pacheco-Hernández, M.L.; Páez-Hernández, M.A.; Rodríguez, J.A.; Galán-Vidal, C.A. Chemical studies of anthocyanins: A review. *Food Chem.* **2009**, *113*, 859–871. [CrossRef]
35. Khoo, H.E.; Azlan, A.; Tang, S.T.; Lim, S.M. Anthocyanindins and anthocyanins: Colored pigments as food, pharmaceutical ingredients, and the potential health benefits. *Food Nutr. Res.* **2017**, *61*, 1361779. [CrossRef]
36. Robert, P.; García, P.; Fredes, C. Drying and preservation of polyphenols. In *Advances in Technologies for Producing Food-Relevant Polyphenols*; Cuevas-Valenzuela, J., Vergara Salinas, J.R., Pérez-Correa, J.R., Eds.; CRC Press, Taylor and Francis Group: Boca Raton, FL, USA, 2017; pp. 281–302.
37. Brito, A.; Areche, C.; Sepulveda, B.; Kennelly, E.J.; Simirgiotis, M.J. Anthocyanin characterization, total phenolic quantification and antioxidant features of some Chilean edible berry extracts. *Molecules* **2014**, *19*, 10936–10955. [CrossRef]
38. Ramirez, J.E.; Zambrano, R.; Sepulveda, B.; Kennelly, E.J.; Simirgiotis, M.J. Anthocyanins and antioxidant capacities of six Chilean berries by HPLC-HR-ESI-ToF-MS. *Food Chem.* **2015**, *176*, 106–114. [CrossRef] [PubMed]
39. Junqueira-Goncalves, M.P.; Yanez, L.; Morales, C.; Navarro, M.; Contreras, R.A.; Zuniga, G.E. Isolation and characterization of phenolic compounds and anthocyanins from murta (*Ugni molinae* Turcz) fruits. Assessment of antioxidant and antibacterial activity. *Molecules* **2015**, *20*, 5698–5713. [CrossRef] [PubMed]
40. Augusto, T.R.; Scheuerman, E.S.; Alencar, S.M.; D'Arce, M.A.; Costa De Camargo, A.; Vieira, T.M. Phenolic compounds and antioxidant activity of hydroalcoholic extracts of wild and cultivated murtilla (*Ugni molinae* Turcz). *Food Sci. Technol.* **2014**, *34*, 667–673. [CrossRef]

41. Ruiz, A.; Mardones, C.; Vergara, C.; Hermosin-Gutierrez, I.; Von Baer, D.; Hinrichsen, P.; Rodriguez, R.; Arribillaga, D.; Dominguez, E. Analysis of hydroxycinnamic acids derivatives in calafate (*Berberis microphylla* G. Forst) berries by liquid chromatography with photodiode array and mass spectrometry detection. *J. Chromatogr. A* **2013**, *1281*, 38–45. [CrossRef] [PubMed]
42. Ruiz, A.; Mardones, C.; Vergara, C.; Von Baer, D.; Gomez-Alonso, S.; Gomez, M.V.; Hermosin-Gutierrez, I. Isolation and structural elucidation of anthocyanidin 3,7-beta-o-diglucosides and caffeoyl-glucaric acids from calafate berries. *J. Agric. Food Chem.* **2014**, *62*, 6918–6925. [CrossRef] [PubMed]
43. Meyer, R.S.; DuVal, A.E.; Jensen, H.R. Patterns and processes in crop domestication: An historical review and quantitative analysis of 203 global food crops. *New Phytol.* **2012**, *196*, 29–48. [CrossRef] [PubMed]
44. Chacon-Fuentes, M.; Parra, L.; Rodriguez-Saona, C.; Seguel, I.; Ceballos, R.; Quiroz, A. Domestication in murtilla (*Ugni molinae*) reduced defensive flavonol levels but increased resistance against a native herbivorous insect. *Environ. Entomol.* **2015**, *44*, 627–637. [CrossRef]
45. Chacon-Fuentes, M.; Parra, L.; Lizama, M.; Seguel, I.; Urzua, A.; Quiroz, A. Plant flavonoid content modified by domestication. *Environ. Entomol.* **2017**, *46*, 1080–1089. [CrossRef]
46. Alfaro, S.; Mutis, A.; Palma, R.; Quiroz, A.; Seguel, I.; Scheuermann, E. Influence of genotype and harvest year on polyphenol content and antioxidant activity in murtilla (*Ugni molinae* Turcz) fruit. *J. Soil Sci. Plant Nutr.* **2013**, *13*, 67–78. [CrossRef]
47. Mariangel, E.; Reyes-Diaz, M.; Lobos, W.; Bensch, E.; Schalchli, H.; Ibarra, P. The antioxidant properties of calafate (*Berberis microphylla*) fruits from four different locations in southern Chile. *Cienc. Investig. Agrar.* **2013**, *40*, 161–170. [CrossRef]
48. Arena, M.E.; Postemsky, P.D.; Curvetto, N.R. Changes in the phenolic compounds and antioxidant capacity of *Berberis microphylla* G. Forst berries in relation to light intensity and fertilization. *Sci. Hortic.* **2017**, *218*, 63–71. [CrossRef]
49. Vvedenskaya, I.O.; Vorsa, N. Flavonoid composition over fruit development and maturation in American cranberry, *Vaccinium macrocarpon* Ait. *Plant Sci.* **2004**, *167*, 1043–1054. [CrossRef]
50. Kulkarni, A.P.; Aradhya, S.M. Chemical changes and antioxidant activity in pomegranate arils during fruit development. *Food Chem.* **2005**, *93*, 319–324. [CrossRef]
51. Wang, S.Y.; Chen, C.-T.; Wang, C.Y. The influence of light and maturity on fruit quality and flavonoid content of red raspberries. *Food Chem.* **2009**, *112*, 676–684. [CrossRef]
52. Parr, A.J.; Bolwell, G.P. Phenols in the plant and in man. The potential for possible nutritional enhancement of the diet by modifying the phenols content or profile. *J. Sci. Food Agric.* **2000**, *80*, 985–1012. [CrossRef]
53. Fredes, C.; Montenegro, G.; Zoffoli, J.P.; Gómez, M.; Robert, P. Polyphenol content and antioxidant activity of maqui (*Aristotelia chilensis* [Mol.] Stuntz) during fruit development and maturation in Central Chile. *Chil. J. Agric. Res.* **2012**, *72*, 582–589. [CrossRef]
54. Arena, M.; Curvetto, N. *Berberis buxifolia* fruiting: Kinetic growth behavior and evolution of chemical properties during the fruiting period and different growing seasons. *Sci. Hortic.* **2008**, *118*, 120–127. [CrossRef]
55. Wang, S.Y.; Chen, H.; Camp, M.J.; Ehlenfeldt, M.K. Genotype and growing season influence blueberry antioxidant capacity and other quality attributes. *Int. J. Food Sci. Technol.* **2012**, *47*, 1540–1549. [CrossRef]
56. Patras, A.; Brunton, N.P.; O'Donnell, C.; Tiwari, B.K. Effect of thermal processing on anthocyanin stability in foods; mechanisms and kinetics of degradation. *Trends Food Sci. Technol.* **2010**, *21*, 3–11. [CrossRef]
57. De Pascual-Teresa, S.; Sanchez-Ballesta, M.T. Anthocyanins: From plant to health. *Phytochem. Rev.* **2008**, *7*, 281–299. [CrossRef]
58. Rhim, J.-W. Kinetics of thermal degradation of anthocyanin pigment solutions driven from red flower cabbage. *Food Sci. Biotech.* **2002**, *11*, 361–364.
59. Mundombe Sinela, A.; Mertz, C.; Achir, N.; Rawat, N.; Vidot, K.; Fulcrand, H.; Dornier, M. Exploration of reaction mechanisms of anthocyanin degradation in a roselle extract through kinetic studies on formulated model media. *Food Chem.* **2017**, *235*, 67–75. [CrossRef] [PubMed]
60. Sharma, H.P.; Sugandha, P.H. Enzymatic added extraction and clarification of fruit juices-A review. *Crit. Rev. Food Sci. Nutr.* **2017**, *57*, 1215–1227. [CrossRef] [PubMed]
61. Reyes, A.; Bubnovich, V.; Bustos, R.; Vásquez, M.; Vega, R.; Scheuermann, E. Comparative study of different process conditions of freeze drying of 'Murtilla' berry. *Dry. Technol.* **2010**, *28*, 1416–1425. [CrossRef]

62. López, J.; Ah-Hen, K.S.; Vega-Gálvez, A.; Morales, A.; García-Segovia, P.; Uribe, E. Effects of drying methods on quality attributes of murta (*Ugni molinae* Turcz) berries: Bioactivity, nutritional aspects, texture profile, microstructure and functional properties. *J. Food Process Eng.* **2017**, *40*, e12511. [CrossRef]
63. Puente-Díaz, L.; Ah-Hen, K.; Vega-Gálvez, A.; Lemus-Mondaca, R.; Di Scala, K. Combined infrared-convective drying of murta (*Ugni molinae* Turcz) berries: Kinetic modeling and quality assessment. *Dry. Technol.* **2013**, *31*, 329–338. [CrossRef]
64. Ah-Hen, K.; Zambra, C.E.; Agüero, J.E.; Vega-Gálvez, A.; Lemus-Mondaca, R. Moisture diffusivity coefficient and convective drying modelling of murta (*Ugni molinae* Turcz): Influence of temperature and vacuum on drying kinetics. *Food Bioprocess Technol.* **2013**, *6*, 919–930. [CrossRef]
65. López, J.; Vega-Gálvez, A.; Bilbao-Sainz, C.; Chiou, B.-S.; Uribe, E.; Quispe-Fuentes, I. Influence of vacuum drying temperature on: Physico-chemical composition and antioxidant properties of murta berries. *J. Food Process Eng.* **2017**, *40*, e12569.
66. Avello, M.; Pastene, E. Actividad antioxidante de infusos de *Ugni molinae* Turcz ("Murtilla"). *Bol. Latinoam. Caribe Plantas Med. Aromat.* **2005**, *4*, 33–39.
67. Rubilar, M.; Pinelo, M.; Ihl, M.; Scheuermann, E.; Sineiro, J.; Nuñez, M.J. Murta leaves (*Ugni molinae* Turcz) as a source of antioxidant polyphenols. *J. Agric. Food Chem.* **2006**, *54*, 59–64. [CrossRef]
68. Delporte, C.; Backhouse, N.; Inostroza, V.; Aguirre, M.C.; Peredo, N.; Silva, X.; Negrete, R.; Miranda, H.F. Analgesic activity of *Ugni molinae* (murtilla) in mice models of acute pain. *J. Ethnopharmacol.* **2007**, *112*, 162–165. [CrossRef] [PubMed]
69. Aguirre, M.C.; Delporte, C.; Backhouse, N.; Erazo, S.; Letelier, M.E.; Cassels, B.K.; Silva, X.; Alegría, S.; Negrete, R. Topical anti-inflammatory activity of 2α-hydroxy pentacyclic triterpene acids from the leaves of *Ugni molinae*. *Bioorg. Med. Chem.* **2006**, *14*, 5673–5677. [CrossRef] [PubMed]
70. Goity, L.E.; Queupil, M.J.; Jara, D.; Alegria, S.E.; Pena, M.; Barriga, A.; Aguirre, M.C.; Delporte, C. An HPLC-UV and HPLC-ESI-MS based method for identification of anti-inflammatory triterpenoids from the extracts of *Ugni molinae*. *Bol. Latinoam. Caribe Plantas Med. Aromat.* **2013**, *12*, 108–116.
71. Arancibia-Radich, J.; Pena-Cerda, M.; Jara, D.; Valenzuela-Bustamante, P.; Goity, L.; Valenzuela-Barra, G.; Silva, X.; Garrido, G.; Delporte, C.; Seguel, I. Comparative study of anti-inflammatory activity and qualitative-quantitative composition of triterpenoids from ten genotypes of *Ugni molinae*. *Bol. Latinoam. Caribe Plantas Med. Aromat.* **2016**, *15*, 274–287.
72. Avello, M.; Valdivia, R.; Mondaca, M.A.; Ordoñez, J.L.; Bittner, M.; Becerra, J. Activity of *Ugni molinae* Turcz against microorganisms with clinical importance. *Bol. Latinoam. Caribe Plantas Med. Aromat.* **2009**, *8*, 141–144.
73. Shene, C.; Reyes, A.K.; Villarroel, M.; Sineiro, J.; Pinelo, M.; Rubilar, M. Plant location and extraction procedure strongly alter the antimicrobial activity of murta extracts. *Eur. Food Res. Technol.* **2009**, *228*, 467–475. [CrossRef]
74. Shene, C.; Canquil, N.; Jorquera, M.; Pinelo, M.; Rubilar, M.; Acevedo, F.; Vergara, C.; Von Baer, D.; Mardones, C. In vitro activity on human gut bacteria of murta leaf extracts (*Ugni molinae* Turcz), a native plant from Southern Chile. *J. Food Sci.* **2012**, *77*, M323–M329. [CrossRef]
75. De Dicastillo, C.L.; Bustos, F.; Valenzuela, X.; Lopez-Carballo, G.; Vilarino, J.M.; Galotto, M.J. Chilean berry *Ugni molinae* Turcz fruit and leaves extracts with interesting antioxidant, antimicrobial and tyrosinase inhibitory properties. *Food Res. Int.* **2017**, *102*, 119–128. [CrossRef]
76. Jofre, I.; Pezoa, C.; Cuevas, M.; Scheuermann, E.; Freires, I.A.; Rosalen, P.L.; De Alencar, S.M.; Romero, F. Antioxidant and vasodilator activity of *Ugni molinae* Turcz. (murtilla) and its modulatory mechanism in hypotensive response. *Oxid. Med. Cell. Longev.* **2016**, 6513416. [CrossRef]
77. Calfío, C.; Huidobro-Toro, J.P. Potent vasodilator and cellular antioxidant activity of endemic patagonian calafate berries (*Berberis microphylla*) with nutraceutical potential. *Molecules* **2019**, *24*, 2700. [CrossRef]
78. Manosalva, L.; Mutis, A.; Urzua, A.; Fajardo, V.; Quiroz, A. Antibacterial activity of alkaloid fractions from *Berberis microphylla* G. Forst and study of synergism with ampicillin and cephalothin. *Molecules* **2016**, *21*, 76. [CrossRef]
79. Manosalva, L.; Mutis, A.; Diaz, J.; Urzua, A.; Fajardo, V.; Quiroz, A. Identification of isoquinoline alkaloids from *Berberis microphylla* by HPLC ESI-MS/MS. *Bol. Latinoam. Caribe Plantas Med. Aromat.* **2014**, *13*, 324–335.
80. Furrianca, M.C.; Alvear, M.; Zambrano, T.; Fajardo, V.; Salazar, L.A. Hypoglycemic effect of *Berberis microphylla* G. Forst root extract. *Trop. J. Pharm. Res.* **2017**, *16*, 2179–2184. [CrossRef]
81. Pitta-Alvarez, S.I.; Medina-Bolivar, F.; Alvarez, M.A.; Scambatto, A.A.; Marconi, P.L. In vitro shoot culture and antimicrobial activity of *Berberis buxifolia* Lam. *Vitr. Cell. Dev. Biol. Plant* **2008**, *44*, 502–507. [CrossRef]

82. Albrecht, C.; Pellarin, G.; Rojas, M.J.; Albesa, I.; Eraso, A.J. Beneficial effect of *Berberis buxifolia* Lam, *Zizyphus mistol* Griseb and *Prosopis alba* extracts on oxidative stress induced by chloramphenicol. *Medicina (Buenos Aires)* **2010**, *70*, 65–70.
83. Reyes-Farias, M.; Vasquez, K.; Ovalle-Marin, A.; Fuentes, F.; Parra, C.; Quitral, V.; Jimenez, P.; Garcia-Diaz, D.F. Chilean native fruit extracts inhibit inflammation linked to the pathogenic interaction between adipocytes and macrophages. *J. Med. Food.* **2015**, *18*, 601–608. [CrossRef]
84. Chang, H.C.; Peng, C.H.; Yeh, D.M.; Kao, E.S.; Wang, C.J. *Hibiscus sabdariffa* extract inhibits obesity and fat accumulation, and improves liver steatosis in humans. *Food Funct.* **2014**, *5*, 734–739. [CrossRef]
85. De Ferrars, R.M.; Czank, C.; Zhang, Q. The pharmacokinetics of anthocyanins and their metabolites in humans. *Br. J. Pharmacol.* **2014**, *171*, 3268–3282. [CrossRef]
86. Zhang, X.; Huang, H.; Zhao, X. Effects of flavonoids-rich Chinese bayberry (*Myrica rubra* Sieb. et Zucc.) pulp extracts on glucose consumption in human HepG2 cells. *J. Funct. Foods* **2015**, *14*, 144–153. [CrossRef]
87. Pavlidou, E.; Giaginis, C.; Fasoulas, A.; Petridis, D. Evaluation of the effect of blueberries consumption on chronic diseases, illness prevention and health promotion. *Nat. Prod. J.* **2018**, *8*, 45–53. [CrossRef]
88. Siddiq, M.; Dolan, K.D.; Perkins-Veazie, O.; Collins, J.K. Effect of pectinolytic and cellulytic enzymes on the physical, chemical, and antioxidant properties of blueberry (*Vaccinium corymbosum* L.) juice. *LWT-Food Sci. Technol.* **2018**, *92*, 127–132. [CrossRef]
89. Speisky, H.; López-Alarcón, C.; Gómez, M.; Fuentes, J.; Sandoval-Vicuña, C. First web-based database on total phenolics and oxygen radical absorbance capacity (ORAC) of fruits produced and consumed within the South Andes Region of South America. *J. Agric. Food Chem.* **2012**, *60*, 8851–8859. [CrossRef]
90. Lila, M.; Ribnicky, D.; Rojo, L.; Rojas-Silva, P.; Oren, A.; Havenaar, R.; Janle, E.; Raskin, I.; Yousef, G.; Grace, M. Complementary approaches to gauge the bioavailability and distribution of ingested berry polyphenolics. *J. Agric. Food Chem.* **2012**, *60*, 5763–5771. [CrossRef] [PubMed]
91. Flores, F.; Singh, R.; Kerr, W.; Pegg, R.; Kong, F. Total phenolics content and antioxidant capacities of microencapsulated blueberry anthocyanins during in vitro digestion. *Food Chem.* **2014**, *153*, 272–278. [CrossRef]
92. Mosele, J.I.; Macià, A.; Romero, M.P.; Motilva, M.J. Stability and metabolism of *Arbutus unedo* bioactive compounds (phenolics and antioxidants) under in vitro digestion and colonic fermentation. *Food Chem.* **2016**, *201*, 120–130. [CrossRef] [PubMed]
93. Ah-Hen, K.S.; Mathias-Rettig, K.; Gomez-Perez, L.S.; Riquelme-Asenjo, G.; Lemus-Mondaca, R.; Munoz-Farina, O. Bioaccessibility of bioactive compounds and antioxidant activity in murta (*Ugni molinae* T.) berries juices. *J. Food Meas. Charact.* **2018**, *12*, 602–615. [CrossRef]
94. Kay, C.D.; Mazza, G.J.; Holub, B.J. Anthocyanins exist in the circulation primarily as metabolites in adult men. *J. Nutr.* **2005**, *135*, 2582–2588. [CrossRef]
95. Bustamante, L.; Pastene, E.; Duran-Sandoval, D.; Vergara, C.; Von Baer, D.; Mardones, C. Pharmacokinetics of low molecular weight phenolic compounds in gerbil plasma after the consumption of calafate berry (*Berberis microphylla*) extract. *Food Chem.* **2018**, *268*, 347–354. [CrossRef]
96. Amin, H.P.; Czank, C.; Raheem, S.; Zhang, Q.; Botting, N.P.; Cassidy, A.; Kay, C.D. Anthocyanins and their physiologically relevant metabolites alter the expression of IL-6 and VCAM-1 in CD40L and oxidized LDL challenged vascular endothelial cells. *Mol. Nutr. Food Res.* **2015**, *59*, 1095–1106. [CrossRef]
97. Warner, E.F.; Zhang, Q.; Raheem, Q.S.; O'Hagan, D.; O'Connell, M.A.; Kay, C.D. Common phenolic metabolites of flavonoids, but not their unmetabolized precursors, reduce the secretion of vascular cellular adhesion molecules by human endothelial cells. *J. Nutr.* **2016**, *146*, 465–473. [CrossRef]
98. Warner, E.F.; Smith, M.J.; Zhang, Q.; Raheem, K.S.; O'Hagan, D.; O'Connell, M.A.; Kay, C.D. Signatures of anthocyanin metabolites identified in humans inhibit biomarkers of vascular inflammation in human endothelial cells. *Mol. Nutr. Food Res.* **2017**, *61*. [CrossRef] [PubMed]
99. Abe, L.T.; Lajolo, F.M.; Genovese, M.I. Potential dietary sources of ellagic acid and other antioxidants among fruits consumed in Brazil: Jabuticaba (*Myrciaria jaboticaba* (Vell.) Berg). *J. Sci. Food Agric.* **2012**, *92*, 1679–1687. [CrossRef] [PubMed]

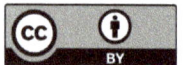

© 2020 by the authors. Licensee MDPI, Basel, Switzerland. This article is an open access article distributed under the terms and conditions of the Creative Commons Attribution (CC BY) license (http://creativecommons.org/licenses/by/4.0/).

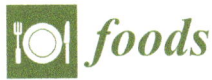

Review

The Pharmacological Effects and Health Benefits of *Platycodon grandiflorus*—A Medicine Food Homology Species

Ming-Yue Ji [1], Agula Bo [1], Min Yang [1], Jin-Fan Xu [1], Lin-Lin Jiang [2], Bao-Chang Zhou [2] and Min-Hui Li [1,2,3,4,5,*]

1. Baotou Medical College, Baotou 014060, Inner Mongolia, China; Jimingyue9@163.com (M.-Y.J.); agula372000@126.com (A.B.); yangmin_0406@aliyun.com (M.Y.); xjf0815@163.com (J.-F.X.)
2. Department of Pharmacy, Inner Mongolia Medical University, Hohhot 010110, Inner Mongolia, China; jianglinlin27@163.com (L.-L.J.); zbc373284882@163.com (B.-C.Z.)
3. Pharmaceutical Laboratory, Inner Mongolia Autonomous Region Academy of Chinese Medicine, Hohhot 010020, Inner Mongolia, China
4. Inner Mongolia Key Laboratory of Characteristic Geoherbs Resources Protection and Utilization, Baotou Medical College, Baotou 014060, Inner Mongolia, China
5. Guangxi Key Laboratory of Medicinal Resources Protection and Genetic Improvement, Guangxi Botanical Garden of Medicinal Plants, Nanning 530023, Jiangxi, China
* Correspondence: prof_liminhui@yeah.net; Tel.: +86-472-716-7795

Received: 15 January 2020; Accepted: 24 January 2020; Published: 31 January 2020

Abstract: *Platycodon grandiflorus* is a widely used edible, traditional Chinese medicinal herb. It is rich in saponins, flavonoids, phenolic acids, and other compounds. It contains a large number of fatty acids such as linoleic acid (up to 63.24%), a variety of amino acids, vitamins, and multiple essential trace elements. *P. grandiflorus* has several biological applications, such as in hypotension, lipid reduction, atherosclerosis, inflammation, relieving cough and phlegm, promoting cholic acid secretion, and as an antioxidant. Further, *P. grandiflorus* is often used in the development of cold mixed vegetables, canned vegetables, preserved fruit, salted vegetables, and cosmetics in northeast China, South Korea, Japan, and Korea. In this paper, the active chemical components and the health benefits of *P. grandiflorus* have been reviewed, providing new ideas for the further development of nutraceutical products to prevent and manage chronic diseases.

Keywords: *Platycodon grandiflorus*; medicinal food; saponins; human health; applications

---

1. Introduction

In recent years, with the gradual enhancement of public health awareness, healthy diets have been recognized as a significant and beneficial health factor. When people keep good healthy diet habits, they also enrich the varieties of food, and take the medicinal plants with therapeutic effect as food into daily life. This kind of "food" not only can satisfy hunger, but also has many functions, such as nutrition, health care, disease prevention, and treatment [1]. The food with this function is defined as a medicine food homology species. The theory of "medicine food homology" was formally put forward in the 1920s and 1930s, and its formation is a long process. *Platycodon grandiflorus* (Figure 1) is a perennial herb belonging to the family Campanulaceae, and it is a medicine food homology species. *P. grandiflorus* has been used as food and medicine for thousands of years in east Asia, such as China, Japan, and Korea. The description of *P. grandiflorus* was first recorded in *Shennong Bencao* in China. Later, it was documented in many other well-known medicinal works in other countries, including *Hanaoka Seishu* (Edo age of Japan, 1760–1835 A.D.) [2,3]. *P. grandiflorus* is rich in amino acids, plant fiber, vitamins, calcium, zinc, potassium, iron, and other trace elements essential in the human diet.

It contains more than 16 amino acids, including 8 essential amino acids [4]. The tender seedlings and roots of *P. grandiflorus* have a broad market in Korea, South Korea, Japan, and northeast Chinese traditional wild vegetables [5]. The method of eating is to process *P. grandiflorus* into pickles, salads. Modern technology can be used for noodles, preserved fruits, and health drinks [6]. In addition, the flower of *P. grandiflorus* is blue, purple or white, and its shape is like a hanging clock, which has a very high ornamental value [4].

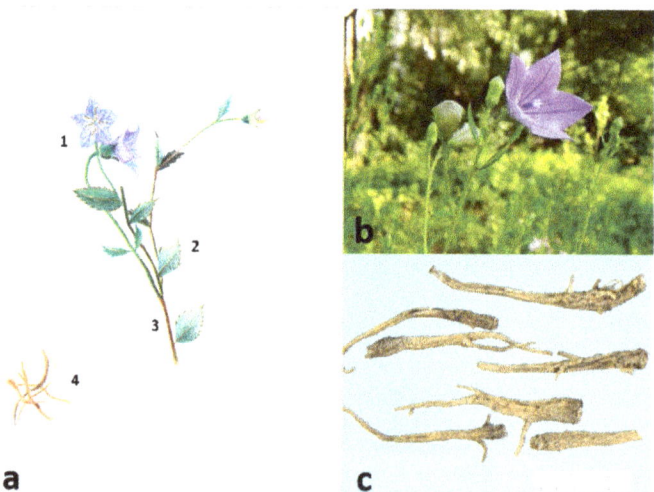

Figure 1. Images of *P. grandiflorus*. (**a**) Line drawing of *P. grandiflorus*: 1. flower; 2. leaf; 3. stem; 4. root. (**b**) Plant of *P. grandiflorus*. (**c**) The medicinal material of *P. grandiflorus*.

The chemical composition of *P. grandiflorus* was first studied by Japanese scholars in the early 20th century [7]. Further studies in modern pharmacology have shown that *P. grandiflorus* contains chemical compounds such as flavonoids, phenolic acids, triterpenoid saponins, polyacetylene, and sterols [8]. These are the main biological components that show significant antitussive, antitumor, antioxidation, anti-inflammatory, hypoglycemic, anti-obesity, and immune enhancement effects. Korean scholars have also found that the alcoholic extract of *P. grandiflorus* has a protective function in mitomycin-induced mutagenesis. *P. grandiflorus* can cause local tissue excitation, contact dermatitis, and hemolysis, and is an inhibitor of the central nervous system, which can reduce blood pressure. *P. grandiflorus* can also reduce tobacco toxicity and control the blood alcohol content in humans; it can thus be made into tobacco additives and alcohol absorption inhibitors [7]. Based on these properties, *P. grandiflorus* is often used in traditional Chinese medicine for respiratory system diseases [9]. In addition to these effects, platycodin D (PD), the main active compound extracted from *P. grandiflorus*, can inhibit lipase activity [10–13]. This property can be utilized in health foods to prevent and treat lipid metabolic disorders [14,15]. Therefore, *P. grandiflorus* can be used to treat various disorders. Most studies on *P. grandiflorus* report the medicinal aspects of the herb, while there are limited studies on medicine food homology.

As a medicine food homology species, *P. grandiflorus* is in great demand in the market. At present, the output in a normal year in China is 1 million kg, of which the export accounts for half. It is reported that 150 thousand kg of *P. grandiflorus* is needed annually in Japan [5]. *P. grandiflorus* as an export vegetable has become a new bright spot in increasing farmers' income and its economic benefit is 2.5 times higher than as medicinal [16]. Many countries demand for *P. grandiflorus* increased stably, the export of fresh *P. grandiflorus* increased sharply; the demand exceeds the supply, the price rises greatly, therefore, *P. grandiflorus* has huge development value and good development prospect.

In this review, the active chemical components and pharmacological activities of *P. grandiflorus* have been summarized based on the literature review. In addition to medicine, alternative applications of *P. grandiflorus* were introduced to provide a new understanding in the homology of medicine and food, with the ultimate goal of using this herb as a naturally-derived therapeutic option.

2. Bioactive Components

2.1. Saponins

Saponin is a type of glycoside whose aglycone is a triterpenoid or spirosterol. Triterpenoid saponins are abundant in *P. grandiflorus* [17,18]. They are the main active component characteristic to *P. grandiflorus*, and are olefin-type pentacyclic triene derivatives. According to the parent nucleus of the saponins, they can be divided into platycodic acid, platycogenic acid, and polygalacic acid [19–21]. According to the Pharmacopoeia of the People's Republic of China, the saponin content should not be less than 6.0% by gravimetric method in order to control the quality of medicinal materials [22]. At present, 75 triterpenoid glycosides have been isolated and identified from *P. grandiflorus*. Among them, platycodin A is considered to be the main saponin of *P. grandiflorus*.

Studies have also confirmed that PD is the main active compound in the extract of *P. grandiflorus* [23]. Guo [24] determined that the PD was present in all parts of the *P. grandiflorus* herb. However, the content of PD in the upper portion of roots and leaves was slightly lower than that of the main root, and the content of PD in the fibrous roots and root bark of the *P. grandiflorus* was higher than that in the aerial parts. PD is both medicinal and nutritional and has high anti-tussive [25], anti-obesity [26], anti-fibrosis [27], anti-inflammatory, and anti-tumor effects [28]. In vitro experiments showed that platycodin D_3 could eliminate phlegm and showed anti-inflammatory activity. In addition, platycodin D_2, platycodin D_3, and PD have significant antitumor activity [29–31]. Platycodin A, platycodin C, deapioplatycodin D, and 16-oxo-PD have been shown to have anti-obesity activities [32–35]. The saponins structures are shown in Figure 2.

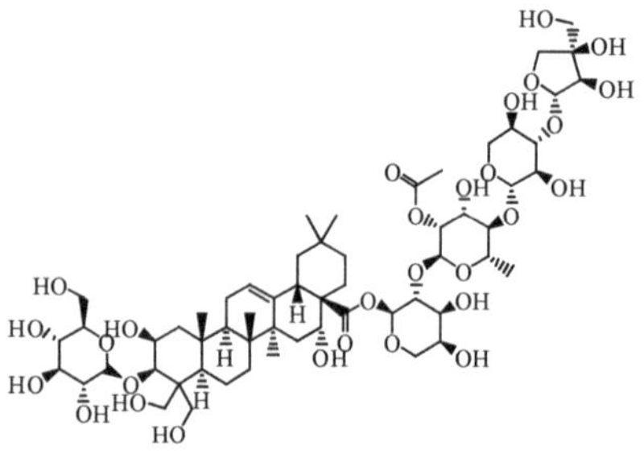

Platycodin A

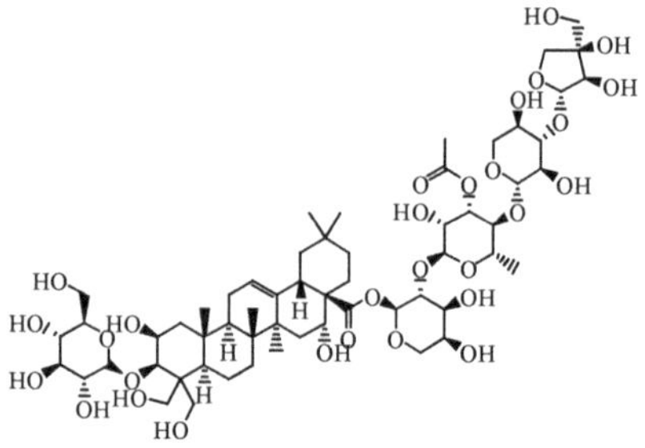

Platycodin C

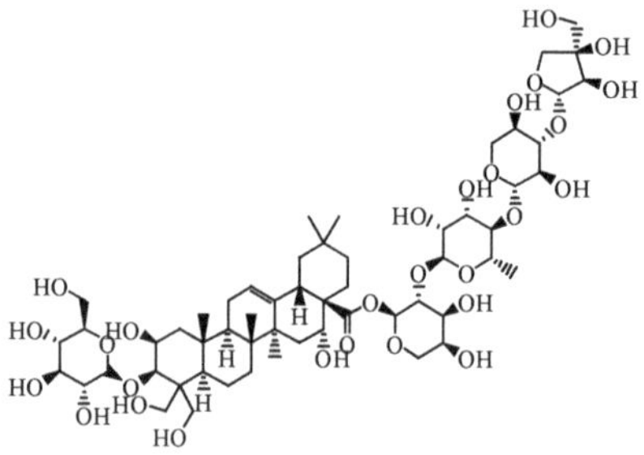

Platycodin D

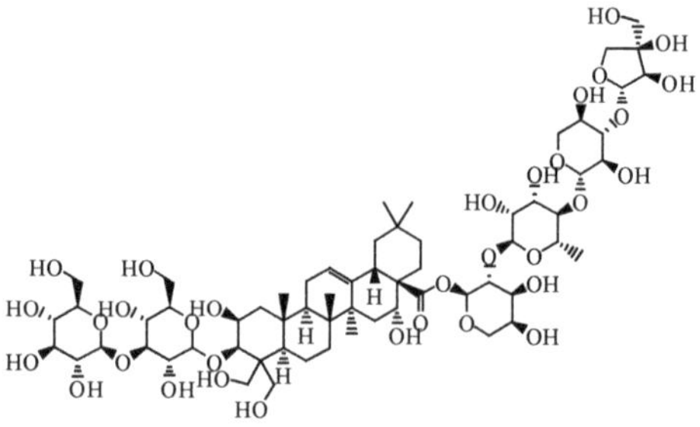

Platycodin D_2

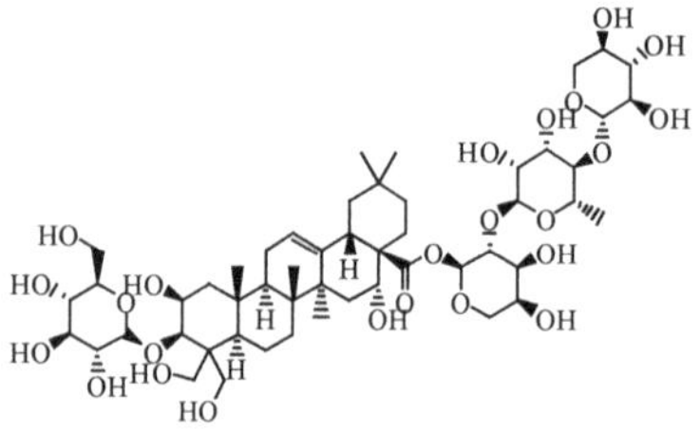

Deapioplatycodin D

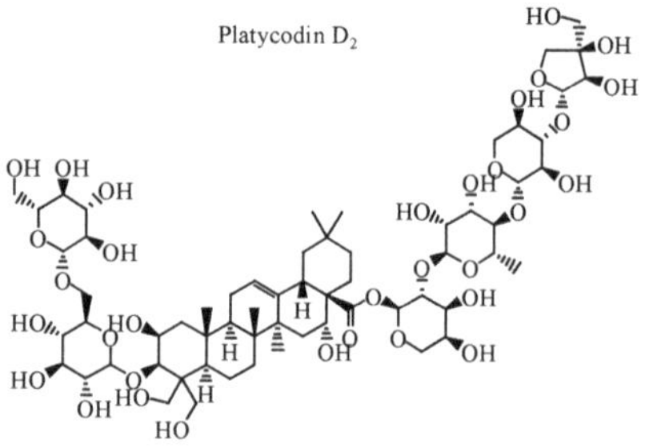

Platycodin D_3

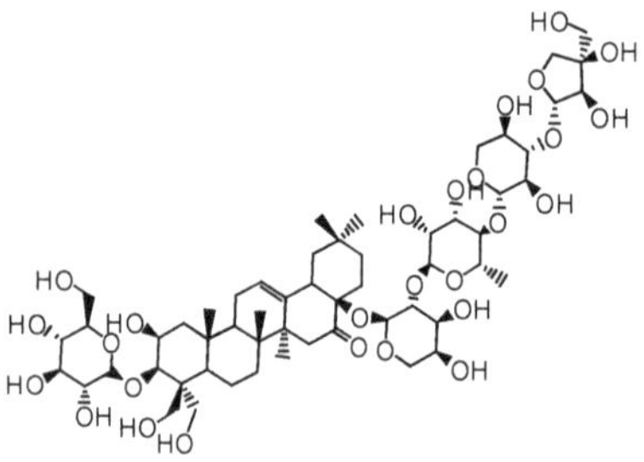

16-oxo-platycodin D

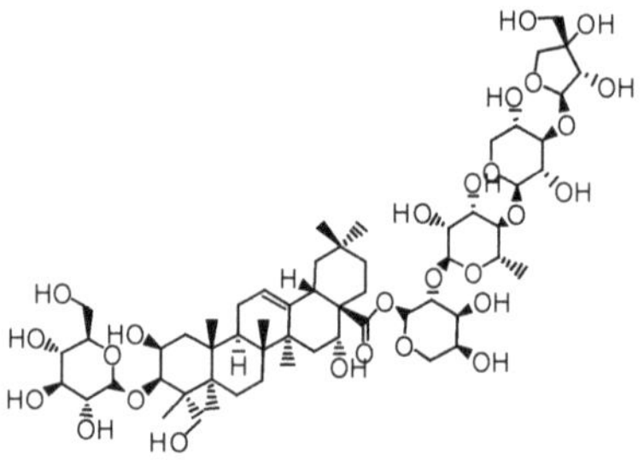

Polygalin D

Figure 2. Active triterpenoid saponins in *P. grandiflorus*.

2.2. Flavonoids

Flavonoids mainly exist in the upper portion of *P. grandiflorus* above the soil, mainly comprising of flavonoids, dihydroflavonoids, and flavonoid glycosides. At present, 11 flavonoids have been isolated and identified from *P. grandiflorus* [36]. It has been shown that six different flavonoids were obtained from the seeds and the flowers of *P. grandiflorus*, while 3 compounds were isolated from the aboveground part of *P. grandiflorus* grown in Poland [37]. Of these flavonoids, luteolin-7-O-glucoside and apigenin-7-O-glucoside exhibit strong antioxidant activity [37,38]. The structures of the flavonoids are shown in Figure 3, and the other nine flavonoids isolated from *P. grandiflorus* are listed in Table 1.

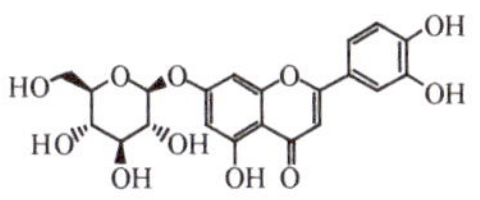

Luteolin-7-O-glucoside 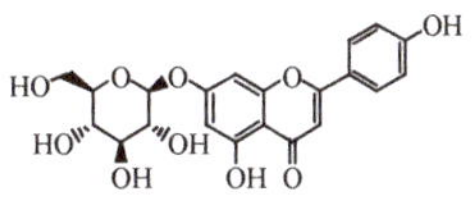   Apigenin-7-O-glucoside

Figure 3. Active flavonoids in *P. grandiflorus*.

Table 1. The other flavonoids components isolated from *P. grandiflorus*.

No.	Name	Ref.
1	Platyconin	[36]
2	Apigenin	[36]
3	(2R,3R)-taxifolin	[36]
4	Luteolin	[36]
5	Quercetin-7-O-glucoside	[36,38]
6	Quercetin-7-O-rutinoside	[36,38]
7	Platycoside	[36,39,40]
8	Delphinidin-3-rutinoside-7-glucoside	[36,41]
9	Flavoplatycoside	[36]

2.3. Other Components

In addition to saponins and flavonoids, *P. grandiflorus* contains other compounds, such as phenolic acids, polyacetylene, sterols, and amino acids [40–44]. Phenolic acids are abundant in the roots and aboveground parts of *P. grandiflorus*; 14 kinds of antioxidant phenolic compounds have been isolated from the *P. grandiflorus* extract. Five polyacetylene compounds have been obtained from *P. grandiflorus*, which is an important criterion for the classification of *P. grandiflorus* [45]. Lobetyol has been found to have an anti-tumor effect.

Macromolecules have also been identified in *P. grandiflorus*. A study showed that *P. grandiflorus* contained 18 amino acids [32]. Among these, gamma-aminobutyric acid is an essential neurotransmitter chemical in the brain's energy metabolism. In addition, the root of *P. grandiflorus* contains fatty acids, which accounted for 88.28% of the total lipids [46]. Inulin, grandoside, and polysaccharides have also been isolated from *P. grandiflorus* [47]. Studies have shown that the polysaccharides of *P. grandiflorus* have strong antioxidant activity [48]. Although the contents of bioactive components of *P. grandiflorus* were different, they all had high efficiency and low toxicity, which provided a scientific basis for characterizing its pharmacological activities. The structures of the other components are shown in Figure 4, and the other non-active components are listed in Table 2.

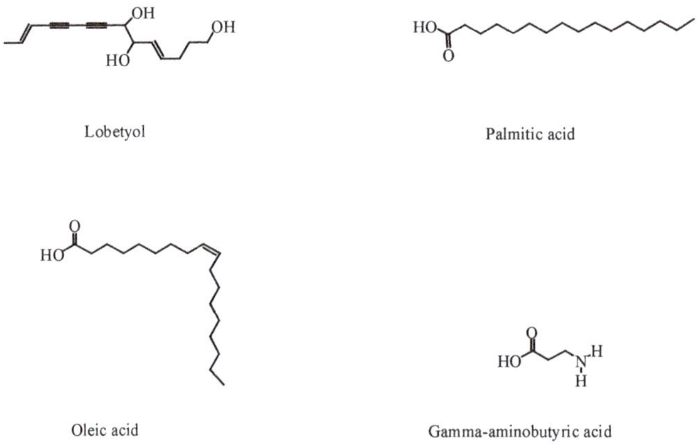

Figure 4. Other active components in *P. grandiflorus*.

Table 2. The others components isolated from *P. grandiflorus*.

Classes	No.	Compound Name	Ref.
Phenolic acids	1	Caffeic acid	[42]
	2	3,4-dimethoxycinnamic acid	[42]
	3	Ferulic acid	[42]
	4	Isoferulic acid	[42]
	5	*m*-coumaric acid	[42]
	6	*p*-coumaric acid	[42]
	7	*p*-hydroxybenzoic acid	[42]
	8	α-resorcylic acid	[42]
	9	2,3-dihydroxybenzoic acid	[42]
	10	2-hydroxy-4-methoxybenzoic acid	[42]
	11	Homovanillic acid	[42]
	12	Chlorogenic acid	[42]
	13	lobetyol	[43]
	14	lobetyolin	[43]
Polyacetylene	15	lobetyolinin	[44]
	16	Lobetyolin	[41]
	17	Platetyolin A	[36,49]
	18	Platetyolin B	[36,49]
Sterols	19	Betulin	[41]
	20	β-sitosterol	[41]
	21	δ-7-stigmastenone-3	[27]
	22	Spinasterol	[36]
	23	α-spinasteryl-3-*O*-β-D-glucoside	[36]
Others	24	Threonine	[36]
	25	Valine	[36]
	26	Phenylalanine	[36]
	27	Methionine	[36]
	28	Isoleucine	[36]
	29	Leucine	[36]
	30	Lysine	[36]
	31	Inulin	[36]
	32	Grandoside	[36]

3. Pharmacological Actions

P. grandiflorus has high edible and medicinal value, contains a variety of active ingredients beneficial to the human body, has relieving cough and asthma activities, anti-tumor, anti-inflammatory and antibacterial, antioxidation, hypoglycemic, liver protection, improves human immunity and other broad pharmacological activities, has good clinical application value and research potential. The main pharmacological activities and the underlying mechanisms are shown in Figure 5.

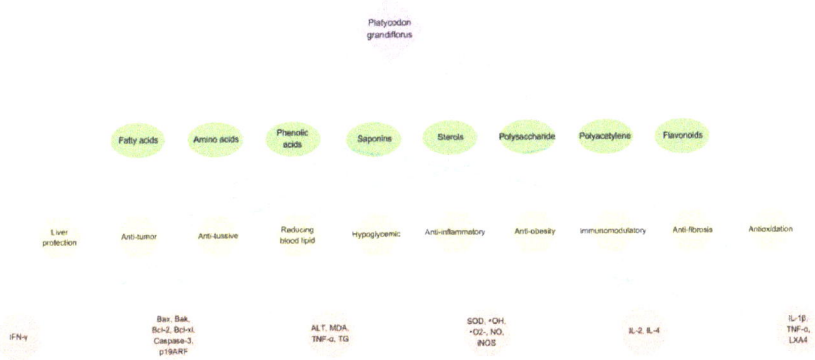

Figure 5. The pharmacological activity mechanism of *P. grandiflorus*. The green ovals represent some activity constituents, yellow polygons represent the common pharmacological activities of *P. grandiflorus*, while represented enzymes and signaling pathways are illustrated by pink polygons. Abbreviations here represent the same meaning as in the body text.

3.1. Relieving Cough and Asthma Activities

P. grandiflorus exhibits strong antitussive, expectorant, and antiasthmatic effects. In an *in vivo* asthma study [50], guinea pigs were randomly divided into five groups: the normal control group, the asthma model group, the dexamethasone group, the *P. grandiflorus* root extract low-dose group, and the *P. grandiflorus* root extract high-dose group. Except for the normal control group, the asthma model was established by ovalbumin in other groups. After successful modeling, the effects of *P. grandiflorus* extract on the levels of serum-related indexes in experimental bronchial asthmatic guinea pigs were observed. The results showed that there was no significant difference in serum-related indexes between the high-dose group and the normal control group ($p > 0.05$) This indicates that the high-dose of the *P. grandiflorus* extract can effectively prolong the latent period of asthma and significantly reduce the generation and release of oxygen free radicals. The extract was also found to simultaneously promote IFN-γ secretion, thereby indirectly playing the role of regulating the Th1/Th2 balance, and promoting the release of lipoxin A4 (LXA4). The LXA4 in the body is adjusted to exert a wide anti-inflammatory and dissipation effect. Therefore, a high-dose extract treatment may be suitable for clinical use in asthma patients.

In another study [51], several animal models were used including chronic bronchitis in mice, guinea pigs with histamine-induced asthma, citric acid-induced cough in guinea pigs, the effects of carrageenin and cotton ball granuloma inflammation in rats. Different doses of platycodin were administered to detect several outcomes, including the number of cells in the alveolar lavage fluid of the slow-branch mice, the histamine-induced asthma reaction, the anti-cough response to the acorn acid and the excretion of the respiratory tract phenol red, the swelling of the foot of the rats, and the weight of the granuloma of the cotton ball. The results of this study suggested that the total number of cells in the alveolar lavage fluid and the number of neutrophils in the lung tissue were significantly lower than that of the control group, while the proportion of the lymphocytes and the macrophages increased and the latent period of the antitussive and cough was prolonged. In addition, cough and asthma was decreased, and the amount of phenol red excretion in the respiratory tract was increased with platycodin administration. This suggested that platycodin has significant antitussive, antiasthmatic, and expectorant effects, and is likely a beneficial for the treatment of chronic bronchitis.

Platycodin can inhibit the activity of nuclear factor kappa B (NF-κB) and downregulate the expression of mucin 5, subtypes A and C (MUC5AC) protein in aldehyde-induced lung cancer cells in a concentration-dependent fashion. This mechanism may be related to the inhibition of NF-κB activation by regulating reactive oxygen species (ROS)—protein kinase C (PKCS)—mitogen-activated protein kinase (MAPK) signaling pathway [52]. PD and platycodin D_3 can also increase the release of respiratory mucin in rats and hamsters. Specifically, the dose of 20 μg/mL platycodin D_3 could effectively promote the release of mucin in rats, and its effect was better than that of the positive control ATP and ambroxol at 200 μg/mL [53].

3.2. Anti-Tumor Activity

Studies have shown that PD, platycodin D_2, and deapioplatycodin D have significant inhibitory effects on the proliferation of A549 (non-small cell lung), SK-OV-3 (ovary), SK-MEL-2 (melanoma), XF498 (central nerve system), and HCT-15 (colon) cell lines in vitro [28]. Kim et al. [54] studied the mechanism of PD induced human leukemia cells (U 937, THP-I, and K 562 cells) for proliferation and cell death. The mechanisms of cell apoptosis were investigated by evaluating cell growth and caspase-3 activity. The effects of different concentrations of PD on synchronous leukemia cells were induced by downregulating Cdc 2/cyclinB-1 and upregulating wee1 expression, resulting in mitotic arrest and endoreduplication, and upregulating CDK-2 protein by downregulating p21. The authors also studied the induction of polyploidy by microtubule polymerization. Their results showed that PD could significantly induce microtubule polymerization in leukemia cells. It revealed that the direct induction of microtubule polymerization in vitro required a high concentration of PD (>200 M). Finally, PD exposure induced apoptosis of U 937 cells by caspase-3 dependent PARP and laminin A. It is therefore logical to assume that the main anti-leukemia activity of PD is to induce internal replication and mitosis, which is caused by the kinetics of compression of the spindle microtubules and the promotion of apoptosis of leukemia cells.

Platycodin D can induce apoptosis in a variety of cancer cells. Yu et al. [55] found that PD activated apoptosis signal regulated kinase 1 (ASK 1) through phosphorylation of threonine ASK 1 and dephosphorylation of serine ASK 1. Moreover, PD induced the activation of endoplasmic reticulum (ER) stress response. The results showed that PD treatment could induce phosphorylation of PKR-like ER kinase (Perk) and eukaryotic initiation factor 2 α (ElF 2α). The expression of glucose regulated protein 78/immunoglobulin heavy chain binding protein (GRP 78/Bip) and CCAAT/enhancer binding protein homologous protein/growth block and DNA damage induced gene 153 (CHOP/GADD 153) were inhibited by N-acetyl-L-cysteine and activated by caspase-4. In addition, the stress responses of ASK 1 and ER induced by PD were also inhibited by N-acetyl-L-cysteine. These results suggest that ROS play a key role in activating ASK 1 and ER stress in PD-treated cancer cells.

Aside from platycodin, *P. grandiflorus* polysaccharides can significantly inhibit the tumor growth of U14 cervical cancer in mice, induce apoptosis of U14 tumor cells, increase the expression of P19ARF and Bax protein, and decrease the expression of mutant p53 protein. It is speculated that *P. grandiflorus* polysaccharides can have an anti-tumor effect by regulating the expression of related genes to promote the apoptosis of tumor cells [56].

3.3. Antioxidation Activity

In addition to antitussive and anti-tumor effects of *P. grandiflorus*, antioxidant effects have also been observed. To this end, the effects of *P. grandiflorus* saponins on the activity of antioxidant enzymes and the concentration of free radicals in lung tissues of mice with chronic bronchitis have been studied. Long-term smoking plus ammonia spray was used to establish chronic bronchitis and superoxide dismutase (SOD) activity of antioxidant enzymes in mice. The authors found that the concentration of free radicals in the lung tissue correspondingly increased, combined with increased activity of iNOS and chronic bronchitis. *P. grandiflorus* saponins significantly increased the activity of the antioxidant enzyme SOD and reduced the activity of the superoxide anion (•O_2), hydroxyl radical (•OH), hydrogen peroxide (H_2O_2), nitric oxide (NO), and other free radicals as well as iNOS. There was an obvious dose-activity relationship, which significantly improved the oxidative stress injury [57].

Gu et al. [58] took H_2O_2-induced PC12 cells as a model of cell oxidative damage. Compared with the model group, *P. grandiflorus* polysaccharide treatment group reduced lactate dehydrogenase (LDH), Malondialdehyde (MDA), and ROS content and enhanced SOD and glutathione peroxidase (GSH-Px) activity in a statistically significant fashion ($p < 0.05$–0.01). In addition, *P. grandiflorus* polysaccharide inhibited the expression of NOX_2, p22phox, and Rac proteins. The results confirmed that *P. grandiflorus* polysaccharide had a protective effect on H_2O_2-induced PC12 cells and could reduce apoptosis. This mechanism may be related to the inhibition of NOX_2 overexpression.

Wang et al. [59] used oxidized low-density lipoprotein (OXLDL) to induce human umbilical vein endothelial cells (HUVECs) to establish its oxidation model. After treatment with different concentrations of the total saponin of *P. grandiflorus*, NO in the culture solution was measured. The level of MDA, and the expression of vascular cell adhesion molecule-1 (VCAM-1) and intercellular cell adhesion molecule-1 (ICAM-1) were used to observe the effects of the total saponin of *P. grandiflorus* on the oxidative damage of oxidized low-density lipoprotein-induced endothelial cells. The results showed that PD was able to significantly reduce the levels of NO and MDA in the cells, reduce the expression of VCAM-1 and ICAM-1 and the adhesion of monocytes and endothelial cells. The authors proposed that the total saponin of *P. grandiflorus* could be a new effective drug with potential antioxidant, lipid-lowering, and anti-atherosclerosis effects.

3.4. Anti-Inflammatory and Antibacterial Activities

Jang et al. [60] studied the anti-inflammatory effect of saponins isolated from *P. grandiflorus* on the production of inflammatory mediators and cytokines in the microglia of BV2 mice stimulated by lipopolysaccharide (LPS). Elevated NO, prostaglandin E (PGE2), and proinflammatory cytokines were detected in BV2 microglia after LPS stimulation. However, *P. grandiflorus* significantly inhibited the excessive production of NO, PGE2, and pro-inflammatory cytokines, including interleukin-1β (IL-1β) and TNF-α in a concentration dependent manner, without causing any cytotoxic effects. In addition, *P. grandiflorus* inhibited NF-κB translocation and LPS-induced phosphorylation of AKT and MAPKs. The results suggest that the inhibition of *P. grandiflorus* on the inflammatory response stimulated by LPS in BV2 microglia is related to the inhibition of the activation of NF-κB and the PI3K/AKT and MAPK signaling pathways. Thus, these findings suggest that *P. grandiflorus* may play a role in the treatment of neurodegenerative diseases by inhibiting the inflammatory response of activated microglia.

Zhu et al. [61] studied the effect of PD on the adhesion of *Candida albicans* to oral mucosal epithelial cells. With the increase in the PD concentration of the *P. grandiflorus* saponin, the change in *C. albicans* from spore phase to mycelium phase was gradually reduced, and the number of adhesive spores and their vitality gradually decreased. Moreover, mRNA levels of IL-8 and human β-defensin (HBD) in supernatant fluid-2 protein and HBD-2 KB cells were gradually reduced, indicating that the characteristics of saponin D reduce *C. albicans* infection of the oral mucosa.

In a separate study [62], a model of chronic bronchitis was established by smoking and ammonia inhalation in mice. Immunohistochemical examination showed that the expression of IL-1β and TNF-α in the lung cells of the model group was significantly higher than that of the normal control group. After 30 days of continuous administration, the expression of IL-1β and TNF-α in lung cells in each treatment group was significantly reduced compared to that in the model group ($p < 0.05$, $p < 0.01$). Western blotting revealed significantly increased levels of IL-1β and TNF-α in lung tissue cells in the model group, compared with normal controls ($p < 0.01$). However, after 30 days of continuous administration, the expression levels of IL-1β and TNF-α in the lung cells of the mice in each treatment group were significantly decreased, with a strong dose-response relationship. The results showed that

P. grandiflorus saponin had a significant inhibitory effect on the expression of inflammatory cytokines IL-1β and TNF-α in the lung tissues of mice with chronic bronchitis. It was speculated that the mechanism of action may have been through inhibiting the production of inflammatory cytokines and free radicals in lung tissues to achieve anti-inflammatory effects.

3.5. Hypoglycemic Activity

Various studies have demonstrated that *P. grandiflorus* shows anti-diabetic activity. The hypoglycemic effect of *P. grandiflorus* extract on diabetic institute of cancer research (ICR) mice was evaluated. The results showed that *P. grandiflorus* ethanol extract could relieve hyperglycemia induced by glucose stimulation. Compared with the model control group, *P. grandiflorus* enhanced the hypoglycemic effect of exogenous insulin without stimulating insulin secretion, suggesting that the insulin sensitivity of diabetic mice increased [63]. Chen et al. [64] treated streptozotocin (STZ)-induced impaired glucose tolerance (IGT) mice with increasing doses of *P. grandiflorus* and found that it had significant inhibitory effect on the activity of α-glucosidase in vitro and in vivo. There was a significant reduction in the blood glucose level of the STZ-IGT mice after oral administration of *P. grandiflorus*. The ethanol extract of *P. grandiflorus* could significantly reduce the blood glucose level in IGT mice at 30 min after meals. This suggested that high doses of ethanol extract of *P. grandiflorus* can significantly decrease blood glucose in IGT mice. It also indicates that reduced blood glucose caused by *P. grandiflorus* is related to the inhibition of α-glucosidase activity.

Qiao et al. [65] believed that for diabetic rats, *P. grandiflorus* can significantly reduce the water intake, food intake, and urine output. The fasting blood glucose in groups administered low, medium, and high doses of *P. grandiflorus* was significantly lower than that in the model group ($p < 0.05$ or $p < 0.01$), and the fasting insulin level, insulin sensitivity index, and glucose tolerance were significantly increased ($p < 0.05$ or $p < 0.01$). *P. grandiflorus* polysaccharides can also increase the activity of superoxide dismutase in liver tissue and decrease the content of malondialdehyde ($p < 0.05$ or $p < 0.01$), indicating that *P. grandiflorus* has a hypoglycemic effect. The mechanism may be to improve fasting insulin levels and antioxidant capacity.

Zheng et al. [66] reported that ethanol extract of *P. grandiflorus* root significantly reduced blood glucose levels in streptozotocin (STZ) diabetic mice, and reduced oral glucose tolerance after 30 min. Though blood glucose levels decreased significantly after combined treatment of STZ diabetic mice, the ethanol extract of *P. grandiflorus* did not affect plasma insulin levels.

3.6. Liver Protection Activity

P. grandiflorus has a therapeutic effect on a variety of drug-induced liver injury models. Khanal et al. [67] studied the protective effects of saponins isolated from the roots of *P. grandiflorus* (Changkil saponins: CKS) on liver injury in mice induced by ethanol. The results showed that levels of serum aminotransferase (ALT) and liver TNF-α increased significantly in the model group, the production of MDA increased, the amount of triglyceride (TG) increased significantly, and the level of GSH in liver tissue decreased significantly, indicating that ethanol induced liver injury in mice. Compared with the model group, the levels of serum ALT, TNF-α, MDA, and TG in the liver of the experimental group were significantly increased, which showed a dose-dependent relationship. Microscopical observation showed that the mice in the model group showed morphological changes such as liver tissue deformation, but on pretreatment with CKS, these changes were significantly inhibited. The above results indicate that CKS may block CYP2E1-mediated ethanol bioactivity and scavenging free-radical inhibition of ethanol-induced liver injury.

Luan et al. [68] observed the effects of total saponins of *P. grandiflorus* on blood glucose, blood lipids, and liver function of type 2 diabetic rats established by tail vein injection of STZ (15 mg/kg) and high glucose and high fat diet for 4 weeks. Total saponins of *P. grandiflorus* (200 mg/kg) for 18 weeks was able to reduce blood sugar, serum cholesterol, triglyceride, low-density lipoprotein levels, and increase serum high-density lipoprotein levels, and improve liver function, thereby reducing type 2 diabetic liver damage in rats.

Hou et al. [69] proved that *P. grandiflorus* and Na_2SeO_3 as raw materials have different degrees of protective effects on liver injury induced by CCl_4 in mice, and the best liver-protecting effect is the high-dose nano-selenium *P. grandiflorus* polysaccharide complex group.

3.7. Other Activities

In addition to the above pharmacological activities, *P. grandiflorus* also has anti-obesity, immune-modulating activity, anti-fatigue, anti-pulmonary damage, and other biological activities.

Zheng et al. [70] found that the water extract of *P. grandiflorus* inhibits the activity of pancreatic lipase, thereby inhibiting the hydrolysis of trioleate and lecithin mixed microparticles, and can reduce the triacyl content in the plasma of rats fed high corn oil. These results suggest that the water extract of Campanulaceae can inhibit the absorption of food fat by the small intestine. Wang et al. [71] found that PD in *P. grandiflorus* showed immunomodulatory activity, stimulating spleen lymphocytes to enhance their proliferative capacity and inducing the secretion of IL-2 and IL-4, and increasing the ratio of $CD4^+/CD8^+$. It suggested that PD could promote the development of splenic lymphocytes from G0/G1 phase to S phase. Yu et al. [72] reported treatment with high, medium, and low doses of an ethanol extract of *P. grandiflorus* could significantly protect against fatigue in mice. Extracts prolonged the mouse climbing rod and swimming time, and significantly increased the reserve of liver glycogen and muscle glycogen after exercise, thus achieving the anti-fatigue effect. Yao et al. [73] also reported that total saponins of *P. grandiflorus* may significantly reduce the inflammatory lesions of lung tissue induced by PM2.5 (PM with aerodynamic diameters ≤2.5 μm) in rats by regulating cytokine and down-regulating the expression of TGF-β and inhibiting the development of fibrosis, which results in the protection and repair on the lung injury of rats caused by PM2.5.

4. Application

4.1. Patent Release of P. grandiflorus

With the improvement of people's living standards and public health awareness, increased attention has been paid to the development of *P. grandiflorus*. There will be increased space for the development of *P. grandiflorus* based on the numerous findings identifying its pharmacological activities. According to the database of Baiten, using *P. grandiflorus* as the key term to search, a total of 15,712 patents were retrieved, including 15,676 Chinese patents. In addition, a total of 37 patents were retrieved from the World Intellectual Property Organization. Figure 6 shows the publication of patents in the last ten years. However, the results show that the number of *P. grandiflorus* patents have declined since 2016. This is likely due to the shortage of *P. grandiflorus*. The decline is likely to continue in the coming years.

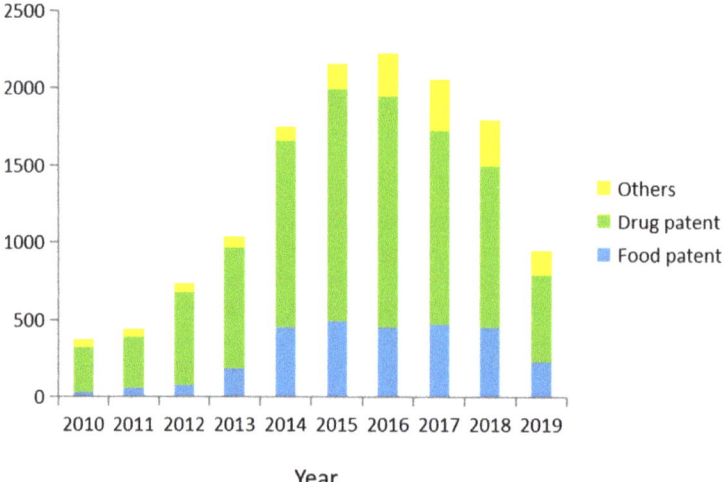

Figure 6. Patent statistics of *P. grandiflorus* from 2010 to 2019.

Through additional analysis, it was found that most of the patents were related to drugs, food, necessities of life, and agriculture. Among them, the number of patents for drugs and food accounted for a larger proportion. Patent statistics show that drugs and foods account for 72.09% and 19.98% of the total patents, respectively. The number of drug patents declined year by year from 2015, while the number of food patents remained relatively stable. With the improvement of public health care awareness, more people focus on the development of health food, not only in the development of drugs. At present, the health food field mainly includes tea, drinks, cakes, noodles, and preserved fruit from *P. grandiflorus*. Among them, the tea from *P. grandiflorus* has the most patents, at 555. In general, *P. grandiflorus* patents have shown a decreasing trend in recent years. Therefore, research on *P. grandiflorus* still needs attention and improvement. The development of medicinal and health care products will undoubtedly be the focus of future research [74]. In the near future, the application of the homologous medicinal herbs will continue to increase.

4.2. Food Application

P. grandiflorus is highly edible and is often used in food in North Korea, South Korea, Japan, and China (Yanbian region). The tender seedlings and roots of *P. grandiflorus* are edible and contain high levels of starch, proteins, and vitamins, and more than 16 kinds of amino acids, including 8 kinds of amino acids necessary for human body. The root of *P. grandiflorus* contains 61.20% sugar and 2.44 mg vitamin B_2 per 100 g. The content of starch, protein, and fiber is 14.00%, 0.19%, and 3.19% in fresh vegetables, respectively. For every 100 g of fresh vegetables, the content of carotene is 8.8 mg and vitamin B_1 is 3.8 mg, which can be made into noodles and other delicious dishes [4]. Fresh roots of *P. grandiflorus* not only preserve its medicinal value, but also the taste and color.

Liu et al. published an invention on nutrient noodles of *P. grandiflorus* [75]. Noodle additives such as wheat oligopeptides and zinc rich arachis oil enhance the taste of the noodles and enhance immunity, thereby promoting the growth and development of children. They are also expected to contribute to anti-oxidation, anti-aging, and improving life expectancy. A *P. grandiflorus* cake with health care functions was invented by Liang et al. [76]. They used processes including raw material handling, mixing, molding, baking, cooling, and packaging to produce the cake. The product is soft, sweet, and delicious, with a flavor of *P. grandiflorus*. This product has a high nutritional value, is low in calories, and is a low-fat green food which integrates nutrition and health care values. In addition, a clear and transparent medicinal liquor was developed, with a unique flavor of *P. grandiflorus*, which retains the efficacy of the traditional Chinese medicine to improve the curative effects of the active ingredients. Tao published the method of making medicinal wine of *P. grandiflorus* [77], a type of health wine that is low in calories, sugar, and fat. It has the effect of relieving cough and resolving phlegm. People can combine the functions of *P. grandiflorus* as a food and medicine, to integrate a medicated diet that aims to keep people fit.

4.3. Clinical Application

In traditional Chinese medicine, the rhizome of *P. grandiflorus* has been widely used. *P. grandiflorus* is mainly used as an expectorant, which has significant effects in treating cough, phlegm, chest tightness, sore throats, and other disorders. It has been documented in many medical books, such as *Shennong Bencao* (Han Dynasty), *Bencao Yanyi* (Song Dynasty, 1116 A.D.), *Bencao Gangmu* (Ming Dynasty, 1590 A.D.), and others. Fortunately, in the Ming Dynasty, Li Shizhen made a systematic summary of *P. grandiflorus* (Jiegeng in Chinese) in *Bencao Gangmu*. In this book, the roots of *P. grandiflorus* could be used to treat cough with chest distress, pulmonary abscesses, and other diseases. In addition, *P. grandiflorus* can usually be used in combination with other herbs, such as *Pinellia ternata*, *Lycium chinense* Mill., *Glycyrrhiza uralensis* Fisch., and others that can increase its therapeutic effect. In the current clinical practice of Chinese medicine, the effects of *P. grandiflorus* are obvious, and with few side effects, its use is very popular. It is widely used as a medicinal compound and Chinese patent medicine in modern clinical medicine, mainly for the treatment of cough, bronchitis, faucitis, and bronchial asthma [78]. In addition, using herbal products as alternative medicines could avoid surgical injury and could also be useful in Western medicine. Researchers have found the advantages of combining Chinese and Western medicine, that can be synergistic and reduce toxicity and side effects, by decreasing drug dosage and extending the adaptive range [79].

Patients with early breast cancer often receive anthracycline-based chemotherapy. However, anthracycline can cause dose-dependent cardiotoxicity. As a traditional Chinese medicine, *P. grandiflorus* has been used for thousands of years to treat cardiovascular diseases. In one study, researchers evaluated the cardioprotective effects and safety of *P. grandiflorus* in patients with early breast cancer receiving anthracycline-based chemotherapy. *P. grandiflorus* may have the potential to prevent anthracycline-induced cardiotoxicity, and also has the advantage of being more affordable [80].

Kikyo-to (KKT) is a formula combination of *Glycyrrhiza uralensis* Fisch. root and *P. grandiflorus* root extracts, which is used for relieving sore throats associated with acute upper respiratory tract infection (URTI) in Japan. This formula is prescribed in primary care. In one study, the therapeutic effect of KKT was sufficient to significantly reduce sore throat, and no side effects were observed [81]. Kikyo-to is a part of Sho-saiko-to-ka-kikyo-sekko. Sho-saiko-to-ka-kikyo-sekko is composed of 9 herbs (gypsum, *Bupleurum* root, *Pinellia* tuber, *Scutellaria* root, *Platycodon* root, jujube fruit, ginseng root, *Glycyrrhiza* root, and ginger rhizome). In some cases, this fixed combination can cure and avert planned surgery to remove tonsils [82].

P. grandiflorus root extracts and *P. grandiflorus* saponin components have been developed by researchers for their antiviral activity. This formula can be used effectively as a preventive or a therapeutic agent for hepatitis C. Moreover, used in clinical practice, this formula is harmless to humans [83].

In addition, apart from the clinical applications mentioned previously, the bioactive components of *P. grandiflorus* also have several other applications. However, chemical methods inevitably produce side-reactions and environmental pollution [84]. There is little research evaluating enzymatic preparation methods to modify triterpene saponins of *P. grandiflorus*. Wie et al. used *Aspergillus niger* crude enzyme extract to transform *P. grandiflorus* to many partially degraded glycosides. This confirms that biotransformation of *P. grandiflorus* has the potential of high efficiency and low toxicity [85].

4.4. Other Applications

P. grandiflorus contains stable anthocyanins, hence it also has the characteristics of a natural pigment. *P. grandiflorus* can thus be used as a natural food pigment in foods and beverages while playing a certain role in regulating physiological functions in the human body. The extract of *P. grandiflorus* has antioxidant effects and eliminates oxygen free radicals. It can be used in the development of anti-oxidation and anti-aging cosmetics. At the same time, the preparation of flavors and pigments from *P. grandiflorus* by acid electrolysis can be used in the production of cosmetics. Recent studies also show that the saponin of *P. grandiflorus* can affect the lipid content in the serum and liver, which has the effect of reducing weight and lipids. Moreover, *P. grandiflorus* has a long flowering period and the colorful flowers are widely used in flower baskets and bouquets [86]. The application of *P. grandiflorus* illustrative figure is shown in Figure 7.

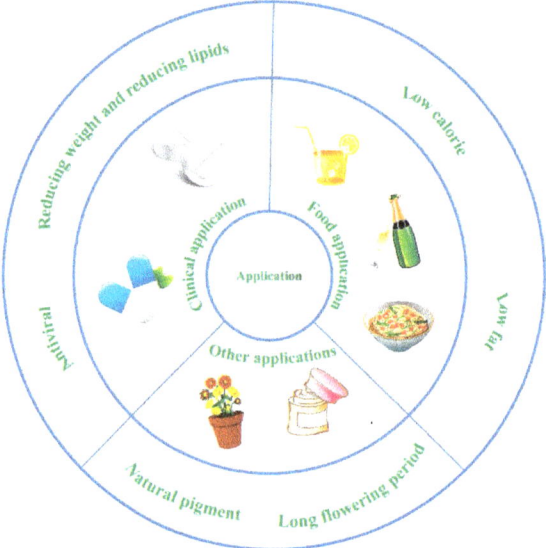

Figure 7. The application of *P. grandiflorus*.

5. Conclusions

P. grandiflorus is a good resource of health food, mainly including proteins, amino acids, trace elements, vitamins, and other substances. In recent years, with the continuous enhancement of people's pursuit of nutritious and healthy food and increasing health care awareness, *P. grandiflorus* has been developed as a medicinal health supplement, functional food, and cosmetic component, especially in the dietary aspect. However, further studies need to be performed to make optimal use of this herb.

At present, studies on *P. grandiflorus* mainly focus on its chemical constituents and pharmacological activities. Modern medical research shows that *P. grandiflorus* has beneficial lung function, clears the throat, moistens the skin, and has preventive effects on respiratory tract diseases. It can also reduce blood pressure and promote blood circulation. *P. grandiflorus* can also regulate the intestines and stomach, promote digestion, and aid in respiratory tract infections. Overall, *P. grandiflorus* has great development potential as a medicine and food homologous variety.

The production process of this herb will also have an impact on its nutritional value. Pickled vegetables are a traditional fermented food in Korea, and its production process determines the quality of the product. The health aspects of pickled vegetables of *P. grandiflorus* are mainly attributed to the saponins and polysaccharides. Some studies have shown that vitamin C, vitamin B, carotene, and the trace element selenium in *P. grandiflorus* can block the synthesis of nitrite and nitrosamine, thereby reducing the content of nitrite. In order to ensure that the properties of *P. grandiflorus* are retained, the existing production process should be optimized to avoid the loss of nutrients during processing.

The pharmacodynamic basis and mechanisms of *P. grandiflorus* are not very clear, and there is a lack of epidemiological investigation data and clinical trials assessing the clinical effects of this herb. Therefore, further systematic and in-depth research is needed. At the same time, as more applications have been found in recent years, the natural resources of wild *P. grandiflorus* can no longer meet the needs. Therefore, it is necessary to strengthen research on cultivation measures to improve the quality of *P. grandiflorus* and promote the development of the industry. These studies will provide new ideas for the development of better therapeutic drugs and health products.

Author Contributions: M.-H.L., A.B., and M.-Y.J. conceived and designed the study; M.-Y.J., A.B., M.Y., J.-F.X., L.-L.J., B.-C.Z. Contributed significantly to the design of the paper, edited and wrote some portion of the paper, compiled the references and analyzed the data; M.-H.L., A.B., and M.-Y.J. wrote the manuscript; All authors have read and agreed to the published version of the manuscript.

Funding: This research was funded by National Natural Science Foundation of China (No. 81760776), National Natural Science Foundation of China (No. 81874336), Natural Science Foundation of Inner Mongolia (No. 2018ZD13), Agriculture Research System of China (No.CARS-21), 2018 Chinese medicine public health service subsidy special "the fourth survey on Chinese materia medica resource" (No. Finance Society (2018) 43).

Conflicts of Interest: The authors declare no conflict of interest.

References

1. Wei, J.X. Application and market of *Platycodon grandifloras*. *Jiangxi Agric.* **2017**, *46*. [CrossRef]
2. Kim, H.R.; Kwon, S.J.; Roy, S.K.; Cho, S.W.; Kim, H.H.; Cho, K.Y.; Boo, H.O.; Woo, S.H. Proteome Profiling Unfurl Differential Expressed Proteins from Various Explants in *Platycodon Grandiflorum*. *Korean J. Crop Sci.* **2015**, *60*, 97–106. [CrossRef]
3. Zhang, L.; Wang, Y.L.; Yang, D.W.; Zhang, C.H.; Zhang, N.; Li, M.H.; Liu, Y.Z. *Platycodon grandiflorus*—An Ethnopharmacological, phytochemical and pharmacological review. *J. Ethnopharm.* **2015**, *164*, 147–161. [CrossRef] [PubMed]
4. Wang, D.; Shu, Y.; Zhao, X.L.; Li, J. Innovation and development value of medicated and edible *platycodon grandiflorum*. *Heilongjiang Agric. Sci.* **2018**, 112–115. [CrossRef]
5. Wang, Y.; Shi, J Y. Research Progress of *Platycodon grandiflorum* in Recent Ten Years. *Food Drug.* **2006**, *8*, 22–24. [CrossRef]
6. Jin, X.; Chen, Q. New progress in pharmacological action of *platycodon grandiflorum*. *Res. Pract. Chin. Med.* **2015**, *29*, 79–82. [CrossRef]
7. Wei, S.Z. The Comprehensive Development and Utilization of Radix Platycodonis. *J. Shanxi Univer. Sci. Technol.* **2005**, 146–148. [CrossRef]
8. Sui, W.X.; Yao, L.; Ma, Y.L. Overview of Pharmacological Research on *Platycodon grandiflorum*. *J. Anhui Agric. Sci.* **2014**, *42*, 4976–4977+5026. [CrossRef]
9. Li, Y.; Wang, J.T.; Gui, S.Y.; Qu, H.H. Progress on Chemical Constituents and Pharmacological Effects of *Platycodon Grondiflonm* (Jacq.) A.DC. *Food Drug* **2016**, *18*, 72–75. [CrossRef]
10. Zhang, Z.Y.; Zhao, M.C.; Zheng, W.X.; Liu, H.Y. Platycodin D, a triterpenoid saponin from *Platycodon grandiflorum*, suppresses the growth and invasion of human oral squamous cell carcinoma cells via the NF-κB pathway. *J. Biochem. Mol. Toxicol.* **2017**, *31*. [CrossRef]
11. Han, L.K.; Zheng, Y.N.; Xu, B.J. Saponins from Platycodi Radix ameliorate high fat diet–induced obesity in mice. *J. Nut.* **2002**, *132*, 2241–2245. [CrossRef] [PubMed]
12. Wang, Y.N.; Zhang, X.; Wei, Z.K.; Wang, J.J.; Zhang, Y.; Shi, M.Y.; Yang, Z.T.; Fu, Y.H. Platycodin D suppressed LPS-induced inflammatory response by activating LXRα in LPS—stimulated primary bovine mammary epithelial cells. *Eur. J. Pharmacol.* **2017**, *814*, 138–143. [CrossRef] [PubMed]
13. Fang, X.X.; Huang, B.T.; Zeng, J.X.; Zhu, J.X.; Wu, B.; Zhong, G.Y.; Liu, F.Q.; Li, H.Z.; Han, F.Y. Content Difference of Total Saponins and Platycodin-D in Platycodonis Radix from Different Origin. *Chin. J. Experimental Tradit. Med. Formulae.* **2016**, *22*, 78. [CrossRef]

14. Zheng, Y.N.; Liu, K.Y.; Xu, B.J.; Han, L.K. Studies on Effects of Platycodi Radix on Lipid Metabolism of Mice with High Fat Diet-Induced Obesity. *J. Jilin. Agric. Univ.* **2002**, *24*, 42–46, 53. [CrossRef]
15. Xu, C.L.; Yang, L.H.; Zheng, Y.N.; Liu, L.X.; Xu, B.J. Determination of platycodin D of radix platycodi in different places by RP-HPLC. *J. Jilin. Agric. Univ.* **1999**, *21*, 35–38.
16. Li, B.F. Cultivation of *Platycodon grandifloras* for export. *Agric. Knowl.* **2003**, *922*, 23.
17. Nikaido, T.; Koike, K.; Mitsunaga, K. Tirterpenoid saponins from root of *Platycodon grandiflorum*. *Nat. Med.* **1998**, *52*, 54–59.
18. Tsuyoshi, S.; Tamotsu, N. Evaluation of saponin properties of HPLC analysis of *Platycodon grandiflorum* A. DC. *Yakugakuzasshi* **2003**, *123*, 431–441. [CrossRef]
19. He, M.L.; Cheng, X.W.; Chen, J.K.; Zhou, T.S. Study on the Components and Quality of *Platycodon grandiflorum*. *Tradit. Chin. Drug Res. Clinical Pharmacol.* **2005**, *16*, 457–460. [CrossRef]
20. Akiyama, T.; Iitaka, Y.; Tanaka, O. Structure of platicodigenin, a sapogenin of *platycodon grandiflorum* a. de candolle. *Tetrahedron Let.* **1968**, *9*, 5577–5580. [CrossRef]
21. Kubota, T.; Kitatani, H.; Hinoh, H. Structure of platycogenic acids A, B and C, further triterpenoid constituents of *platycodon grandiflorum*. *J. Chem. Society D: Chem. Commun.* **1969**, *22*, 1313–1314. [CrossRef]
22. Zhao, X.L. Research progress in chemical constituents, biological activities and exploration utilization of *Platycodon grandiflorum*. *Chin. Condiment* **2012**, *37*, 5–8+24. [CrossRef]
23. Tian, Y.H. Study on the chemical composition and biological activity of *Platycodon Grandiflorum*. Master's Thesis, Jilin Agricultural University, Jilin, China, 2017.
24. Guo, L. Study on quality Standard of *Platycodon grandiflorum*. Master's Thesis, China Academy of Chinese Medical Sciences, Beijing, China, 2007.
25. Zhu, J.X.; Zeng, J.X.; Zhang, Y.M.; Zhong, G.; Liu, F.; Li, H. Comparative Study on Antitussive and Expectorant Effects of *Platycodon grandiflorum* from Different Areas. *Modernization Tradit. Chin. Med. Mater. Medica-World Sci. Technol.* **2015**, *17*, 976–980. [CrossRef]
26. Han, L.K.; Xu, B.J.; Kimura, Y.; Zheng, Y.N.; Okkuda, H. Platycodi radix affects lipid metabolism in mice with high fat diet-induced obesity. *J. Nutr.* **2000**, *130*, 2760–2764. [CrossRef] [PubMed]
27. Lee, K.J.; Choi, C.Y.; Chung, Y.C.; Kim, Y.S.; Ryu, S.Y.; Roh, S.H.; Jeong, H.G. Protective effect of saponins derived from roots of *Platycodon grandiflorum* on tert-butyl hydroperoxide-induced oxidative hepatotoxicity. *Toxicol. Lett.* **2004**, *147*, 271–282. [CrossRef]
28. Kim, Y.S.; Kim, J.S.; Choi, S.U.; Kim, J.S.; Lee, H.S.; Roh, S.H.; Jeong, Y.C.; Kim, Y.K.; Shi Yong Ryu, S.Y. Isolation of a new saponin and cytotoxic effect of saponins from the root of *Platycodon grandiflorum* on human tumor cell lines. *Planta Med.* **2005**, *71*, 566–568. [CrossRef]
29. Ishii, H.; Tori, K.; Tozyo, T. Structures of polygalaein-D and-D_2, platyeodin-D and -D_2 and their monacetates, saponins isolated from *platycodon grandiflorum* A. DC. determined by carbon-13 nuclear magnetic resonance spectroscopy. *Chem. Pharm. Bull.* **1978**, *26*, 674–677. [CrossRef]
30. Wang, C.; Levis, G.B.S.; Lee, E.B. Platycodin D and D_3 isolated from the root of *platycodon grandiflorum* modulate the production of nitric oxide and secretion of TNF-α in activated RAW 264.7 cells. *Int. Immunopharm.* **2004**, *4*, 0–1049. [CrossRef]
31. Hwang, Y.L.; Ahn, H.J.; Ji, G.E. Fermentation of Platycodi Radix and bioconversion of platycosides using co-cultures of Saccharomyces cerevisiae KCTC 7928 and Aspergillus awamori FMB S900. *Food Sci. Biotechnol.* **2015**, *24*, 183–189. [CrossRef]
32. Zhou, Y. Research Progress of Platycodon Grandiflorum. *World Latest Med. Inf. (Electronic Version)* **2017**, *17*, 19+22.
33. Ma, X.Q.; Li, S.M.; Chan, C.L. Influence of sulfur fumigation on glycoside profile in Platycodonis Radix (Jiegeng). *Chin. Med.* **2016**, *11*, 32. [CrossRef] [PubMed]
34. Fukumura, M.; Iwasaki, D.; Hirai, Y. Eight new oleanane-type triterpenoid saponins from platycodon root. *Heterocycles* **2010**, *81*, 2793–2806. [CrossRef]
35. Choi, Y.H.; Yoo, D.S.; Cha, M.R. Antiproliferative effects of saponins from the roots of *Platycodon grandiflorum* on cultured human tumor cells. *J. Nat. Prod.* **2010**, *73*, 1863–1867. [CrossRef] [PubMed]
36. Deng, Y.L.; Ren, H.G.; Ye, X.W.; Xia, L.T.; Zhu, J.; Yu, H.; Zhang, P.Z.; Yang, M.; Zhang, J.L.; Xu, S.B. Progress of Historical Evolution of Processing, Chemical Composition and Pharmacological Effect of Platycodonis Radix. *Chin. J. Exp. Tradit. Med. Formulae* **2019**. [CrossRef]

37. Mazol, I.; Glensk, M.; Cisowski, W. Polyphenolic compounds from *Platycodon grandiflorum* A.DC. *Acta Pol. Pharm.* **2004**, *61*, 203–208. [PubMed]
38. Inada, A.; Murata, H.; Somekawa, M. Phytoehemieal Studies of seeds of Medicinal Plants II. A New Dihydroflavonol Glycoside and a New 3-Methyl-l-butanol Glycoside from Seeds of *Platycodon grandiflorum* A.DC. *Chem. Pharm. Bull.* **1992**, *40*, 3081–3083. [CrossRef]
39. Fu, W.W.; Fu, J.N.; Zhang, W.M.; Sun, L.X.; Pei, Y.H.; Liu, P. Platycoside O, a new triterpenoid saponin from the roots of *Platycodon grandiflorum*. *Molecules* **2011**, *16*, 4371–4378. [CrossRef]
40. Yoo, D.S.; Choi, Y.H.; CHA, M.R. HPLC-ELSD analysis of 18 platycosides from balloon flower roots (Platycodi Radix) sourced from various regions in Korea and geographical clustering of the cultivation areas. *Food. Chem.* **2011**, *129*, 645–651. [CrossRef]
41. Xie, X.X.; Zang, C.; Zeng, J.X.; Zhang, C.H.; Mao, Z.; He, J.W.; Wang, H.L.; Zhong, G.Y.; Zhang, S.W.; Han, H.F. Research progress on chemical constituents and pharmacological activities of *platycodon grandiflorum*. *Tradit. Chin. Med. J.* **2018**, *17*, 66–72+13. [CrossRef]
42. Zuo, J.; Yin, B.K.; Hu, X.Y. Research Progress in the Chemical Constituents and Modern Pharmacology of Platycodon. *J. Liaoning Univ. TCM* **2019**, *21*, 113–116. [CrossRef]
43. Ahn, J.C.; Hwang, B.; Tada, H.; Ishimaru, K.; Sasaki, K.; Shimomura, K. Polyacetylenes in hairy roots of *Platycodon grandiflorum*. *Phytochem.* **1996**, *42*, 69–72. [CrossRef]
44. Tada, H.; Shimomura, K.; Ishimaru, K. Polyacetylenes in *Platycodon grandiflorum* hairy root and campanulaceous plants. *J. Plant Physiol.* **1995**, *145*, 7–10. [CrossRef]
45. Sun, Q.; Meng, Y.L.; Wu, B.C.; Zhu, D.; Wang, W.M. Chemical constituents and pharmacological effects of *platycodon grandiflorum*. *Heilongjiang J. Tradit. Chin. Med.* **2017**, *46*, 64–65.
46. Gong, X.; Wang, J.G. Study on the Fatty Acid Compositions of *Platycodon grandiflorum* A. DC by GC-MS. *J. Anhui Agr. Sci.* **2010**, *38*, 11780–11782. [CrossRef]
47. Liu, Z.H.; Liang, B.; Tian, J.K. Advances in chemistry and pharmacology of plants in *Platycodon grandiflorum*. *Asia-Pac. Tradit. Med.* **2006**, *7*, 9–63.
48. Dong, Z.; Cao, W.G.; Duan, H.; Zhang, X.T.; Chen, J.; Zhang, K. Study on Extraction, Isolation, Purification and Biological Activity of Polysaccharides from *Platycodon grandiflorum*. *Genomics Appl. Biol.* **2018**, *37*, 3534–3539. [CrossRef]
49. Chen, B.; Li, X.P.; Huo, X.H.; Li, Z.M.; Li, W.; Sun, Y.S. HPLC method for simultaneous determination of three polyacetylenes in Platycodonis Radix from different habitats. *Chin. J. Pharm. Anal.* **2018**, *38*, 22–27.
50. Yu, W.Y.; Zhu, H.J. Study on pharmacological mechanism of *platycodon grandiflorum* in treating bronchial asthma. *Acta Chin. Med. Pharmacol.* **2012**, *40*, 38–40. [CrossRef]
51. Sun, R.R.; Zhang, M.Y.; Chen, Q. Study on anti-inflammatory and antitussive and antiasthma effects of *Platycodon grandiflorum* saponins capsule. *Pharmacol. Clin. Chin. Mater. Med.* **2010**, *26*, 27–29.
52. Choi, J.H.; Hwang, Y.P.; Han, E.H.; Kim, H.G.; Park, B.H.; Lee, H.S.; Park, B.K.; Lee, Y.C.; Chung, Y.C.; Jeong, H.G. Inhibition of acrolein-stimulated MUC5AC expression by *Platycodon grandiflorum* root derived saponin in A549 cells. *Food Chem. Toxicol.* **2011**, *49*, 2157–2166. [CrossRef]
53. Shin, C.Y.; Lee, W.J.; Lee, E.B.; Choi, E.Y.; Ko, K.H. Platycodin D and D_3 Increase Airway Mucin Release in vivo and in vitro in Rats and Hamsters. *Planta Med.* **2002**, *68*, 221–225. [CrossRef] [PubMed]
54. Kim, M.O.; Moon, D.O.; Choi, Y.H.; Lee, J.D.; Kim, N.D.; Kim, G.Y. Platycodin D induces mitotic arrest in vitro, leading to endoreduplication, inhibition of proliferation and apoptosis in leukemia cells. *Int. J. Cancer* **2008**, *122*, 2674–2681. [CrossRef] [PubMed]
55. Yu, J.S.; Kim, A.K. Platycodin D Induces Reactive Oxygen Species–Mediated Apoptosis Signal–Regulating Kinase 1 Activation and Endoplasmic Reticulum Stress Response in Human Breast Cancer Cells. *J. Med. Food* **2012**, *15*, 691–699. [CrossRef] [PubMed]
56. Lu, W.F.; Yang, Y.L.; Jia, G.F.; Zhao, C. Anti-tumor activity of polysaccharides isolated from *Radix platycodonis*. *Northwest J. Pharm.* **2013**, *28*, 43–45. [CrossRef]
57. Chen, C.; Zhang, M.Y.; Sun, R.R.; Zhang, Z.Z.; Chen, Q. Effects of Kikyosaponin Capsule on Antioxidases Activities and Free Radical Concentration of Lungs of Chronic Bronchitis Mice. *Chin. J. Tradit. Med. Sci. Technol.* **2010**, *17*, 323–324. [CrossRef]
58. Gu, C.Y.; Chen, Q.L.; Li, H.T. Protective Effects and Mechanism of Polysaccharide from Platycodon Grandiflorum on Damage of PC12 Cells Induced by H_2O_2. *J. Nanjing Univ. Tradit. Chin. Med.* **2017**, *33*, 268–272. [CrossRef]

59. Wang, M.S.; Wu, J.T. Effect of Platycodin D on OxLDL-induced Oxidative Injury of Endothelial Cells. *Food Sci.* **2013**, *34*, 293–296. [CrossRef]
60. Jang, K.J.; Kim, H.K.; Han, M.H.; Oh, Y.N.; Yoon, H.M.; Chung, Y.H.; Kim, G.Y.; Hwang, H.J.; Choi, Y.H. Anti-inflammatory effects of saponins derived from the roots of *Platycodon grandiflorus* in lipopolysaccharide-stimulated BV2 microglial cells. *Int. J. Mol. Med.* **2013**, *31*, 1357–1366. [CrossRef]
61. Zhu, L.F.; Wang, B. Platycodin D protects oral epithelial cells against infection of Candida albicans. *Chin. J. Pathophysiol.* **2017**, *33*, 161–165. [CrossRef]
62. He, L.L.; Chen, Q.; Peng, S.M.; Cao, Y.G.; Li, Y.; Zhu, M. The Effect of Kikyosaponin on Expression of IL-1β and TNF-α from Pneumonocyte of Chronic Bronchitis (CB) Mice. *Chin. J. Cell Biol.* **2013**, *35*, 23.
63. Zheng, J.; Ji, B.P.; He, J.G.; Li, B.; Li, Y.; Zhang, X.F. Influence of *Platycodon grandiflorum* in Blood Glucose of Streptozotocin-induced Diabetic ICR Mice. *Food Sci.* **2006**, *27*, 525–528. [CrossRef]
64. Chen, M.J.; Yu, B.; Zhao, Y.R.; Wu, H.P. Inhibitory effect of *Platycodon grandiflorum* on α-glucosidase activity and glucose tolerance in IGT mice. *Pharmacol. Clin. Chin. Mater. Med.* **2009**, *25*, 60–62.
65. Qiao, C.H.; Meng, X.S. Hypoglycemic effect of *Platycodon grandiflorum* Polysaccharide and its Mechanism. *Chin. J. Gerontol.* **2015**, *35*, 1944–1946. [CrossRef]
66. Zheng, J.; He, J.G.; Ji, B.P.; Li, Y.; Zhang, X.F. Antihyperglycemic effects of *Platycodon grandiflorum* (Jacq.) A. DC. extract on streptozotocininduced diabetic mice. *Plant Food Hum. Nutr.* **2007**, *62*, 7–11. [CrossRef]
67. Khanal, T.; Choi, J.H.; Hwang, Y.P.; Chung, Y.C.; Jeong, H.G. Saponins isolated from the root of *Platycodon grandiflorum* protect against acute ethanol-induced hepatotoxicity in mice. *Food Chem. Toxicol.* **2009**, *47*, 530–535. [CrossRef]
68. Luan, H.Y.; Zhang, J.H.; Zhao, X.L.; Zhang, X.S.; Ou, Q. Effect of total glycosides of *Platycodon grandiflorum* on glycolipid metabolism in rats with type 2 diabetic liver disease. *Chin. Tradit. Patent Med.* **2013**, *35*, 1307–1309. [CrossRef]
69. Hou, W.; Hou, L.Y.; Zhang, Y.J.; Zheng, X.F.; Li, G.S.; Peng, X.; Gao, J.B. Protective effects of nano–selenium/*platycodon* polysaccharides complex on CCl_4-induced liver damage in mice. *Sci. Technol. Food Ind.* **2018**, *39*, 308–311, 317.
70. Zheng, Y.N.; Liu, K.Y.; Xu, B.J.; Han, L.K. Experimental Study on Anti-obesity Mechanism of *Platycodon grandiflorum*. *J. Jilin Agric. Univ.* **2002**, *24*, 42–46. [CrossRef]
71. Wang, M.; Han, J.Q.; Zhang, F.; Yu, Y.; Li, J.S. Immunomodulatory activity of platy saponin D on mouse spleen lymphocytes. *Chin. Vet. Sci.* **2018**, *48*, 93–100. [CrossRef]
72. Yu, T.; Li, X.D.; Jin, Q.K.; Yan, H.S.; Li, S.J.; Cui, C.B. Anti-fatigue effects of extract of *Platycodon grandiflorum* on mice. *Sci. Technol. Food Ind.* **2012**, *33*, 394–396. [CrossRef]
73. Yao, L.; Zhang, J.W.; Meng, Q.J.; Dong, K.; Wang, W.M. Study on the effects of PM2.5 on lung injury and total saponins in *Platycodon grandiflorum*. *Chin. J. Inform. TCM* **2017**, *24*, 38–41. [CrossRef]
74. Ge, D.; Wang, J.T.; Gui, S.Y.; Qu, H.F. Review on Chemical Constituents, Biological Activity and Comprehensive Utilization of *Platycodon grondiflonm* A. DC. *Guangzhou Chem. Ind.* **2015**, *43*, 7–9. [CrossRef]
75. Liu, J.H.; Tian, J.J. A wheat oligopeptide rich in zinc *Platycodon grandiflorum* nutritive noodles. China, CN 105581242A, 18 May 2016.
76. Liang, P.; Wang, N.Y.; Jin, G.Q.; Chen, H.S.; Zhang, D.W. A Method for Making Platycodon grandiflorum Health Cake. China, CN 105145760A, 16 December 2015.
77. Tao, F. A Method for Making Medicinal Herbs of Campanulate. China, CN 105861219A, 17 August 2016.
78. Liu, X.G. Treatment of 56 cases of chronic pharyngitis with *Platycodon grandiflorum* Powder and gargle. *J. Med. Forum.* **2005**, *26*, 57. [CrossRef]
79. Nyakudya, E.; Jeong, J.H.; Lee, N.K.; Jeong, Y.S. Platycosides from the Roots of *Platycodon grandiflorum* and Their Health Benefits. *Prev. Nutr. Food Sci.* **2014**, *19*, 59–68. [CrossRef] [PubMed]
80. Hao, W.; Liu, S.; Qin, Y.N.; Sun, C.P.; Chen, L.Y.; Wu, C.Y.; Bao, Y.J. Cardioprotective effect of *Platycodon grandiflorum* in patients with early breast cancer receiving anthracycline-based chemotherapy: study protocol for a randomized controlled trial. *Trials* **2017**, *18*, 1–7. [CrossRef]
81. Ishimaru, N.; Kinami, S.; Shimokawa, T.; Kanzawa, Y. Kikyo-to vs. Placebo on Sore Throat Associated with Acute Upper Respiratory Tract Infection: A Randomized Controlled Trial. *Int. Med.* **2019**, *58*, 2459–2465. [CrossRef]
82. Goto, F.; Asama, Y.; Ogawa, K. Sho-saiko-to-ka-kikyo-sekko as an alternative treatment for chronic tonsillitis to avoid surgery. *Complement. Ther. Clin. Pract.* **2010**, *16*, 216–218. [CrossRef]

83. Kim, J.W.; Lee, S.W.; Park, S.J.; Shin, J.C.; Yang, J.W.; Lim, J.H. Pharmaceut composition for preventing or treating hepatitis C, comprising the root extracts of Platycodon grandiflorum or Platycodon grandiflorum saponin components. US, US 2011027.4656A1, 8 January 2011.
84. Li, W.; Zhao, L.C.; Wang, Z.; Zheng, Y.N.; Liang, J.; Wang, H. Response surface methodology to optimize enzymatic preparation of Deapio-Platycodin D and Platycodin D from *Radix Platycodi*. *Int. J. Mol. Sci.* **2012**, *13*, 4089–4100. [CrossRef]
85. Wie, H.J.; Zhao, H.L.; Chang, J.H.; Kim, Y.S.; Hwang, I.K.; Ji, G.E. Enzymatic modification of saponins from *Platycodon grandiflorum* with *Aspergillus niger*. *J. Agric. Food Chem.* **2007**, *55*, 8908–8913. [CrossRef]
86. Kim, Y.P.; Lee, E.B.; Kim, S.Y.; Li, D.; Ban, H.S.; Lim, S.S.; Shin, K.H.; Ohuchi, K. Inhibition of Prostaglandin E2 Production by Platycodin D Isolated from the Root of *Platycodon grandiflorum*. *Planta Med.* **2001**, *67*, 362–364. [CrossRef]

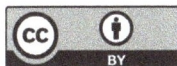 © 2020 by the authors. Licensee MDPI, Basel, Switzerland. This article is an open access article distributed under the terms and conditions of the Creative Commons Attribution (CC BY) license (http://creativecommons.org/licenses/by/4.0/).

MDPI
St. Alban-Anlage 66
4052 Basel
Switzerland
Tel. +41 61 683 77 34
Fax +41 61 302 89 18
www.mdpi.com

Foods Editorial Office
E-mail: foods@mdpi.com
www.mdpi.com/journal/foods

www.ingramcontent.com/pod-product-compliance
Lightning Source LLC
LaVergne TN
LVHW070410100526
838202LV00014B/1432

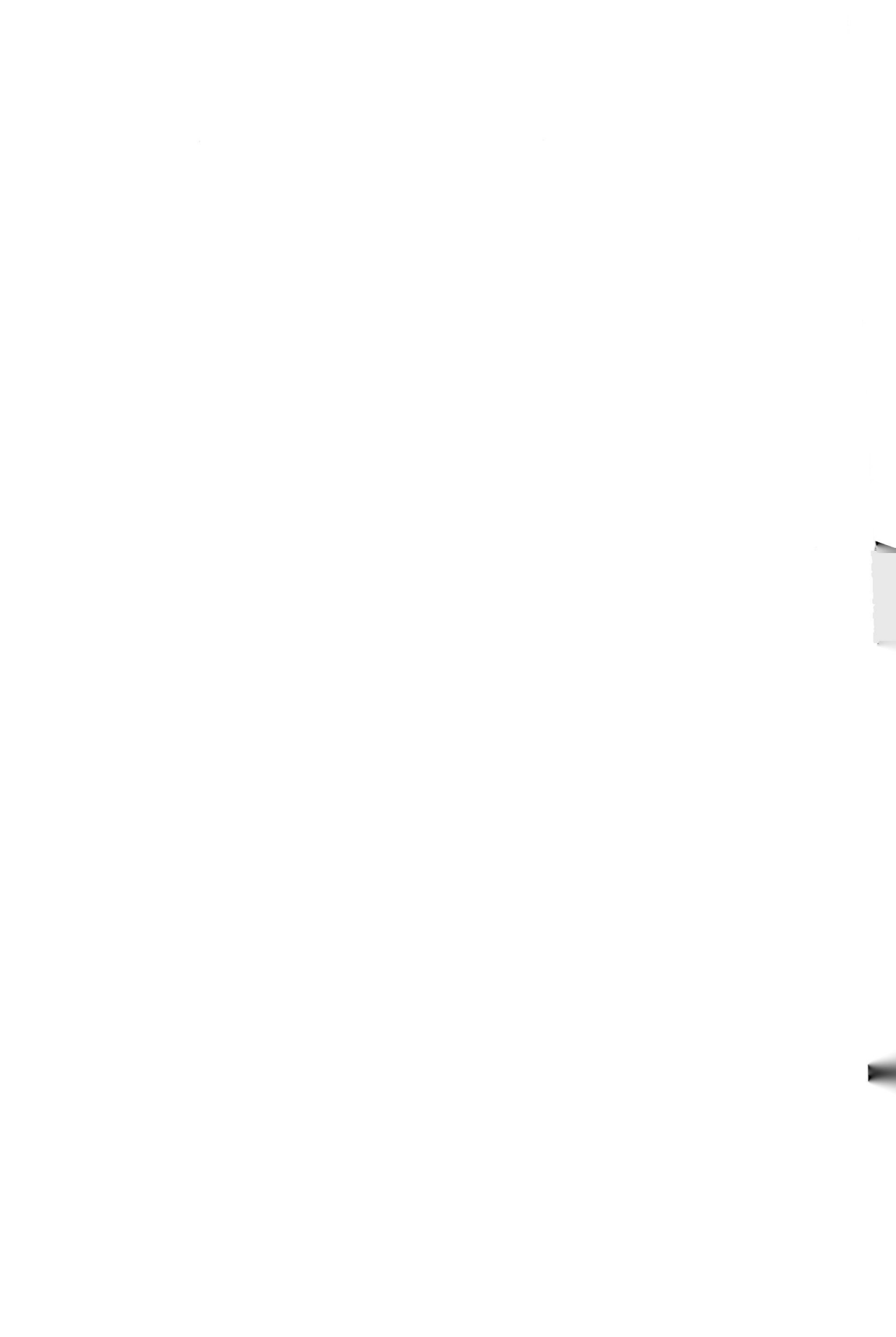